Psychopharmacogenetics

Psychopharmacogenetics

Edited by
Basil E. Eleftheriou
The Jackson Laboratory
Bar Harbor, Maine

PLENUM PRESS • NEW YORK AND LONDON

Library of Congress Cataloging in Publication Data

Main entry under title:

Psychopharmacogenetics.

Includes bibliographies and index.
1. Psychopharmacology. 2. Behavior genetics. I. Eleftheriou, Basil E. [DNLM: 1.
Psychopharmacology. 2. Pharmacogenetics. QV77 P962]
RC483.P777   615'.78   75-23100
ISBN 0-306-30881-9

©1975 Plenum Press, New York
A Division of Plenum Publishing Corporation
227 West 17th Street, New York, N.Y. 10011

United Kingdom edition published by Plenum Press, London
A Division of Plenum Publishing Company, Ltd.
Davis House (4th Floor), 8 Scrubs Lane, Harlesden, London, NW10 6SE, England

Printed in the United States of America

PREFACE

This short volume of an apparently double hybrid science deals with major pharmacologic effects on behavior in genetically defined animal and, to a lesser extent, human populations. Thus, a new name, psychopharmacogenetics, was coined to designate its contents.

The necessity for such compilation of some of the major data has become increasingly urgent. For some time now, there has been available information dealing with pharmacogenetics and behavior genetics. Recently, with ever-increasing frequency, however, data have been accumulating that deal with the effects of specific drugs on behavior and behavioral responses in animals with known genetic background. Initially, the data were gathered in various species and in a number of strains within given species of animals. With the availability of mutations, inbred strains, segregating strains of various types, recombinant inbred strains and congenic lines, the experimental approach to psychopharmacogenetics has now reached a new peak of sophistication. This volume attempts to present some of the major experiments in this area, along with comprehensive survey of the status of a given drug.

It is hoped that reading of the information that has been compiled herein will ultimately lead to a stimulus for further research in the areas outlined, as well as make the reader acquainted with new approaches to drug:behavior:genetic research.

June, 1975   Basil E. Eleftheriou

CONTENTS

PSYCHOPHARMACOGENETICS: AN INTEGRATIVE APPROACH TO THE STUDY OF GENES, DRUGS AND BEHAVIOR

Basil E. Eleftheriou, Ph.D.

Senior Staff Scientist

The Jackson Laboratory, Bar Harbor, Maine 04609

Pharmacogenetic research deals with differences in drug response between responding units, whether they are comparative in nature or possess a known, genetically defined background. On the other hand, psychopharmacology is the study of a class of behavior altering drugs in animals and humans that ultimately deals with the effects of pharmacologic agents upon these systems. Behavior genetics is another area which deals with the changes in behavioral response of certain defined genetic systems. All three areas, at one time or another, have overlapped and merged to study behavioral responses in genetically defined systems when certain pharmacological agents that alter behavior have been employed. Because of this general overlap, which at times is also quite specific, the necessity arises for a new field of study with the specific approach of studying the behavioral altering drugs in well defined genetic systems. This double hybrid science should properly be called psychopharmacogenetics. Thus, the area which is being specifically created in this presentation is an area which deals with pharmacologic agents that alter a given behavior in controlled genetic systems. It offers an honest and precise conceptualization of the hybrid scientific approach that is involved, and defines the manner in which this approach should be employed in ultimately clarifying the complexities involved in studies dealing with this hybrid area.

Basically, the reader may wonder whether this is something new and may question its novelty. By no means do we state that we have a novel presentation. Rather, the reader should focus his attention to interpreting the various contributions in view of psychopharmacogenetic research, rather than with research dealing with psychopharmacology, pharmacogenetics, or behavior genetics. It is

the ultimate hope of the editor that the redefinition of the bound-
aries of this type of research may ultimately eliminate some of the
competition among the three areas that are involved which will
ultimately serve to unite in a common cause of research approach,
the study of psychopharmacogenetics. It is also hoped that the
reader will find this volume useful and helpful in reviewing the
available information in the major areas within this field from
the point of view of pertinent references, evaluation by some of
the contributors of specific areas, and, hopefully, the utilization
of this information in teaching others the proper technique of approach in the study of psychopharmacogenetics.

Fuller and Hansult's presentation emphasizes the well-known
findings that different genomes may respond quite differently to
equal doses of the same drug, and they may also respond differentially to the same drug in what has been oftentimes called paradoxical responses. Such inherited differences in the response of different genotypes to the same drug are of great significance in determining individual vulnerability to drug abuse, and individual response to therapeutic agents. Thus, in some cases, the genotype may
place strong constraints upon the use of certain drugs and their
efficacy for certain types of treatment. Generally, Fuller and
Hansult emphasize the often ignored, but significant fact that contraindications which are not heeded may produce psychological consequences which ultimately are as serious, and oftentimes more
serious than physical ones. These contributors further emphasize
the importance of the new scientific heterozygote and the area of
psychopharmacogenetics which has the complexity of a triple parenthood, and may add some difficulties for the experimenter in carrying out certain types of experiments. Nevertheless, from the viewpoint of psychology and pharmacology this area presents interesting
parallels between the mode of action of drugs and gene substitutions
upon behavior. Fuller and Hansult present some discussion into the
possible animal models that can be used for carrying out research
in this area.

The presentation by Kalow and LeBlanc underscores some of the
implications of psychopharmacogenetic research, especially when
dealing with genetic variation in the disposition of psychoactive
drugs, and the genetic variation of the drug effects. The therapeutic implications of psychopharmacogenetic information is also
discussed in this contribution. Additionally, the non-pharmacolog-
ic implications of psychopharmacogenetic research are also presented in relation to the use of various psychoactive drugs by different societies and acceptance, control, and regulation of various
pharmacological agents. It gives us some "food for thought" when
we consider psychopharmacogenetic research with certain types of
pharmacological agents.

Eleftheriou and P. K. Elias present a novel approach to the

genetic study of drugs which induce behavioral alterations. This
new genetic approach deals with the recombinant-inbred strains of
mice. These strains were derived from a cross of two unrelated but
highly inbred progenitor strains, and then maintained independently
from the F_2 generation under a regimen of strict inbreeding. This
procedure genetically fixed the chance recombination of genes as
full homozygosity was approached in the generations following the
F_2 generation. The resulting battery of strains can be looked upon,
in one sense, as a replicable recombinant population. The utility
of such strains for analyzing gene systems is described in detail.
In addition, disucssion is made of the congenic lines (which are
not to be confused with the recombinant-inbred strains) that were
developed independently from an initial cross of C57BL/6By to
BALB/cBy by a regimen of skin-graft testing, and then backcrossed
to C57BL/6By for a number of generations. This procedure resulted
in congenic C57BL/6By, each of which differ from the C57BL/6By itself by only an introduced chromosomal segment including a BALB/cBy
strain allele at a distinctive histocompatibility (H) locus. Each
of these congenic lines has been tested against RI strains by means
of skin-graft to find which of the RI strains carry the BALB/cBy
strain allele and which the C57BL/6 allele at a particular H-locus,
thereby establishing their strain distribution patterns. Thus, the
pattern in which the RI strains exhibit low or high response to a
given drug-induced beahvior is compared to the strain distribution
patterns already determined for the H-loci. The matching strain
distribution pattern indicates possible identity or close linkage
to genes. To emphasize their presentation, Eleftheriou and P. K.
Elias have analyzed statistically a large amount of data dealing
with various pharmacologic agents and their behavioral induced alteration in these genetically defined mice. These analyses were
conducted in order to develop hypotheses regarding similar genetic
models for different drugs, different doses of the same drug and
effects of different drugs on a variety of behaviors. Their presentation emphasizes the utility of such genetically defined strains
of mice, and their significance in application to psychopharmacogenetic research in general. The availability of such strains
makes it economically feasible for genetic analyses and linkage of
loci responsible for particular drug responses in an efficient and
short period of time which far surpasses the existing genetic analyses in any species.

The presentation by Shuster, regarding the genetic analysis
of morphine effects in relation to its activity, analgesia, tolerance and sensitization, relates some of the more interesting and
novel approaches in the psychopharmacogenetic role of morphine.
It is clear that while it has not yet been possible to define the
exact number and location of the genetic determinants that control
the response to narcotic drugs in mice, a good start has been made.
The way is now clear for additional measurements with suitable backcrosses or by use of appropriate congenic lines, in order to present

us with a genetic model for morphine effects which can be ultimately used to clarify the manner in which morphine imparts its pharmacologic effect upon the central nervous system, and the subsequent
alteration of certain of the behaviors. But, even without complete
genetic definition, it is clear that we now have "model" strains
that can be used to examine the neurochemical basis of narcotic tolerance and sensitization. A beginning has also been made in relating to analgesic response to the number of narcotic receptors in
the brain. The necessity for additional experiments along these
lines is emphasized by Shuster. Certainly, this breakthrough in
obtaining genetic strains with extremes in the effects of morphine
facilitates further research.

Lapin presents some interesting and certainly new data regarding the effects of apomorphine in several strains of mice. Quanti-
tators and qualitators of strain differences in responses to apomorphine were noted in spontaneous locomotion and reelings in all
of the strains examined. Additionally, it was noted that apomorphine produced hypothermia in all strains, although there was a
differential quantitative response to this phenomenon. It appears
that, in the strains examined, there were no causal relationships
between lowering of motor activity and hypothermia induced by apomorphine. Whether this indicates that different genetic factors
are involved in the two phenomena is not clear at this time, but
certainly merits further research into this field. Of considerable
interest was the finding that apomorphine hypothermia was antagonized in all strains by pretreatment with haloperidol or desmethylimipramine. The accumulated data certainly indicates the involvement of monaminergic mechanisms, particularly dopaminergic and
serotonergic, which need further clarification.

The use of inbred strains, recombinant inbred strains, and
congenic lines, as well as within strain behavioral homogeneity and
biochemical differences, are discussed by Oliverio and Castellano.
Extensive discussion is presented on strain specific differences in
the relationship of the adrenergic system, electroencephalographic
responses and brain lesion studies to various pharmacological agents.
Further presentation is made of some of the newer and more novel
genetic analyses into the effect of drugs and behavior by the use
of recombinant-inbred strain technique. Exploratory activity is
discussed in terms of its modification by scopolamine, amphetamine,
and ethanol, as well as the interaction of pharmacologic agents with
various environmental factors which may face a particular experimenter at a given time. Thus, extensive discussion is presented which
attempts to clarify the finding that genetic mechanisms are not the
sole source of variation when the individual reactivity to various
drugs is considered. These variables are further confounded when
the environment appears to be differentially interacting upon a
particular genotype to its response to a given pharmacological agent
which ultimately affects various behaviors in animals and in humans.

The complexities of well formulated experimental designs are discussed for those who deal in the area of psychopharmacogenetics.
The complex environmental factors which interact with a particular
genotype in a response to a given drug are discussed in terms of
learning, prior experience, and activity, all of which interact in
a complex manner. However, Oliverio and Castellano attempt pains-
takingly to clarify some of these factors and offer some unique
alternatives.

The contribution of M. F. Elias and C. A. Pentz directs our
attention to the necessity of an understanding of the relationship
between genotype and behavioral effects of anesthetics and anesthesia which may be ultimately facilitated by increasing utilization
of behavior or genetic techniques and methods that go beyond the
repeated demonstration that genotype interacts with environmental
factors. In this particular area of drug-behavior-genetic interaction, there seems to be clear evidence for the fact that anesthesia results in retrograde amnesia when it is present during a
critical period after information input. The critical period may
reflect consolidation of an electrophysiological memory trace.
However, more precise control of anesthetic dosages in combination
with systematic and programmatic studies will be necessary to characterize the mechanisms which intervene between genes and behavioral response to anesthetic agents. One may question whether there
is anything further to be gained from studying the time course of
memory consolidation in a behavior:genetic study employing the
retrograde amnesia paradigm. This approach may reveal little about
the underlying mechanisms of memory. A more profitable strategy
may be to capitalize on data which implicate the neurotransmitter
substances as an important link between genes and memory processes.
Excellent examples of this research strategy, employing the behav-
ior:genetic context, is provided in recent works of some investigators. Generally, Elias and Pentz recommend that increased research
efforts be directed toward the use of drugs which have been implicated in learning and memory processes as a means of exploring the
genetic basis of memory with genetic models. This, however, does
not preclude or imply that descriptive studies (strain comparisons)
have no value, or that studies of effects of anesthetics and behavior should be discontinued. On the contrary, studies which relate
differences in genotype to behavioral and structural alterations resulting from chronic exposure to trace doses of anesthetics should
be particularly worthwhile if they were to be done in life-span context. Strain difference studies would also be a useful first step
in studies designed to separate effects of premedication, hyperventilation, surgical stress, and various combination of anesthetics
which influence behavior. In short, these contributors emphasize
the necessity for reorienting experimental approaches to some of
the underlying causative mechanisms dealing with the psychopharmacogenetic effects of anesthetic agents. They also emphasize the
need for increased sophistication in the application of the genetic

methodology that is now available in studying behavior that is altered by anesthesia.

Eriksson presents a detailed and inclusive description of some
of the major causative determinants of alcoholism in humans, and
alcohol preference and drinking behavior in animals. For some time
now, a common misconception has been that the cause of alcoholism
must be either genetic or environmental; that if genetic influences
were accepted, then environmental ones would have to be eliminated.
Actually, in phenomena such as alcoholism, the phenotype is determined through interactions between the genotype and the environment.
It has been shown, in animals, that the metabolism of alcohol and
alcohol drinking behavior are controlled by polygenic systems, that
is, the inheritance is quantitatively influenced by the additive influences of many genes and their respective alleles. Thus, traits
controlled by such systems tend to follow a normal distribution.
Even in animals, measuring the phenotype of drinking behavior in a
simple self-selection situation is very difficult: various measures
can be used, each with its own advantages and limitations. With
humans, there are even more major problems in determining the phenotype. Eriksson emphasizes that the most common methods have utilized questionnaires, or the selection of subjects who have suffered
certain social consequences of excessive drinking, such as hospitalization or even incarceration. Although the phenotypic measurement
procedures are not perfect, they are major criticism against most
human studies. This is the inherent difficulty in separating genetic from environmental influences. Eriksson points to some of the
attempts that have been made to find genetic markers for alcoholism
with ABO blood group types and with color vision defects. Finally,
a discussion is presented with some of the recent animal research
which attempts to reproduce, in animals, some of the major characteristics of human alcoholism such as imbibing voluntarily to the
level of extreme intoxication. Generally, his discussion brings us
up-to-date on this major social affliction of our society.

In all instances, the reader should keep in mind that each con-
tributor attempts to consolidate data that are oftentimes somewhat
contradictory due to the nature of experimental design used, philo-
sophical approach, possible seasonal, diurnal or environmental effects,
as well as various other uncontrollable variables that plague each
experimenter. Some of the latter variables and their possible interaction with specific experimental approaches are discussed by
Oliverio and Castellano. Human behavioral interactions with pharmacogenetics and the difficulties encountered in their assessment are
exemplified by the presentations especially of Eriksson. Particular
social bias may enter and oftentimes cloud some of our more objective
evaluation attempts. Nevertheless, the psychopharmacogenetic approach
may ultimately lead us to clear thinking and eventual solutions.

The present status of the work dealing with audiogenic seizures and acoustic priming is discussed in detail by Schlesinger and Sharpless. This is a field which, early in its development, has encompassed major aspects of psychopharmacogenetics. Historically, this came about by the early genetic linkage of a locus which in mice exerts an influence on audiogenic seizures and the study of which dealt extensively with the behavioral effects and possible alteration, and its influence by various pharmacological agents. Recently, comprehensive studies have been undertaken, and results emphasize the significant role of biogenic and indole amines in this phenomenon. This is a phenomenon which has been exhaustively studied from various points of interest: genetic and ontogenetic; acoustic priming and laterality; relations between sound-drug and electrically-induced seizures; morphological correlates dealing with the cortex, thalamus, inferior colliculus and the ear; neurophysiological correlates dealing with cochlear microphonic and auditory thresholds, and biochemical correlates dealing especially with serotonin, norepinephrine, and γ-aminobutyric acid, as well as pharmacologic manipulations dealing with levels of serotonin, norepinephrine, and alterations by reserpine and tetrabenzedrine, and various monoamine oxidase inhibitors. One of the more novel approaches to this subject is the recent emphasis that has been applied to the circadian rhythm susceptibility to audiogenic seizures and the accompanying drug effects. Finally, a clarification of the theory regarding the role of serotonin, norepinephrine and, to a lesser extent, dopamine, is presented in relation to their role in audiogenic seizures. Generally, the presentation of all the data falls into two types: (1) correlational data which suggests a relationship between these brain amines and seizure susceptibility to genotype, and (2) pharmacological and dietary manipulations of levels of these brain amines which appear to alter seizure susceptibility in the directions predicted from the model which the authors present. In short, it is a comprehensive compilation of the psychopharmacogenetic events dealing with audiogenic seizures and acoustic priming in genetically defined species of mice.

Omenn and Motulsky present a detailed discussion of some of the major clinical syndromes that are encountered by clinicians dealing with drug therapy. They detail the approaches to the study of these various syndromes, especially dealing with genetic background, in treatment of these syndromes, and the differential responses of various drugs which alter behavior. These authors begin with the method of analyses in human populations which are: (a) population surveys, (b) family studies, and (c) twin studies. In all of these methods, the recent focal point of initiating studies of drug response revolved around biochemical evaluative diagnosis. Thus, based on biochemical diagnosis, Omenn and Motulsky present to us the gene-determined differences in the metabolism of specific drugs such as succinylcholine, phenothiazine, ethanol, aryl hydrocarbons,

phenelzine, isoniazide, dilantin, and many others. In addition, a
detailed discussion is presented on the new approach of clinical
evaluation of the genetically determined differences in tissue
sensitivity to various groups of drugs, and aspects of their metabolism and influence in various human populations. These studies
include caffeine-induced wakefulness, taste sensitivity, reactions
of the autonomic nervous system to various drugs, malignant hyperthermia from anesthetics, susceptibility to cyanosis from methemoglobinemia monoamines, and their role in platelets and the brain,
and susceptibility of red blood cells to hemolysis by various oxidizing agents. Finally, the pharmacogenetic basis of major behavioral disorders is presented in a detailed discussion of schizophrenia, alcoholism, affective disorders, seizure disorders, and minimal brain dysfunction such as hyperactivity syndrome. Thus, in
this latter discussion, the psychopharmacogenetic relationship is
presented. In this logical developmental approach, Omenn and
Motulsky finally delineate the application and meaning of psychopharmacogenetics to humans which consist of investigations of
differences among individuals in a therapeutic and adverse effects
of behavior-modifying drugs. Clinically significant examples of
well-defined, genetically-determined differences in metabolism of
such drugs and in tissue sensitivity to drug action are discussed
extensively. Although single gene mechanisms are prominent among
these examples, it should be emphasized that polygenic inheritance
appears to be the more common manner in which genes influence the
absorption, metabolism, and tissue action of many drugs. Approaches
to the study of particular drugs in humans is presented in detail.

The presentations by Fann and colleagues emphasizes the great
need of knowledge in the pharmacology and treatment of various disorders in the human population. The first presentation deals with
neuroleptic-induced movement disorders, and it typifies the great
necessity for cataloguing the psychopharmacogenetic responses in
human populations in terms of well documented and controlled population studies. The second presentation further underscores the
major problems encountered in the treatment of human populations,
and the problems encountered with interactions of some pharmacologic agents. Fann points the direction of needed future research to
help clarify and elucidate the basis for the variation in response
to these agents.

The contribution by Ellinwood and Kilbey details the differential response to amphetamine for several parameters in various
species of animals and in the human. Although there are species-
-specific patterns in the stereotyped behavioral responses to
amphetamine, it is difficult, at this time, to identify genetic components and control due mainly to the lack of genetic research in
this area. An additional complicating factor in this particular
research area is that the biochemical predictors of some specific
neurobiochemical events involved in amphetamine responses have not

been established genetically. Furthermore, the relation of some
known genetic factors to behavior and pharmacological actions of
amphetamine have not been consolidated in a combined experiment
with the psychopharmacogenetic approach. Generally, based on the
available information, it appears that amphetamine determined behavioral responses are polygenic. Thus, this complex situation
presents some difficulties in establishing animal models for the
study of amphetamine induced behavioral changes. However, all the
possible genetic analyses have not been exhausted, and some specific
mouse strains exist which exhibit profound differences in their
responses to amphetamine. The use of such strains in future genetic
studies should provide the basis for psychopharmacogenetic research.

Finally, the chapter on statistics, contributed by M. F.
Elias, points out the necessity of applying the appropriate statistical analysis when dealing with psychopharmacogenetic research.
This chapter may be a deviation from the accepted normal contribution in volumes such as this, but it underscores and emphasizes the
necessity for experimenters in this area to be highly selective in
their approach to statistical analyses where optimum derivation of
the genetic model which they wish to propose is concerned. Generally, most of us utilize routinely the available statistics of standard deviation, chi-square, Student's t-test, and one-way or two-
-way analyses of variance. Few of us bother to go beyond this
routine statistical approach in analyzing complex data with such
newly devised techniques as multivariate analysis of variance, or
even application of the covariance analysis when dealing with complex systems. Elias does an excellent job of informing us of possible alternative statistical analyses which can be employed profit-
ably to analyze our complex experimental evidence when dealing with
hybrid areas such as psychopharmacogenetics. Experimenters in this
area should carefully glean the available information from these
statistical analyses and consider their application.

Discussion of species specific or divergent responses to the
same pharmacologic agent is presented by several contributors to
this volume, and detailed presentation here will only lead to re-
dundancy. The point to be made here, however, is that, in most
experimental or clinical situations, the unexpected response to a
particular drug is termed paradoxical. Thus, the inhibitory effect
of amphetamine in hyperkinetic children, the stimulatory effects of
scopolamine, the non-analgesic effects of morphine in 35% of patients
are all considered paradoxical, since they do not follow the generally established response pattern of these drugs. In view of recent experimental evidence in well-defined genetic systems, these
opposite responses should no longer be considered paradoxical.
Rather, these responses are undoubtedly due to different alleles of
the major locus responding to a given pharmacological agent. Whether
we should consider one (most prevalent), or the other (least prevalent

or "paradoxical") as dominant or recessive is of no importance to
our argument. The important consideration is that we reassess our
established concepts of what constitutes "paradoxical responses"
when dealing with the genetics of a given population, be it animal
or human. Realistically, however, in order to evaluate individuals
for their particular responses to a given drug, so that risks are
reduced, we must devise adequate tests, albeit a lofty but difficult
goal. Aspects of this approach are discussed in this volume.

Generally, it is hoped that the contributions in this short
volume on the hybrid science of psychopharmacogenetics helps to re-
orient our way of thinking and approach to this complex research
area. It is hoped that students and experimenters alike will find
this contribution of immense value in their approach to research,
or in teaching courses related to psychopharmacogenetics. If this
is done, the editor feels a certain comfort in having accomplished
most of his objectives in the preparation of this contribution.

GENES AND DRUGS AS BEHAVIOR MODIFYING AGENTS

John L. Fuller, Ph.D., Chairman

and

Carole D. Hansult, Ph.D.

Department of Psychology
State University of New York at Binghamton
Binghamton, New York   13901

CONTENTS

INTRODUCTION

Hybrid sciences are not uncommon. The status of psychopharmacology and behavior genetics is attested by the existence of
specialty journals, textbooks and organized associations. Pharmacogenetics is less well defined as a separate area, but various
books and reviews testify to its vigor. Now, we have a book on
psychopharmacogenetics which is clearly the offspring of three
parental sciences, genetics, pharmacology and psychology. Is this
simply an area of overlap between three established areas or does

11

it have characteristics of its own, even a touch of heterosis or hybrid vigor?

Only time will provide the answer to this question. The present paper attempts to summarize what each parent might contribute to the triple hybrid based upon the accomplishments of the accepted double hybrids. We shall also consider from the viewpoint of psychology the similarities and differences between the effects of genetic variation and drug administration upon behavior.

Psychopharmacogenetics properly must employ the fundamental concepts of its three parents, not simply their techniques. One does not become a biophysicist by using an electrocardiograph to monitor heart rate, or a behavior geneticist by demonstrating that two strains of mice have different behavioral reactions to amphetamine. The justification for this book lies in the assumption that persons acquainted with the basic ideas of psychology, genetics and pharmacology will design and execute better experiments in the field.

Naturally, approaches to pharmacological effects upon behavior and their relationship to heredity vary with the training of the investigator. Pharmacologists tend to be most concerned with the chemical dynamics of drugs in living systems. The behavioral effects of a drug and the genome of the subjects are either not noted, or are regarded as barriers to interpreting drug activity in molecular terms. By standardizing the strain of animal and the behavioral procedures used, the pharmacologist increases the possibility of obtaining meaningful data related to differences in dosage or changes in chemical side groups of his favorite psychotropic drug.

The geneticist (behavioral variety) finds his rewards in discovering variability in the behavioral effects of drugs attributable to genetic manipulation. He may follow up the demonstration of such effects by working backward towards RNA and DNA, thus becoming molecular like the pharmacologist, or he may concentrate on a biometrical analysis of his data, and problems of mode of inheritance. If single-locus control of significant variation is indicated, the possibilities of success in the molecular approach are enhanced. The important point is that a geneticist cannot standardize on one genome; he must test many, even though this means that statements on the behavioral effects of a drug must be written separately for each genome tested.

Psychologists insist on studying the behavioral effects of drug administration in a variety of contexts and often with multiple indices of response. These range through effects on synaptic transmission, general activity, and rate of learning to territorial

defense. For psychologists, standardization of drug and genome
are convenient means of attaining reliability of behavioral data.

Superficially, then, there appears to be little or no formal
agreement concerning the best way to get on with the business of
research in psychopharmacogenetics. The objectives of the three
most interested groups are diverse and their optimal conditions
are in some instances antithetical. A look at the record, however, is less discouraging. There are impressive research accomplishments by persons from each of the ancestor disciplines. Investigators have been able to adhere to their basic concerns related to their home discipline, and at the same time become involved with variables which are ordinarily left to others. Before briefly mentioning some examples to illustrate this point,
we shall look at some similarities and differences between the
effects of gene substitutions and drug administration upon behavior.

GENES, DRUGS AND BEHAVIORAL CHANGE

Genes and drugs are both chemicals, though very different
in structure, and potentially the actions of both are explicable
in molecular terms. Behavior, of course, is not defined in molecu -
lar units, but is a series of events over time. Genes and drugs,
therefore, modify behavior through intermediary physical processes.

An important characteristic of genes is pleiotropy which means
that a gene substitution produces a diverse set of phenotypic ef -
fects. Presumably, all these are related in some way to one specific
gene product, but the complex pathways are often very difficult to
follow. Albino mice, for example, lack melanin, have abnormal
visual pathways, are less active in open field tests and, in certain
circumstances, show reduced alcohol intake. The reduction in pig-
ment can be related to lack of tyrosinase, and reduced sensitivity
to the inhibitory effect of bright illumination upon an eye not
protected against excessive radiation. The deviant optic nerve
fibers and the changes in alcohol intake are less easily explained
by the primary gene action.

Drugs possess specificity sufficient to classify many of them
as cholinergic, monoamine oxidase inhibitors and the like, Because
neurotransmitters are involved in so many neural functions, the effects of drugs upon behavior are also pleiotropic. Chemical specificity does not necessarily result in psychological specificity,
and so-called side effects are comparable to the pleiotropic actions of genes.

Both genes and drugs are tissue and cell specific to a degree.

All cells have the same complement of DNA, but the active portion differs in neurons, gland cells and hematopoetic cells. Neurotropic drugs have slight effects upon gland cells. Such specificities are explicable in chemical terms.

It is common knowledge that a drug may have different quantitative, and even qualitative, effects depending upon the genome of the recipient. It is less often recognized that a gene substitution modifies metabolism differently depending upon the background on which it is expressed. An example is the variable expression of the viable yellow (A^{vy}) gene in the mouse (Wolff, 1971). In one cross (C57BL/6 x VY) 88% of the offspring were mottled yellow; 12% were agouti. In an AKR x VY cross only 42% were agouti. Pleiotropic effects of this dominant gene include differences in rate of growth, food and water intake, level of serum insulin and general activity. The point to be emphasized is that the phenotypic expression of A^{vy} varies unpredictably within genomes and predictably between them. The background genome also influences the effects of the A^{vy} gene upon liver enzymes (Wolff & Pitot, 1973). Apparently, this locus is concerned with regulatory functions, and its manifestations are background-dependent to a high degree.

In a way, this pervasive presence of a variable background genome is a handicap to both the behavior geneticist and the psychopharmacologist. How much simpler it would be if a gene or a drug could always be counted upon to behave in the same way. One might even ask whether a lawful science of psychopharmacogenetics can exist, if so many variables must be considered in every experiment. The optimistic view is that genetic variation offers an opportunity, and that the right kinds of experiments will lead to the formulation of general principles which will apply across genomes.

BEHAVIOR GENETICS OF DRUG ADDICTION

Probably, the most widely used and often overused psychotropic drug is ethyl alchohol. Although no one doubts the significance of social factors in the etiology of alcoholism, there is strong evidence that inherited predispositions significantly affect the risk of this condition (Schuckit, 1972). Nichols (1972) has hypothesized, largely on the basis of animal research, that there may be a general trait of addictability which is operative in many drug dependencies. Inherited variations in physiological reactions to ethanol have been demonstrated in twin studies (Partanen et al., 1966; Vesell, 1972), racial comparisons (Fenna et al., 1971; Wolf, 1972), and by animal research (Kakihana et al., 1966). This kind of knowledge has practical applications in the use of medication for detoxification and rehabilitation of addicts.

The clincial administration of drugs in cases of acute overdose

of alcohol as well as for long term rehabilitation are now standard
hospital procedures. But not all medications which produce sympto-
matic relief are used. In the treatment of alcoholics for delirium
tremens, for instance, the phenothiazines usually are not administered
because they have low cross tolerence to alcohol (Jaffe, 1965) and
possess eleptogenic properties (Victor, 1970). Since such patients
already run a high risk of convulsions, drugs which lower the seizure
threshold naturally are to be considered with caution. The use of
barbiturates is less of a hazard, but is in question because these
drugs supress REM as does alcohol, and patients who already exhibit
dreaming deficits are unable to make them up (Greenberg & Pearlman,
1967). At present, other drug classes such as the benzodiazepines
are preferred. This class of anti-anxiety muscle relaxants has high
cross-tolerence to alcohol, is not eleptogenic and does not substantially reduce REM (Reggiani, in Garattini et al., 1973).

But drugs act on many systems and at many levels. If a patient
is showing signs of acute alcohol overdose but blood alcohol levels
are low, the attending physician must consider genetic constitution
as a possible causative factor. A history of cutaneous hepatic or
acute intermittent porphyria predisposes a patient to alcohol intolerence (Goldberg, 1962). Such persons are also highly sensitive
to barbiturates so that under no circumstances should those drugs
be given during ethanol detoxification.

In addition, if any CNS depressant is to be used as a postalco-
hol anti-anxiety drug, the clearence rates for ethanol must be determined for each patient. Since, as mentioned earlier, it has been
demonstrated that certain racial groups differ in rates of alcohol
metabolism (Fenna et al., 1971), this factor should be kept in mind
during chemotherapy for acute overdose. Particular genotypes clear
alcohol very slowly. When there is a history of long-term drinking,
however, the problem is less immediate because these patients possess
a substantial ability to induce the necessary enzymes after prolonged exposure to alcohol.

It seems, then, that there is a broad range of behaviors from
complete alcohol intolerence with inadequate enzyme induction (porphyria) to impressive alcohol tolerence and enzyme induction with or
without physical dependence. Naturally, varying degrees of toxic
reaction are arrayed between these extremes. Underlying the phenotypic pictures are specific predisposing genotypes. In addition to
the biological factors, there are of course strong social and personal influences upon behavior. It would be naive to think that all
porphyrics admitted for acute toxic alcohol reaction were unaware of
their condition. For whatever reasons, these patients drink despite
or because of their intolerance. Genetic predisposition itself may
be used as a tool for self-descruction.

PSYCHOLOGICAL ASPECTS OF DRUG-GENE INTERACTION

Up to now only immediate physical and behavioral aspects of
gene-drug interaction have been discussed. There are, however,
long-term psychosocial consequences of being deviant, even if the
deviance is brought about by the administration of drugs. Through
contact with their culture, people develop attitudes some of which
modify definitions of, and conduct toward the unusual as well as
the familiar. Everyone is eventually introduced to these, including persons who are defined as "different". Such people must in
turn develop opinions of themselves, and of others which invariably
reflect the influence of their own anomalies. Those with whom we
are now concerned only come to understand their problem after a
toxic reaction of some kind. For example, many subclinical myopath-
ies are dominantly inherited (Moulds & Denenborough, 1974a). The
difficulty arises when affected subjects are given the general
anaesthetic, halothane or large doses of caffeine. Such treatment results in malignant hyperpyrexia and often death (Moulds &
Denenborough, 1974b). Psychosocial adjustment in survivors is
necessary, but the transition from "normal" to "not normal" can be
traumatic. It is especially difficult for those who confuse con-
formity with excellence, and variation with inferiority. For those
whose disorder did not come as a surprise, there are other problems.

Illustrations are not hard to find. Patients suffering from
glucose-6-phosphate dehydrogenase deficiency are plagued from
birth with severe anaemia. This is usually diagnosed early, but
they also have inherited an intolerance for several drugs. These
include 8-aminoquinoline based antimalarials, sulfonamide antibi-
otics, furan derivitive antibacterials (Beutler, 1971a; Beutler,
1971b), the analgesic, acetanalide (Prankherd, 1963) and the anti-
microbial, chloramphenicol (Weinstein, in Goodman & Gilman, 1970).
These medications which are safely used in much of the general
population cause rapid haemolysis resulting in severe haemolytic
anaemia when administered to patients with G-6-PD. Already weak
and listless, those affected become weaker and develop palpitations,
systolic murmurs and shortness of breath until the cell rupturing
has returned to its usual rate.

When such a debilitating response is superimposed upon a
life which includes frequent hospitalizations and restriction of
normal activity. the total impact of the illness increases. Under these circumstances children are especially vulnerable to depression (Whitten & Fischoff, 1974). They may become frustrated
and ashamed. Those with sickle cell anaemia or haemophilia are
further burdened with repeated episodes of extreme pain. Where
the symptoms are exacerbated by drugs, the psychosocial outlook
worsens. Sadly, up to this writing, very little research has been
done on the impact that gene-drug interaction has on psychosocial

development and functioning, but the area is certainly of great importance and must eventually be investigated.

SUMMARY

In summary, the hybrid science of psychopharmacogenetics requires the simultaneous manipulation of three kinds of independent
variables. From the viewpoint of psychology there are interesting
parallels between the mode of action of drugs and gene substitutions
upon behavior.

Different genomes may respond quite differently to equal doses
of the same drug. Such inheritied differences are important in
determining individual vulnerability to drug abuse, and individual
response to therapeutic agents. In some case, genotype may place
strong constraints upon the use of certain drugs. When the genetic
contraindications are not heeded, the psychological consequences
may be as serious as the physical one.

We believe that this scientific heterozygote has the potential
for a long and healthy life. The complexity of triple parenthood
adds difficulties for the experimenter, but it also increases the
probability of innovative approaches to problems which neither
parent science can solve by itself.

REFERENCES

BEUTLER, E., 1970a, Annotation. Brit. J. Haemat. 18:117.

BEUTLER, E., 1970b, Glucose-6-phosphate dehydrogenase deficiency,
    In: "The Metabolic Basis of Inherited Disease" (E. Stanbury,
    J. B. Wyngaarden & D. S. Fredrickson, eds.) McGraw Hill, London.

FENNA, A., MIX, L., SCHAEFER, O. & GILBERT, J. A. L., 1971, Ethanol
    metabolism in various racial groups, Canad. Med. Ass. J., 105:
    472.

GOLDBERG, A., 1962, "Diseases of Porphyrin Metabolism," Charles C.
    Thomas, Springfield, Ill., pp. 373.

GREENBERG, R. & PEARLMAN, C., 1964 Delirium tremens and dream de-
    privation, Report of the Ass. for Psychophys. Study of Sleep,
    Palo Alto.

KAKIHANA, R., BROWN, D. R., MCCLEARN, C. E. & TABERSHAW, I. R., 1966,
    Brain sensitivity to alcohol in inbred mouse strains, Science
    154:1574.

MOULDS, R. F. W. & DENENBOROUGH, M. A., 1974a, Biochemical basis of malignant hyperpyrexia, Brit. Med. J., 4 May, 241-244.

MOULDS, R. F. W. & DENENBOROUGH, M. A., 1974b, Identification of susceptibility to malignant hyperpyrexia, Brit. Med. J., 4 May, 245-247.

NICHOLS, J. R., 1972, The children of addicts: what do they inherit? Ann. N. Y. Acad. Sci., 197:60.

PARTANEN, J., BRUUN, M. & MARKKANEN, K., 1966, Inheritance of drinking behavior. A study in intelligence, personality and use of alcohol in adult twins. The Finnish Foundation for Alcohol Studies.

PRANKERD, T. A. J., 1963, Hemolytic effects of drugs and chemical agents. Clin. Pharmac. Ther., 4:334.

SCHUCKIT, M. A., 1972, Family history and half-sibling research in alcoholism. Ann. N. Y. Acad. Sci., 197:121.

VESELL, E. S., 1972, Ethanol metabolism: regulation by genetic factors in normal volunteers. Ann. N. Y. Acad. Sci. 197:79.

VICTOR, M., 1970, The alcohol withdrawal syndrome, Postgrad. Med., 47:68.

WEINSTEIN, L., 1970, Miscellaneous microbial, antifungal and antiviral agents. In: "The Pharmacological Basis of Therapeutics" (L. S. Goodman and A. Gilman, eds.), MacMillan, London.

WHITTEN, C. F. & FISCHOFF, J., 1974, Psychosocial effects of sickle cell disease, Arch. Inter. Med., 133:681.

WOLFF, G. L., 1971, Genetic modification of homeostatic regulation in the mouse, Amer. Naturalist, 105:241.

WOLFF, C. L. & PITOT, H. C., 973, Influence of background on enzymatic characteristics of yellow ($A^y/-$, $A^{vy}/-$) mice. Genetics, 73:109.

WOLFF, P. H., 1972, Ethnic differences in alcohol sensitivity, Science, 175:449.

EFFECTS OF APOMORPHINE IN MICE OF DIFFERENT STRAINS

I. P. Lapin, Chief

Laboratory of Psychopharmacology
Bekhterev Psychoneurological Research Institute
Leningrad, USSR

CONTENTS

INTRODUCTION

Studies on the pharmacology of apomorphine as an adrenergic drug were initiated in this laboratory in January of 1964, subsequent to the presentation of an exciting paper by Professor M. L. Belenky (1964) at the meeting of the Presidium of All-Union Pharmacological Society in Leningrad. In this paper, we were informed, for the first time, concerning the role of apomorphine as an a-drenergic drug. Even the usage of these two words, namely "apomorphine" and "adrenergic" was never encountered prior to this time. M. L. Belenky (1964) reported the potentiation of the pressor effect of adrenaline and noradrenaline by apomorphine in cats, and hyperthermic and excitatory effects of this drug in rabbits. The latter effects of apomorphine were compared with those of amphetamine. In this initial paper, M. L. Belenky suggested that apomorphine inhibits catechol-0-methyltransferase (COMT), because it has two OH groups in the 0-position, the feature common for various COMT inhibitors such as pyrogallol or quercetin. Shortly thereafter, these and other adrenergic effects of apomorphine in cats and rabbits were reported in detail (Belenky et al., 1965; Belenky, 1966), as well as the inhibition in cats of COMT in vivo (Belenky et al., 1966). These series of experiments formed the background for further search for new derivatives of apomorphine and amphetamine exhibiting adrenergic central and peripheral activity (Belenky, 1966).

Recently, hyperthermic effect of apomorphine in rabbits was once again described (Hill & Horita, 1972), and the involvement of dopaminergic (Hill & Horita, 1972; Horita & Quock, 1974) and serotonergic (Quock & Horita, 1974) mechanisms was suggested. Evidence for a presynaptic action of apomorphine (Ferris et al., 1974) and for inhibition of COMT by apomorphine (McKenzie, 1974), two actions suggested by M. L. Belenky, were published in 1974. The latter investigator also mentioned some similarities and dissimilarities between effects of apomorphine and amphetamine, and when asked whether he agrees that our laboratory should continue our studies on amphetamine in mice and rats by comparing this drug with apomorphine, he agreed, and thus we began these comparative studies focusing our attention mainly on body temperature, motor activity and aggressiveness because only these effects of amphetamine were studied previously in isolated and grouped mice and rats.

In some initial experiments, we have observed that, in contrast to rabbits, in mice, apomorphine produced hypothermia and inhibition of locomotion. The former effect seemed to be the most intfiguing and unknown and, therefore, it was studied pharmacologically in detail. Results of our studies on pharmacological effects of apomorphine in comparison with pyrogallol and amphetamine in mice, rats, and rabbits were reported at the 36th Meeting of the Leningrad

Pharmacological Society (December 15, 1964). In tests of hypothermia in mice, interaction of apomorphine with adrenergic (antidepressant, neuroleptics, etc.), serotonergic (BOL-148 and MCE),
and cholinergic (atropine, benactyzine) drugs was described (Lapin,
Samsonova, 1968a, Lapin, 1969a), and activation of adrenergic and
serotonergic processes by apomorphine as well as its direct action
on thermoregulation was suggested. Apomorphine hypothermia in
mice was used in this laboratory as an end point to study pharmacological activity of antidepressants (Lapin, 1969b) and to differentiate them, anticholinergic and neuroleptics (Schelkunov,
1968). Species differences in pharmacological effects of apomorphine were also reported (Lapin & Samsonova, 1968b).

Apomorphine hypothermia in mice was again described some
years later (Bartlett et al., 1972; Fuxe, Sjövist, 1972) and possible dopaminergic effect of this drug in agreement with the idea
of Ernst (1966, 1967) in this phenomenon was suggested. In our
studies on apomorphine (1964-69), as well as in those of M. L.
Belenky and his collaborators, the possible role of dopamine was
not suggested. This idea, as is presently circulating, appeared
after the papers of Ernst (1966, 1967) were published.

As pharmacological effects of amphetamine appeared to be
strain-dependent in mice (Lapin, 1974), it is natural that we
were interested in the comparative effects of apomorphine in mice
of different strains. Results of these comparative studies, which
we consider as preliminary approaches to further psychopharmacogenetic studies, are reported in the present chapter.

METHODS

Male mice of five strains (SHR, inbred from the Swiss strain,
BALB/cJ, C57BR, C57BL/6J, and C3H/A), weighing 18-22 g were sup-
plied by Rappolovo Farm (Leningrad). Mice were housed in animal
rooms of the Laboratory in groups of 30 mice per cage (30x27x28 cm).
Standard diet and cow milk were given ad libitum. Prior to the experimental testing, the mice were kept in the laboratory in groups
of 8-10 mice, in metal cages of 20x15x10 cm with a wire mesh cover.
While in the laboratory, mice were not fed. Room temperature was
maintained at 19-20°C. Experiments were carried out in May-June.

Locomotion and rearing behavior were measured visually, not in
the automatic electronic integrator used in the previous studies
(Lapin, 1974). This was done in order to observe general behaviour
during the testing period. This seemed to be of importance in a
study of apomorphine which had not been administered previously to
these strains. A single mouse was placed in an open-field type of
metal cage of 20x15x10 cm for two minutes, and the number of lines

crossed (locomotion) and the rearings were counted by means of digit counters. Effect of apomorphine on locomotion and rearings was tested 30 minutes after injection.

Body temperature was measured by an electrothermometer (TPEM-Im). A thermistor was inserted in the rectum to a depth of 1.5 cm. In experiments with apomorphine, rectal temperature was measured before injection and then 30, 60, 90, and 120 minutes after injection. When in the same experiment locomotion and rearings were counted, body temperature was measured immediately after removing a mouse from the box. Apomorphine hypothermia was determined in the majority of experiments as a difference (t^o) between temperature of a given mouse 30 minutes after injection and the temperature immediately prior to the injection. It has been observed (Lapin & Samsonova, 1968a) that fall of body temperature in apomorphine-treated mice is maximal 30 minutes after injection. In some experiments (e.g., with threshold and subthreshold doses of apomorphine) cumulative thermic index (sum of t for each measurement as compared with the initial temperature) was used.

Intensity of apomorphine stereotype behavior was rated according to the method of Ernst (1967). The difference consists in the presence of sniffing without compulsive gnawing. Stereotype during the first hour after the injection of apomorphine was rated every 15 minutes.

Apomorphine hydrochloride was injected i.p. in a form of fresh water solution (powder was dissolved not more than 15 minutes prior to the last injection of a group in a volume of 10 ml/kg. In controls, distilled water was injected. Additionally, to test antagonism to apomorphine, aqueous solutions of haloperidol and desmethylimipramine were injected i.p. 60 minutes before apomorphine (the latter in doses of 10 or 20 mg/kg). Statistical treatment of data was made according to the Student's "t" test.

RESULTS

Spontaneous motor activity

There are considerable differences in locomotion and rearings in intact mice of the various strains that were tested (Table 1). Generally, motor activity is highest in C57BR mice and lowest in BALB/cJ mice. The decreasing order of strains for locomotion and rearing is as follows: C57BR C57BL/6J and SHR C3H/A BALB/cJ.

The principal difference with data previously obtained (Lapin, 1974) consists in higher activity of the C57BL/6J strain which has previously been the strain that has exhibited both locomotion and

rearings. This strain seems to rather inconsistent when comparison is made between previous observations (Lapin, 1974) and the present study. Unlike earlier studies, in the present one mice were
much more active and excitable and more aggressive (they frequently
bit each other and the fingers of an experimenter). In previous
studies, C57BL/6J mice were lacking in both spontaneous and shock-
induced aggressive behavior.

Table 1

Locomotion, rearings and body temperature in mice of different
strains examined. (Groups of 16 intact mice. Experiment was carried out in a single day at 10:00 a.m. - 1:00 p.m.).

No.	Strain	Locomotion mean ± S.E.M.	p<	Rearings mean ± S.E.M.	p<	Body Temp.
1.	SHR	23.1 ± 2.7		15.5 ± 2.1		38.2
2.	BALB/cJ	18.4 ± 2.3	2 vs 4 .002	8.0 ± 1.7	2 vs 4 .001	38.3
3.	C57BL/6J	24.4 ± 1.1	3 vs 2 .05	15.4 ± 0.9	3 vs 2 .01	37.9
4.	C57BR	29.3 ± 1.6	4 vs 5 .002 4 vs 3 .05	18.5 ± 0.9	4 vs 5 .01 4 vs 3 .02	38.0
5.	C3H/A	20.0 ± 2.1	5 vs 3 ns	12.0 ± 1.2	5 vs 3 .02	38.1

When measured for the second time, 7-9 days later, locomotion
and rearings were rather similar in all strains (see controls in
Tables 2 and 3). However, mice were more active than during the
first measurement. This decline in strain differences may be due
to dissimilar rates of extinction of locomotion and rearings and/or
dissimilar responses to housing, handling, etc. Previously, it has
been observed (Lapin, 1974) strain differences in the intensity of
extinction of rearings under short time intervals (in C57BR mice
the rate of extinction was the highest). Rectal temperature was
similar in all strains examined (Table 1).

Effect of apomorphine on locomotion

Apomorphine in doses of 5, 10, and 20 mg/kg decreased locomotion in C3H/A mice and increased it in C57BL/6J mice (Table 2). In
all other strains, there was no significant effect on locomotion.
In this dose range of apomorphine, there was no dose-response relationship in C3H/A and C57BL/6J strains.

Table 2

Effect of apomorphine on locomotion of mice of different
strains tested. (Groups of 8 mice. Statistical significance of
the difference compared with control of the respective strain. ●
p<0.05; o p<0.02; ■ p<0.01; □ p<0.002; ▲ p<0.001; mean ± S.E.M.)

No.	Strain	Control	Locomotion Apomorphine (mg/kg)		
			5	10	20
1.	SHR	12.7 ± 2.1	7.8 ± 2.4	15.2 ± 1.7	9.2 ± 1.9
2.	BALB/cJ	10.0 ± 1.6	7.1 ± 1.9	6.2 ± 1.6	10.0 ± 1.8
3.	C57BL/6J	11.0 ± 1.5	21.3 ± 2.3 ■	8.6 ± 2.1	21.1 ± 3.6 ○
4.	C57BR	18.5 ± 5.0	20.0 ± 3.3	17.4 ± 2.3	10.0 ± 1.6
5.	C3H/A	22.1 ± 3.5	7.3 ± 1.4	8.8 ± 1.6 □	7.3 ± 1.8 □

In a dose of 50 mg/kg apomorphine significantly decreased locomotion in all strains examined.

Effect of apomorphine on rearings

Rearings were inhibited by apomorphine in C3H/A and BALB/cJ
strains (Table 3). There was no dose-response relationship in this
action of apomorphine.

Table 3

Effect of apomorphine on rearings of mice of different strains
tested. Mean ± S.E. M. (Statistical significance according to
Table 2).

No.	Strain	Control	Rearings Apomorphine		
			5	10	20
1.	SHR	10.8 ± 3.1	3.8 ± 1.3	9.2 ± 1.7	7.0 ± 1.5
2.	BALB/cJ	5.0 ± 1.5	2.2 ± 1.2	4.1 ± 1.3	5.2 ± 1.5
3.	C57BL/6J	8.0 ± 1.7	11.1 ± 0.6	2.4 ± 1.3	11.2 ± 2.9
4.	C57BR	7.6 ± 2.1	7.5 ± 1.1	9.3 ± 1.6	11.3 ± 1.4
5.	C3H/A	15.4 ± 2.5	1.5 ± 0.3 ▲	3.5 ± 1.7 ■	4.1 ± 1.1 ■

In a dose of 50 mg/kg apomorphine, inhibited rearings significantly and about equally in all strains except SHR.

Apomorphine hypothermia

Apomorphine lowered body temperature in all five strains. Threshold dose was 0.5 for SHR, 0.75 for BALB/cJ, and 1.0 mg/kg for C57BL/6J, C57BR and C3H/A. Maximal hypothermia, as reported previously (Lapin & Samsonova, 1968a) was registered 30 minutes after injection of the drug. For this reason, apomorphine hypothermia was compared in the various strains at this time interval.

Considerable differences between strains were observed in apomorphine hypothermia (Table 4). These differences were most clear with a dose of 5 mg/kg. The decreasing order of strains for the intensity of apomorphine hypothermia was as follows: BALB/cJ SHR = C3H/A C57BR C57BL/6J. Dose-response relationship was observed within a dose range of 5-20 mg/kg only in the C57BR strain.

Table 4

Apomorphine hypothermia in mice of different strains examined. Mean $\pm$ S.E.M. [In C57BL/6J mice, hypothermia after 5 mg/kg of apomorphine (-1.0 $\pm$ 0.5) in the present experiment was smaller than in other experiments where fall of temperature was statistically significant. Data on Table 4 belong to the same animals whose locomotion and rearings are represented on Tables 2 and 3.]

No.	Strain	Control	Hypothermia $(- t^{o}_{30})$ Apomorphine (mg/kg)			
			5	p<	10	20
1.	SHR	0.2 $\pm$ 0.4	4.9 $\pm$ 0.3	1 vs 2 .02	4.4 $\pm$ 0.2	4.3 $\pm$ 0.2
2.	BALB/cJ	0.5 $\pm$ 0.3	5.7 $\pm$ 0.1	2 vs 3 .01	5.3 $\pm$ 0.2	5.3 $\pm$ 0.3
3.	C57BL/6J	0.1 $\pm$ 0.1	1.0 $\pm$ 0.5	3 vs 4 .01	4.1 $\pm$ 0.8	4.3 $\pm$ 0.9
4.	C57BR	1.1 $\pm$ 0.1	3.8 $\pm$ 0.3	4 vs 2 .01	4.8 $\pm$ 0.2	6.4 $\pm$ 0.2
5.	C3H/A	0.1 $\pm$ 0.2	4.8 $\pm$ 0.4	5 vs 4 .05 5 vs 2 .05	5.5 $\pm$ 0.5	5.1 $\pm$ 0.3

At a dose of 50 mg/kg, apomorphine induced the about equal reduction in body temperature in all strains (-5.9 to -7.4^{o}C).

Increase of apomorphine of a dose range of 5-20 mg/kg resulted in prolongation of hypothermia in all strains, i.e., dose-response relationship.

Diminution of apomorphine hypothermia by most typical antagonists of apomorphine such as haloperidol and desmethylimipramine was not equal for all strains tested (Table 5). For both antagonists, BALB/cJ strain was the most sensitive, and C57BL/6J the least sensitive. In fact, after administered doses of desmethylimipramine, antagonism to apomorphine was not even observed in C57BL/6J mice. In C3H/A strain, both haloperidol and desmethylimipramine were less effective than in all other strains except C57BL/6J. In all strains examined, haloperiodl induced ten-fold more activity (based on comparison of effective doses in mg/kg) than desmethylimipramine.

Table 5

Diminution of hypothermic effect of apomorphine by pretreatment with haloperidol or desmethylimipramine. Each letter represents a result of one experiment (mean value for a group of 8 mice). o - there was no significant diminution of apomorphine hypothermia (as compared with control in the same strain): a - $p < 0.05$; a - $p < 0.01$; A - $p < 0.002$; A - $p < 0.001$ (a - A = degrees of antagonism to apomorphine).

Strain	Antagonism to apomorphine						
	Haloperidol (mg/kg)			Desmethylimipramine (mg/kg)			
	0.05	0.25	0.5	0.5	1.0	2.5	5.0
SHR	0	a	A	0	a	0	A
BALB/cJ	A	a	A	0	0	a	a
C57BL/6J	0	0	A	0	0	0	0
C57BR	0	a	a	0	0	A	a
C3H/A	0	0	A	0	0	a	0

Apomorphine stereotypies

Injections of apomorphine in doses of 10 mg/kg and higher resulted (1-2 minutes later) in strong excitement with squealing, aggressive vertical postures and attacks. The emotional component of excitement was much more pronounced in C57BR and

C57BL/6J strains, than in the other strains tested. Typical
stereotypies were observed 5-7 minutes after injection. There
was a tendency for a dose-response relationship (Table 6). This
relationship was more evident for the duration of stereotypies
than for the intensity. For instance, in SHR mice, 60 minutes
after injection of a dose of 10 mg/kg of apomorphine, stereotypies were observed only in 2 mice of 7 (mean score for the group
was 0.3); after a dose of 20 mg/kg, in 7 mice out of 7 (mean
score 1.1); and after a dose of 40 mg/kg, in 7 mice of 7 (mean
score 1.9). Response data for BALB/cJ mice were as follows:
at 10 mg/kg - 2/7 (mean score 0.3); at 20 mg/kg - 6/7 (mean
score 0.7); at 40 mg/kg - 7/7 (mean score 2.1). This observation suggests that the prolongation of apomorphine stereotypes
can be used as a criterion of enhancement of the respective
action of apomorphine and, conversely, the shortening of apomorphine stereotypies - as a criterion of diminution of the action
of apomorphine. The same principle for measuring effects of
drugs on amphetamine stereotypies was offered by Dr. E. L. Schelkunov (1964) of this laboratory. Of the five strains tested,
C57BL/6J and C3H/A differed by being significantly less intensive
stereotypies (Table 6).

Table 6

Apomorphine stereotypies in mice of different strains tested.
(Mean scores for 60 min. ± S.E.M.)

		S t e r e o t y p i e s[1]					
No.	Strain	Apomorphine (mg/kg)					
		10	p<	20	p<	40	p<
1.	SHR	5.0 ± 1.0		6.5 ± 0.4		7.6 ±	
2.	BALB/cJ	6.0 ± 0		7.9 ± 0.4		10.4 ± 0.6	
3.	C57BL/6J	3.4 ± 0.2	.001	3.0 ± 0	'.001	4.6 ± 0.5	*.001
4.	C57BR	6.0 ± 0		8.0 ± 0		8.0 ± 0	
5.	C3H/A	3.1 ± 0.2	.001	4.1 ± 0.4	'.001	6.7 ± 0.3	**.01

1. Statistical significance of the differences: ε - with groups
   2 and 4; ' - with groups 1, w and 4 ($p_{5-1} < .01$); $p_{3-5} < .02$;
   *with groups 1, w and 4; ** - with groups 2, 3 and 4.

Qualitative characteristics of stereotypes were not identical in all strains. Leaning against a wall was predominant posture in SHR, BALB/cJ, and C3H/A strains. It was lso observed in some mice of C57BL/6J strain, but not in C57BR. The latter almost always remained in a vertical posture. It is worth noting that all strains exhibited practically one type of stereotyped behavior, namely that of sniffing. In some mice licking of wall and wire ceiling was also observed. However, no gnawing and/or biting the wire, grooming, nor any other type of stereotype, such as exhibited by amphetamine-treated mice (Ther, Schramm, 1962), were present. Although all strains were rather similar in their general appearance (i.e., vertical posture and compulsive sniffing, and increased excitability to external stimuli), they were different in their locomotion which interrupted, on occasion, their vertical posture. BALB/cJ and C57BR strains were inhibited, exhibited cataleptic posture, and moved very slowly, whereas C57BL/6J and SHR were excited and moved very quickly reminiscent of amphetamine-intoxicated grouped mice. Rushes of C3H/A mice look similar to those of control (no apomorphine mice.

DISCUSSION

Apomorphine in doses of 5, 10, and 20 mg/kg either decreased locomotion and rearings or did not change them in mice of 5 strains tested. The only exception was the C57BL/6J strain in which significant stimulation of locomotion was registered (Table 2). It has been reported previously (Lapin & Samsonova, 1968a; 1968b; Lapin, 1969a; Maj et al., 1962) that apomorphine in mice only decreased locomotion, whereas there is an opposite effect in rats (Lapin & Samsonova, 1968b; Grabowska et al., 1973). There is only a single paper (Frommel, 1965) which reports the stimulant effect of apomorphine (1 mg/kg) in mice. As it has been pointed out previously (Lapin & Samsonova, 1968b), observations made by means of a vibrograph may be based on more frequent vibrations of a box caused by stereotypies and not by locomotion. We have also obtained increased numbers of counts using an electronic integrator (Lapin & Samsonova, 1968b), a device principally similar to a vibrograph, used by Frommel. Since locomotion is enhanced during the first 30 minutes after injection of apomorphine and then stereotypies predominant, continuous registration (during 2 hours) in a vibrograph, such as that used by Frommel measures probably mainly stereotypies. It is important, therefore, to point out that stimulation of locomotion in C57BL/6J mice, in the present study, was registered by measuring the cross-overs and not vibrations of the floor.

Observations that a dose of 50 mg/kg apomorphine caused a decline in both locomotion and rearings in all strains of mice including C57BL/6J suggest that, in mice, the basic effect of this drug on motor activity is one of inhibition. Lack of the dose-response relationship in inhibitory action of apomorphine on locomotion of male albino-Swiss mice was reported elsewhere (Maj et al., 1972).

Apomorphine hypothermia, to varying degrees, was observed in all 5 strains; it decreased (C3H/A), increased (C57BL/6J) or did not change (SHR, BALB/cJ and C57BR) in correlation with motor activity. This observation can be considered as an argument supporting the idea that apomorphine hypothermia and inhibition of motor activity in mice are not causally mutally related. It has been suggested (Maj et al., 1972) that the depression of locomotor activity produced by apomorphine is coreelated with the hypothermizing action of the drug. It is also possible that, in the mouse, a species with body temperature highly dependent on general motor activity, a decrease of locomotion can result in lowering of body temperature. Strain differences in the effect of apomorphine on locomotion provide, in our opinion, crucial data on the relationship between these two effects of apomorphine in mice.

In the present study, previous observations that apomorphine hypothermia in a dose range of 1 - 100 mg/kg (Lapin & Samsonova, 1968a) or 0.8 - 50 mg/kg (Maj et al., 1972) is not dose-dependent were confirmed. The only exception was seen in C57BR mice.

It is of great interest whether monoaminergic processes involved in the action of apomorphine are responsible for strain differences in effects of this drug in mice. Dopaminergic mechanisms are suggested to be involved in apomorphine hypothermia in mice (Fuxe & Sjövist, 1972; Barnett et al., 1972). Strain differences in mice (NMRI and C3H) in temperature responses (both hyper- and hypothermic) to d-amphetamine are suggested to be related to the turnover of dopamine in striatum (Caccia et al., 1973). Antagonistic action of haloperidol (Table 5), a strong blocker of dopamine receptors, suggests that stimulation of dopaminergic receptors by apomorphine can take place in all mouse strains examined. Recent data and hypothesis about a secondary stimulation of the striatal dopamine receptors by apomorphine (Grabowska et al., 1973; Grabowska, 1974) give rise to the question of whether or not strain differences in effects of apomorphine, in particular hypothermia, are related to serotonergic mechanisms. This question is reinforced by data on differences in serotonin metabolism in two strains of mice (C57BL/6J and BALB/cJ) accompanied by differences in sleep patterns (Mitler et al., 1973). There was evidence for the relatively mild role of serotonergic component in the hypothermic effect of apomorphine in mice (Lapin, 1971). However, the problem requires furthur study and experiments are now in progress in our laboratory

to answer the question regarding the involvement of serotonergic
mechanisms in effects of apomorphine in different strains of mice.

SUMMARY

    Spontaneous locomotion and rearings and effects of apomorphine
were compared in adult male mice of 5 strains: SHR (inbred from
Swiss), BALB/cJ, C57BL/6J, CC57BR, and C3H/A. Strain differences
were registered in spontaneous locomotion and rearings. Apomorphine
in doses of 5-20 mg/kg produced hypothermia in all strains, whereas motor activity was lowered only in one strain (C3H/A), and increased in C57BL/6J mice. This observation suggests that in the
strains examined, there are no causal mutual relationships between
lowering of motor activity and hypothermia induced by apomorphine.
Apomorphine hypothermia was antagonized in all strains by pretreatment with haloperidol or desmthylimipramine (the only exception
was inactivity of desmethylimipramine in doses of 0.5 - 5.0 mg/kg
in the C57BL/6J strain). Quantitative and qualitative strain differences in apomorphine stereotypies are described. Data obtained
stimulated further experiments which are now in progress on involvement of monoaminergic mechanisms (particularly dopaminergic and
serotoninergic) in strain differences in effects of apomorphine.

REFERENCES

BARNETT, A., GOLDSTEIN, J., & TABER, R. I., 1972, Apomorphine-induced
    hypothermia in mice: a possible dopaminergic effect. Arch.
    Int. Pharmacodyn. 198:242.

BELENKY, M. L., Some results of studies on problems of pharmacology
    of adrenergic processes. Abstr. of papers of the Meeting of
    the Presidium of the All-Union Pharmacol. Soc. (January 10-11,
    1964), Leningrad, 1964, 15-18 (In Russian).

BELENKY, M. L., 1966, On some new possible ways of pharmacological
    action on regulation of activity of cardio-vascular system.
    Vestnik. Akad. Med. Nauk. (Moscow), 1966, 4:54 (In Russian).

BELENKY, M. L., VITOLINA, M. A., & VITOLINA, R. O., 1965, On the
    probable importance of competetive inhibition of COMT in the
    mechanism of action of apomorphine. In: "Problems of General
    Pharmacology and Toxicology", Leningrad, 15-24 (In Russian).

BELENKY, M. L., VITOLINA, M. A., & BAUMANIS, E. A., 1966, Effect of
    apomorphine on inactivation of adrenaline in cats. Bull. Exp.
    Biol. Med. (Moscow), 64:54. (In Russian).

CACCIA, S., CECCHETTI, G., GARATTINI, S., & JORI, A., 1973, Inter-
     action of (+)-amphetamine with cerebral dopaminergic neurons in
     two strains of mice, that show different temperature responses
     to this drug. Brit. J. Pharmacol. 49:400.

ERNST, A. M. & SMELIK, P. G., 1966, Site of action of dopamine and
     apomorphine on compulsive gnawing behaviour in rats. Experientia
     22:837.

ERNST, A. M., 1967, Mode of action of apomorphine and dexamphetamine
     on gnawing compulsion in rats. Psychopharmacologia, 10:316.

FERRIS, R. M., TANG, F. L. M., & RUSSEL, A. V., 1974, In vitro evi-
     dence for a presynaptic action of apomorphine. Pharmacologist,
     No. 2, 16:328.

FROMMEL, E., 1965, The cholinergic mechanism of psychomotor agita-
     tion in apomorphine-injected mice. Arch. Int. Pharmacodyn.,
     154:231.

FUXE, K., & SJÖVIST, F., 1972, Hypothermic effect of apomorphine in
     the mouse. J. Pharm. Pharmacol., 24:702.

GRABOWSKA, M., 1974, On the role of serotonin in apomorphine-induced
     locomotion stimulation in rats. Pharmacol. Biochem. Behav. 2:263.

GRABOWSKA, M., ANTKIEWICZ, L., MAJ, J., & MICHALUK, J., 1973, Apomor-
     phine and central serotonin neurons. Pol. J. Pharmacol. Pharm.
     25:29.

HILL, H. F., & HORITA, A., 1972, A pimozide-sensitive effect of
     apomorphine on body temperature of the rabbit. J. Pharm. Pharmac.
     24:490.

HORITA, A., & QUOCK, R. M., 1964, Dopaminergic mechanisms in drug-
     induced temperature effects. Proc. 2nd Symp. Pharmacology of
     Thermoregulation (Paris, 1974), Karger, Basel, 129-137.

LAPIN, I. P., 1969a, Biochemical Pharmacology of Metabolism of Cate-
     cholamines. In: "Chemical Factors of Regulation of Activity
     and Biosynthesis of Enzymes" (ed. V. N. Orekhovitch), Medicina,
     Moscow, 216-247 (In Russian).

LAPIN, I. P., 1969b, Pharmacological Activity of Quaternary Deriva-
     tives of Imipramine and Diethylaminopropinyl-iminodibenzyl.
     Pharmakopsychiatrie-Neuropsychopharmakologie, 2:14.

LAPIN, I. P., 1971, Is there a serotoninergic component in the hypothermic effect of apomorphine in mice? In: Problems of Pharmacology of Neurotropic Drugs (abstr. of the conference, Riga, May 1971), Zinatne, Riga, 23-26 (In Russian).

LAPIN, I. P., 1974, Behavioral effects of psychoactive drugs influencing the metabolism of brain monoamines in mice of different strains. In: The Genetics of Behavior (ed. J. H. F. van Abeelen), North-Holl. Publ. Co., Amsterdam, Chapter 17, 417-432.

LAPIN, I. P., & SAMSONOVA, M. L., 1968a, Apomorphine-induced bypothermia in mice and the effect on thereon of adrenergic and serotoninergic agents. Farmakol. Toxikol. (Moscow), 31:563, (In Russian).

LAPIN, I. P., & SAMSONOVA, M. L., 1968b, Species differences in the effects of apomorphine as an adrenergic agent. Bull. Exp. Biol. Med. (Moscow) 66-63 (In Russian).

MAJ, J., GRABOWSKA, M., GAJDA, L., & MICHALUK, J., 1972, On the central action of apomorphine in mice. Dissert. Pharm. Pharmacol. 24:352.

MCKENZIE, G. M., 1974, The effects of COMT inhibitors on behavior and dopamine metabolism. Psychopharmacology Bull., 10:31.

MITLER, M. M., COHEN, H. B., GRATTAN, J., DOMINIC, J., DEGUCHI, T., BARCHAS, J. D., DEMENT, W. C., & KESSLER, S., 1973, Sleep and serotonin in two strains of Mus. musculus. Pharmacol. Biochem. Behav. 1:501.

QUOCK, R. M., & HORITA, A., 1974, Apomorphine: Modification of its hyperthermic effect in rabbits by p-chlorophenylalaine. Science 183:539.

SCHELKUNOV, E. L., 1964, Method of "amphetamine stereotypy" for testing the action of drugs on central adrenergic processes. Farmakol. Toxikol. (Moscow) 27:628 (In Russian).

SCHELKUNOV, E. L., 1968, Pharmacological effects of apomorphine in mice as tests to differentiate antidepressants, anticholinergics and neuroleptics. Farmakol. Toxikol. (Moscow), 31:559 (In Russian).

THER, L., & SCHRAMM, H., 1962, Apomorphin-Synergismus (Zwangsnagen bei Mäusen) als Test zur Differenzierung Psychotroper Substanzen. Arch. Int. Pharmacodyn. 138:302.

IMPLICATIONS OF PSYCHOPHARMACOGENETICS RESEARCH

W. Kalow, M.D.

and

A. E. LeBlanc, M.D.

Department of Pharmacology
University of Toronto
Addiction Research Foundation
Toronto, Canada

CONTENTS

INTRODUCTION

Comparisons are the essence, the beginning and the end, of every research effort. In pharmacogenetic research, (Who, 1973) the items of comparison are differences in drug response (or parameters related to drug response) between responding units which may be human subjects, animals, or even isolated cells. Pharmacogenetic research in man is possible only if there are person-to-person difference in drug response, and the research is worthwhile only if the differences are substantial. On the other hand, if there are differences, every effort to account for these will remain incomplete unless the genetic element is evaluated.

Psychopharmacological agents are a particularly important class of drugs that may alter behavior, and individual differences in response (Propping & Kopun, 1973; Omenn & Motulsky, 1974) to them are often striking. Therefore, it is not surprising that these should be subjected to intense pharmacogenetic studies.

In looking at the implications of these studies, one finds that these may differ greatly in breadth, significance and area of human activity which might be affected. A review of these implications may be organized by recognizing three different spheres which one may designate as pharmacological implications, implications for health care, and implications for social policies. Regarding pharmacological implications, the subject matter is divided naturally by the fact that the expression of genetic differences may depend on drug metabolism, ability to respond and tendency to self-medication. Implications for health care hinge on whether pharmacogenetic research will lead to idiosyncratic medication, or will at least enhance the possibility to individualize drug therapy. There are secondary implications regarding cost of research and of therapy, and consequences for medical teaching. Finally, the sociopolitical implications are concerned with legal consequences, and questions regarding the burden of proof for psychopharmacogenetic information.

The following pages attempt to give a brief overview of these different areas of concern.

PHARMACOLOGICAL IMPLICATIONS

Genetic variation in the disposition of psychoactive drugs

The implications of pharmacogenetic investigations into the fate of drugs in the body, are in principle the same for psychoactive as for other drugs. The clinical significance of such in-

vestigations may be greater for the former since psychoactive drugs
must be lipid-soluble in order to reach the brain, and they depend
on metabolism for excretion from the body because of their lipid-
solubility. Furthermore, exposure of a given person to psychoactive drugs tend to be chronic. Under these circumstances, if
there is a deficiency in the ability to metabolize a drug, there
may be a cumulative effect which could magnify an initial dis-
similarly into a 20-or 30-fold difference in blood levels (Sjöqvist
& Von Bahr, 1973).

A strong genetic component in drug metabolism would suggest
that the metabolizing capacity of a given subject for a given
drug would tend to remain constant over long periods of time
(Alexanderson, 1972). Since drug metabolism may lead to the formation of unstable intermediates which react irreversibly with
cell constituents, the drug metabolizing capacity of an individual may well be associated with susceptibility to serious drug
toxicities, such as hepatotoxicity or carcinogenicity (Gillette,
1974).

Furthermore, since the number of drug metabolizing pathways
in man seems to be limited, one can expect to observe that persons
with a poor capacity to metabolize drug A may also be poor in
metabolizing drug B, while there may be no such relationship to
drug C (Kadar et al., 1973). For instance, although nortriptyline
and desmethylimipramine are metabolized at rather different rates,
a slow metabolizer of one drug is slow for the other, so that
therapeutic failures are not corroected by a change from one of
these drugs to the other (Alexanderson, 1972). Dose adjustment
of the given drug is the logical course of action. Further research into the genetics of the metabolism of psychopharmaca are
bound to lead to similar relevations.

Any successful genetic investigation in this area can open
important insights into biochemical relationships. A past example
is the discovery that some subjects have a variant form of alcohol dehydrogenase which oxidizes ethanol in vitro at 5 times the
normal rate (Edwards & Evans, 1967) while there is no difference
in vivo (Von Wartburg,& Schürch, 1968). This observation led to
the important conclusion that it is not the enzyme itself, but the
supply of the co-factor NAD which determines the rate of alcohol
metabolism in man. This has numerous implications; for instance,
it explains the clinically important link between alcohol metabolism and lactic acid levels.

Enzyme induction is a well-known cause of an enhanced rate of
drug metabolism, but not all individuals respond to all inducers
(Vesell, 1974). Studies into the genetics of human susceptibility
to induction of drug-metabolizing enzymes are still scarce, but

future studies may well prove to have far-reaching biological implications. Of the many adaptation phenomena, including drug tolerance or dependence, (Kalant et al., 1971) at least some will
surely depend on the induced formation of one or other kind of
enzyme.

Genetic variation of drug effects

In theory, the presence or absence of a therapeutic response
to a drug may serve to distinguish between different diseases
which are not differentiated at present because they have a similar symptomatology. However, before one can begin to realize
this possibility, one has to be able to tell whether the failure
of drug therapy in a given patient is due to a lack of compliance
of the patient, or due to faulty drug absorption or other factor
which reduces the drug concentration at the receptor site. In
short, the determination of drug levels in plasma or urine, and a
pharmacokinetic interpretation of these levels, are prerequisites
for genetic studies into the drug response of nerve cells or
other affected structures. So far, these prerequisites were
not often realized for psychopharmacological agents except for
alcohol. Many of these agents are so potent that they require
minute amounts which escape detection in body fluids by all but
highly specialized methods.

The data which are available tend to confirm the old suspicion that much of the variation in response to psychoactive
drugs cannot be accounted for by differences in drug disposition.
For instance, there are no close correlations between plasma
levels of chlorpromazine and its antischizophrenic action (Curry,
1974) nor between those of nortriptyline and its antidepressant
action (Asberg, 1974). Thus, there is a variation which cannot
be fruitfully studied without genetic consideration. One can
hope that future research in these areas will pay off handsomely
in the understanding of mental illnesses or pathological behaviour
patterns.

The research into this area of drug effects may be aided by
studies in biochemical genetics, if it can be shown that a particular enzyme defect is associated with deviant drug effects. For
instance, it will be interesting to see whether the discovery of
at least 2 different forms of monoamine oxidase in man (Nies et
al., 1974) and the demonstration of the genetic control of the
activities of this enzyme, will provide an explanation for deviant
effects of drugs which are known to be inhibitors or substrates of
monoamine oxidase.

Genetic variation in the propensity
to self-medication

Several modern studies strongly suggest that there is a genetic component in the propensity to become an alcoholic (Partanen et al., 1966; Goodwin et al., 1973). Yet it is questionable whether these studies will ever be useful for the amelioration of drug dependence or habituation on a large scale, since there will always be an environmental component in drug taking. It is likely that control of undesirable self-medication will be always more effective via this environmental component than via the genes. Thus, within limits and considering the feasibility of choices, the most effective way to reduce the rate of alcoholism in a population seems to be to reduce availability of alcohol through social policy action (Popham et al., 1975). This does not mean that genetic studies into the propensity of drug misuse are redundant. If tendencies to abuse or to improperly use drugs are inherited, the therapist, and for that matter, the affected individual, may use this information to blunt the consequences.

In addition, such studies may have great value as curiosity-oriented research. A spin-off of such research is for instance, the recognition that liver dysfunctions can affect colour vision in a clincially significant way (Thuline, 1972). Another example is the recognition by Winokur and his associates (Winokur et al., 1970) of a genetic association between depressive illness and propensity to alcoholism, which may provide the basis for new insights into the cause of a mental aberration or disease.

THERAPEUTIC IMPLICATIONS OF
PSYCHOPHARMACOGENETIC INFORMATION

It should be clear from the foregoing that research in psychopharmacogenetics can have numerous consequences and may help to solve various problems. However, it is possible to arrive at one generalization: Pharmacogenetic research is an indispensable tool for the exploration of idiosyncratic medication, i.e. individualization of drug therapy. Once it is known which steps in the numerous interactions between body and drug are genetcially controlled, one will know to what extent therapeutic and toxic effects of drugs are stable characteristics and thereby predictable in individual subjects. Predictability is an important element in true individualization of drug therapy.

Once predictability has been established through research, predictions may become a service requirement. In some case, enzyme tests using blood or cells, or neurological or behavioural

tests, could be the most suitable means of predicting an individual's drug response; perhaps more often, the past response to a
drug will be used to forecast future responses to the same and/or
to some other drugs. For this purpose, good records would have
to be established in order to preserve a history of drug intake
and response, and other relevent information in a population.
Modern technology would permit this to occur. For instance,
records like the Danish Government's registry of psychiatric
data or the Boston Collaborative Drug Surveillance Programme,
(Jick et al., 1970) could be models for a drug registry.

When one thinks of individualization of drug therapy at the
present time, one is inclined to consider only individual dose
adjustment, or at best, some trial and error in the choice of
drugs. However, one should not forget that the current practices
of drug therapy and drug development are based on statistical
concepts. If a new drug causes harm to a small percentage of
patients, the drug may be discarded and thereby withheld from the
majority of subjects who could benefit from it. If one would be
able to predict on the basis of the known biochemical make-up
of individual patients who would or would not respond adversely
to that drug, the drug could remain available. In short, idiosyncratic medication could greatly increase the treasure chest
of available drugs.

The implementation of the findings of research in this area
will depend totally on the levels of knowledge of medical prac-
titioners. At the present time, medical training emphasizes a
medicine of statistical norms. The notion that each patient is
different will have to be amplified from a maxim into a practical
procedure for routine medical practice. This is essential, though
difficult, given the already crowded medical curriculum.

One may hold that at the present time in the Western world,
the most serious shortcoming in drug therapy is not lack of
knowledge, but deficiencies in the application of available
knowledge. This is certainly true in many areas of medicine.
However, in the field of pharmacogenetics of psychoactive drugs,
lack of knowledge is a crippling defect. There is reason to believe that a significant number of hospitalized mental patients
are in fact correctable therapeutic failures. In other words,
how many patients are given inappropriate dosage regimens or
due to ignorance, are being denied a more effective medication?

This type of questioning has become urgent since scarce
research funds tend to favor allocation to those areas of research where the gain in improved quality of life and reduction
of health costs will be maximal. Psychopharmacogenetic research
appears to be such an area. At the present cost of hospitaliza-

tion, the additional release of only a few patients a year, would more than take care of the costs of psychopharmacogenetic research.

NON-PHARMACOLOGICAL IMPLICATIONS
OF PSYCHOPHARMACOGENETIC RESEARCH

From the work of Angst (1961) it has been known for many years that there is a genetic component in determing the response to antidepressants, but the data did not have any clinical impact. One reason may be that they are merely descriptive. A deeper reason may be the resurgence of mind-body dichotomy in modern society.

Any suggestion that the mind can be subject to the same variations as are height, eye colour, etc., will be understood by some people and yet provoke a great outcry in the general populace. This concern has been given considerable piquancy in examining questions of intelligence. (Dobzhansky, 1973; Jensen, 1973). It serves no purpose to debate the pros and cons of the research data but it does provide a number of lessons.

The first is that the whole genetic area has been politicized by the concept of race. While most geneticists would see "races" merely as statistical entities representing higher than usual concentrations of or higher proportion of certain configurations of genetic information, (Montagu, 1969) the general public does not share this view.

The second lesson is that the burden of proof in research is not the same in all situations. It has been recognized for some time that there is need for statistical treatment of data, and the need for replication and use of several test systems. An application of this philosophy is well exemplified in the introduction of new drugs into the medical system. In the case of genetic research into mental functions, the burden is probably greater than in many other areas of biological research.

It is clear that societies generally use psychoactive drugs. It is almost a definition of man that he actively alters his mental state with exogenous chemicals. This use has, by its widespread nature, become to most people a right. Also, drug use has a very important ritual function in most societies. To comment on it genetically creates many emotional problems which are translated into a variety of social problems. For example, the notion of the Indian having special alcohol problems due to genetic consideration has been used as an argument for special court response. This same question has been raised for other genetical abnormalities associated with violence.

This type of thinking raises a special problem with the law.
The law, though it does have a capacity to change, operates for
the most part on statistical norms. As the great jurist Oliver
Wendell Holmes said: "Difficult cases make bad laws." It must be
remembered that a great many laws deal directly with drugs (impaired driving) or are affected by drug effects (mitigation of
sentence for criminal acts). Thus, increased knowledge of psychopharmacogenetics may ultimately affect many important social
systems which are by their nature fragile.

CONCLUSIONS

Psychopharmacogenetics has already had an impact on concepts
of drug responses. The future is likely to bring substantial advances. First, because in the time scale of biological science,
this is a young field and much remains to be done. Secondly, the
burgeoning amount of important animal data has laid the foundation
for rapid advances in the clinical area. As the field continues
to develop, it will be important to recognize the impact on the
non-pharmacological areas.

REFERENCES

ALE ANDERSON, B., 1972, Pharmacokinetics of desmethylimipramine
    and nortriptyline in man after single and multiple oral
    doses - A cross-over study, Europ. J. Clin. Pharmacol.

ANGST, J., 1961, A Clinical Analysis of the effects of tofranil
    in depression. Longitudinal and follow-up studies. Treat-
    ment of blood-relations. Psychopharmacologia 2:381.

ASBERG, M., 1974, Plasma nortriptyline levels - relationship to
    clinical effects. Clin. Pharmacol. Ther. 16:215.

CURRY, S. H., 1974, Concentration-effect relationships with major
    and minor tranquilizers. Clin. Pharmacol. Ther. 16:192.

DOBZHANSKY, T., Race, intelligence and genetics - difference are
    not deficits. Psychology Today, 7, #7, 97-101, December 1973.

EDWARDS, J. A. & E ANS, D. A. P., 1967, Ethanol Metabolism in subjects
    possessing typical and atypical liver alchol dehydrogenase.
    Clin. Pharmacol. Ther. 8:824.

GILLETTE, J. R., 1974, Commentary - A perspective on the role of
    chemically reactive metabolites of foreign compounds in
    toxicity - II. Alterations in the Kinetics of covalent
    binding. Biochem. Pharmacol. 23:2927.

GOODWIN, D. W., SCHULSINGER, F., HERMANSEN, L., GUZE, S. B., & WINOKUR, G., 1973, Alcohol problems in adoptees raised apart from alcoholic biological parents. Arch. Gen. Psychiatry. 28:238.

JENSEN, A., Race, intellignece and genetics - the differences are real. Psychology Today, 7, #7, 80-86, December 1973.

JICK, H., MIETTINEN, O. S., SHAPIRO, S., LEWIS, G. P., SISKIND, V., & SLONE, D., 1970, Comprehensive drug surveillance. JAMA 213:1455.

KADAR, D., INABA, T., ENDRENYI, L., JOHNSON, G. E., & KALOW, W., 1973, Comparative drug elimination capacity in man-glutethimide, amobarbital, antipyrien, and sulfinpyrazone. Clin. Pharmacol. Ther. 14:552.

KALANT, H., LEBLANC, A. E., & GIBBONS, R. J., 1971, Tolerance to and dependence on some non-opiate psychotropic drugs. Pharmacol. Rev. 23:135.

MONTAGUE, A., 1969, The Concept of race. Collier Books, London.

NIES, A., ROBINSON, D. S., HARRIS, L. S., & LAMBORN, K. R., 1974, Comparison of monoamine oxidase substrate activities in twins, schizophrenics, depressives, and controls. Neuro-psychopharmacology of monoamines and their regulatory enzymes. E. Usdin, (ed). Raven Press, New York. pp. 59-70.

OMENN, G. S., & MOTULSKY, A. G., 1974, Pharmacogenetics and mental disease. Psychol. Med. 4:125.

PARTANEN, J., BRUUN, K., & MARKKANEN, T., 1966, Inheritance of drinking behavior. Finnish Fdn. for Alcohol Studies, Helsinki.

POPHAM, R. E., SCHMIDT, W., & DELINT, J., 1975, Prevention of Hazardous drinking: Implications of research on the effect of government control measures. Symposium on law and drinking behavioral proceedings. Eds. J. A. Ewing & B. A. Rouse, Nelson-Hall, Chicago.

PROPPING, P. & KOPUN, M., 1973, Pharmacogenetic aspects of psycho-active drugs: Facts and fancy. Humangenetick 20:291.

SJÖQVIST, F. & VON BAHR, C., 1973, Interindividual differences in drug oxidation: Clinical importance. Drug. Metabo. Dispo. 1:469.

THULINE, H. C., 1972, Considerations in regard to a proposed
   association of alcoholism and color blindness. Ann. N. Y.
   Acad. Sci. 197:148.

VESELL, E. S., 1974, Factors causing interindividual variations
   of drug concentrations in blood. Clin. Pharmacol. Ther.
   16:135.

VON WARTBURG, J. P. & SCHÜRCH, P. M., 1968, A typical human liver
   alcohol dehydrogenase. Ann. N. Y. Acad. Sci. 151:936.

WINOKUR, G., REICH, T., RIMMER, J. & PITTS, F. N., JR., 1970,
   Alcoholism. III. Diagnosis and familial psychiatric illness
   in 259 alcoholic patients. Arch. Gen. Psychiat. 23:104.

WHO - Scientific Group. Pharmacogenetics. Wld. Hlth. Org.
   Techn. Report Ser. #524, 1-40, 1973.

RECOMBINANT INBRED STRAINS: A NOVEL GENETIC APPROACH FOR

PSYCHOPHARMACOGENETICISTS[1]

Basil E. Eleftheriou and Penelope K. Elias

The Jackson Laboratory, Bar Harbor, Maine   04609
and Department of Psychology, Syracuse University,
Syracuse, New York

CONTENTS

---

[1] Preparation of this chapter and data presented have been variously
supported by grants HD 05860, and HD 05523 to B. E. Eleftheriou
and 08220 to Penelope K. Elias from the National Institute of
Child Health and Human Development.

INTRODUCTION

Historically, species variation in drug responses was one of the primary pharmacological phenomena noted by various investigators dealing with drug responses. Extensive research was conducted into the responses of various species of animals to an identical drug. Thus, it was noticed early in the area of comparative pharmacology that all stimulant agents did not uniformly stimulate, all depressant agents did not uniformly depress and all analgesics did not uniformly induce analgesia in all species examined.

With the increased availability of inbred strains within given species, the logical procedure within the area of comparative pharmacology was the study of strain variations and their F_1 hybrids within a given species. Thus, the realization was created that the genotype of a given animal is of primary importance in its respective response to a given pharmacological agent. Once researchers in this area became cognizant of this strain variation, the area of pharmacogenetics was created.

Pharmacogenetics is the study of individual responses in a particular species, and research in this area is worthwhile only if divergent responses are established. Additionally, our ability to account for these differences will remain incomplete unless the genetic elements are evaluated.

In a similar fashion to the development of pharmacogenetics, the area of behavior genetics was also created. Sometime during the early 1960's both pharmacogeneticists and behavior geneticists initiated programs of strain comparison of various behavior-altering drugs in inbred strains of rabbits and rats, but particularly in inbred strains of mice. This particular approach attracted and still attracts the fascination of a great number of distinguished comparative scientists dealing in these areas of behavior genetics and pharmacogenetics. The generation of this type of comparative data in drugs, behavior and genetics is now in geometric relationship to the number of investigators participating. Even within a given species, however, this extensive accumulation of data has not helped substantially in elaborating causative or controlling mechanisms with appropriate genetic models that can be studied further.

THE GENETIC APPROACH

An alternative to the comparative approach is the use of strains of a given species whose background is known. This approach offers a unique insight into the genetic controlling mechanisms of drugs and subsequent behavior, as well as the genetic control of drug induced behaviors which may, in turn, influence physiological events. Unfortunately, the availability of such strains is limited to a few species. Among these, the one species where such availability is high and where genes have been mapped is the house mouse, Mus musculus. In this chapter, a brief discussion will be presented on the availability of strains of mice that can be used for behavior--drug-genetic experiments. In short, because of the obvious advantages of mouse populations, the discussion will concentrate on three available genetic systems of breeding: (a) inbred strains; (b) recombinant-inbred strains; and (c) congenic lines. With these three basic genetic procedures, an experimenter wishing to avail himself of these genetic tools can enhance and further his research objectives dealing with drugs and behavior. Actually, an excellent and rather comprehensive survey of these systems has been recently compiled by Green (1974).

INBRED STRAINS

The experimental approach of using various strains in comparative studies is used widely in the area of behavior and drugs. Usually, the subjects can come from strains chosen with respect to the same trait used in the comparison study. More frequently, the

strains were developed for quite different traits, oftentimes not
related to drugs and behavior. Inbred strains are maintained not
by selection, but by adherence to a particular mating system. Comparisons between non-inbred stocks are also useful in drugs and
behavior. For example, the laboratory albino rat is significantly
different from those caught in the wild. Nevertheless, the genetic
homogeneity achieved by inbreeding provides a research tool for
which there is no substitute.

Inbreeding is the mating of animals more closely related than
the average, and its quantitative expression is in relative terms
which have reference only to a specified foundation stock in genetic equilibrium. All of the individuals of a given species are
related to some extent, but usually only the closer degrees of relationship bear significance for the problem of inbreeding. Inbreeding is a relative concept, and its intensity varies over a wide
range because of the different types of inbreeding regimens that
are used. However, the brother-sister and parent-offspring matings
represent the most intense form possible with animals incapable of
self-fertilization, such as the mouse. Breeding to other families
within a strain, represents outbreeding with relation to the family group, but inbreeding (if families are related) with respect to
the species as a whole. The primary goal of inbreeding is to enhance the probability that offspring will inherit the same genes
from both parents. Thus, it leads to a decline in heterozygosis
and the fixation of genotypes. The rate of fixation is a function
of inbreeding intensity, and Wright's (1923) coefficient of inbreeding is designed to express the expected decrease of heterozygosis in relation to the original foundation stock. In contrast,
there is no way of expressing the degree of heterozygosis of a
random-bred stock in terms of the number of loci involved, although
knowledge of the origin and phenotypic variability of a group may
enable the experimenter to judge it as relatively great or small.
For clarification and theoretical treatment of the various inbreeding regimens, the reader is referred to any basic text in genetics.

Intense inbreeding over a long period of time leads to the
production of very homozygous stocks. Whether such stocks or
strains ever attain a completely isogenic state is quite unknown.
Usually, inbreeding is accompanied by a decline in vigor and reproductive capacity, although some strains are fertile and active after 50 or more generations of brother-sister matings. It is possible that the necessity of selecting for viability results in the
maintenance of some heterozygosity, but it must be relatively small

and can usually be neglected. The experimenter who uses these
strains, however, cannot assume that the removal of genotypic variants necessarily eliminates phenotypic variants. There is ample
evidence that homozygous individuals are less well buffered against
minor environmental agents and inbred animals may be no more uniform in response than random-bred subjects (McLaren and Michie,
1956). The use of F_1 hybrids between any given inbred strains re-
tains the advantages of genetic uniformity, while adding the advantages of superior developmental and physiological homeostasis.
Most of the evidence to support this view is derived from physiological and morphological studies (Lerner, 1954). Unfortunately,
however, there are a few complications in applying the concept of
developmental homeostasis to behavioral characters, that can also
be indirectly associated to behaviors affecting hormones (Mordkoff
and Fuller, 1959). An increase in behavioral variability which may,
in turn, effect hormones or drugs may actually facilitate aspects
of physiological homeostasis. An organism must develop in only
one of a number of possible patterns, and it can behave successfully in a multitude of ways while affecting differentially the
same hormones. Thus, by necessity, this phenomenon of differential
effects upon the same hormones by different behaviors must be
explained on the basis of thresholds or related membrane phenomena.
This complicates the genetic approach to behavior and drugs considerably.

    A hybrid between two inbred strains may actually be more var-
iable than either parent if the hybrid genotype happens to fall in
a critical range for determination of a given trait. For example,
almost all C57BL/6J mice are resistant to audiogenic seizures, and
almost all DBA/2J mice are susceptible. Their F_1 hybrid is intermediate, hence much more variable from individual to individual
(Fuller and Thompson, 1960). However, in spite of this reserva-
tion, F_1 hybrids are highly recommended for general experimental
purposes. In one instance, Meier (1964) has found less variability among F_1 hybrids than their respective inbred parents. Once
homozygosity has been reached, inbred lines retain their genetic
characters for long periods of time in the absence of outcrossing.
Over many generations, mutations will undoubtedly occur, and the
characteristics of the strain can change. However, general experience in biological research suggests that the drift is usually
small and unimportant over a given experimenter's lifetime. There
are some instances, however, wherein an occasional investigator
has described a cryptic mutation which altered the behavior of
mice of a line separated from the main one for 30 generations

(Denenberg, 1959).

It is imperative that the cautious investigator dealing in
genetic research with drugs and behavior should take steps to
prevent subline differentiation where possible. However, in reali-
ty, this is inevitable when stocks are separated over a period of
generations or by geographic necessity. A case in point is the
recently found differences in open-field behavior, corticosterone,
and hypothalamic norepinephrine levels in the subline C57BL/6J and
C57BL/6By which have been separated from each other for some time
(Eleftheriou, unpublished). To prevent such variability and a subline differentiation, comparisons with other workers will be facilitated if a breeding stock is regularly replaced from a mammalian
genetics center. Workers using the same source will have genetically nearly identical subjects. On a small scale, a controlled
mating system may be used to prevent diversification within a single
colony. Generally, however, the experimenter using inbred strains
from a genetic center should also be aware of the major effects
upon mice of different strains due to transportation, season of the
year, and general handling and housing within a given laboratory.
Thus, extreme caution should be applied to obtain results which
approximate given environmental conditions. Different laboratory
conditions may affect behavioral responses and, consequently, drug
responses due to hitherto unknown factors in a given experimental
laboratory (Sprott and Eleftheriou, 1974; Oliverio, Eleftheriou
and Bailey, 1973a).

Genetic uniformity among animals within inbred strains implies
that differences in a given phenotype of individual mice of the same
strain are almost exclusively non-genetic in origin, except for the
necessary sex and occasional mutation dimorphism. Differences between strains which exceed the variability observed within them
indicate phenotypic differences attributable to a difference in
heredity. Therefore, the amount of genetic determination can be
estimated statistically by comparing phenotypic variants between
and within inbred strains. This knowledge has been applied extensively in the area of behavior genetics, to a limited extent in
the area of genetics and hormones, but it has almost never been
applied to the area of behavior and drugs. Unfortunately, however, even comparative studies of given inbred strains that are not
followed by further crossbreeding or backcrossing of a given trait
provide, at best, the limited information that variation in a particular trait characteristic is affected by genotype. In short, it
is not sufficient to study given traits in a number of inbred strains.

Rather, for a true genetic approach one must pursue the problem
further by attempting to isolate the genetic determinants of the
particular trait. In order to accomplish this, crossing and backcrossing of various strains, that usually exhibit the extremes of
a given trait, is necessary. This procedure of crossing and backcrossing is time-consuming and the average investigator may find it
not only experimentally unfeasible, but tedious and expensive. As
a consequence, many investigators have avoided the pursuit of characterizing genetic controlling mechanisms of particular traits
which to them were of great interest.

In short, the detection of differences between pure breeding
stocks is only the first step of a genetic analysis. Segregation
and linkage analyses are additional necessary steps. Particular
investigators doing genetic research have found the majority of the
more interesting strain differences are usually controlled by more
than one pair of alleles, or are influenced by uncontrollable environmental variation, or both. This situation usually prevents
Mendelian analysis of given traits. Even in instances where
Mendelian segregation ratios have been observed, linkage tests are
usually laborious and uncertain. A given investigator who has
ample animal housing facilities, finances, and considerable time
on his hands can pursue the genetic characterization of a particular trait of his interest in order to obtain linkage. Unfortunately, however, usually only geneticists exhibit the patience required for this time-consuming approach. The average investigator
interested in the area of drugs and behavior would rather have a
tool which will offer him an answer in a rather short period of
time since his major interest is not genetics.

RECOMBINANT INBRED STRAINS: A NEW APPROACH
IN GENETIC ANALYSIS

In recent years, the number of potentially useful single-gene
markers has increased as a result of the discovery of isozyme and
immunological polymorphisms (Roderick et al., 1971; Snell and
Cherry, 1971). These developments have increased the number of
loci that can be followed in a linkage test, thus enhancing the
probability of linkage detection (Hutton and Coleman, 1969). Unfortunately, however, typing individuals with respect to these loci
is generally more laborious than typing for visible markers. Such
typing is frequently destructive, precluding additional observations
on the test animal. Recently, Bailey (1971) had developed a method
of segregation and linkage analysis, the recombinant inbred strains
(RI), that capitalizes very effectively on the existence of these
cryptic genetic markers. This method offers a simple and unique
approach to the detection of strain differences regarding segrega-

tion and linkage analysis. The method is generally applicable to
otherwise difficult traits. The RI method's utility relies upon
the fact that polymorphic variation is very extensive in cross
fertilizing species (Lewontin and Hubby, 1966; Harris, 1966), a
fact that is reflected in multiple genetic differences between inbred strains. Mammals have sufficient DNA to code for thousands
of genes, and a significant proportion of loci exhibits polymorphic
variation. Thus, unrelated strains differ by hundreds, possibly
thousands, of genetic loci. The usual test for segregation and
linkage analyses are limited since they only have a few loci that
can be followed in a single segregant individual. The recombinant-
inbred method developed by Bailey (1971) circumvents this difficulty by developing a number of inbred lines from the F_2 generation
produced from the cross of two unrelated but highly inbred strains
(Fig. 1). The recombinant inbred strains comprise a genetically
fixed population of segregants at hundreds of loci that has contin-
uity in space and time. Thus, this method, developed by Bailey,
differs in principle from traditional approaches to linkage studies
in that data gathered at different times and at different places
are cumulative. Furthermore, this approach offers a workable procedure for extending segregation and linkage analysis to complex
characters.

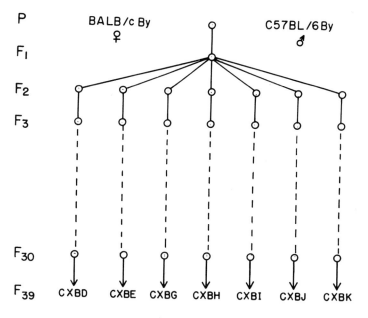

Fig. 1. Derivation of the recombinant-inbred strains from the inbred progenitor strains BALB/cBy and C57BL/6By. In the generations
following the F_1, each RI strain was independently developed and
maintained by a brother-sister mating regimen.

The method is remarkably and uniquely simple. The RI strains were derived from the cross of two unrelated, but highly inbred progenitor strains, and then maintained independently from the F_2 generation under strict regimens of brother-sister inbreeding. This procedure genetically fixes the chance recombination of genes as full homozygosity is approached in the generations following the F_2 generation. The resulting battery of strains can be looked upon in one sense as a replicable recombinant population. The utility of such strains for analyzing gene systems is described elsewhere (Bailey, 1971). Of the several original RI strains developed, seven are now in existence (CXBD, CXBE, CXBG, CXBH, CXBI, CXBJ, and CXBK). These were derived from a cross of strains, BALB/cBy (C) by C57BL/6By (B6), followed by over 40 generations of full-sib matings. The letters D through K were arbitrarily chosen to denote the different strains, while the letters C and B denote the original progenitor strains which were crossed. Additionally, two reciprocal F_1 hybrids (B6CF$_1$ and CB6F$_1$) are also available. The rationale for the development of this genetic procedure is that linked genes will tend to become fixed in the same combinations (progenitor) as they entered the cross. Unlinked genes are randomly assorted in the F_2 generation and are, therefore, equally likely to be fixed in progenitor or recombinant phases. Such a group of inbred strains may be thought of as a fossilized segregating population.

In the actual use of these RI strains for segregation analysis, it is expected that for a given trait which is controlled by a single pair of segregating genes, two classes of RI strains will be apparent in equal frequency, the two classes resembling the two progenitor strains. Generally, if the trait is controlled by more than one pair of genes, intermediate or more extreme classes are expected. In cases of epistasis, types to be expected may be beyond and/or below the progenitor strains. If many segregating loci influence the given trait, with small additive effects, a continuous distribution of RI phenotypes is expected. Environmental factors and incomplete penetrance can be reduced to insignificance by measuring numerous individuals from each strain. Whereas, the number of subjects required for a strain will depend on the heritability of a given trait, the number of RI strains required depends on the genetic complexity of that trait. If the goal is to distinguish between one- and two-locus models with the several types of epistasis possible, as many as 20 RI strains are usually desirable. Those traits which are controlled by more than two segregating loci are probably beyond the practical limits of complete analysis, although it may be possible to detect a major locus even when numerous minor loci are segregating. Detection of a major locus in such cases will usually depend on the close linkage of the major locus to a suitable marker.

The most important use of the RI strains is in the linkage analyses per se. Once fixation is attained, no genetic changes occur save mutation. Consequently, each RI strain needs to be typed only once for a given character. Typing of the group RI strains for a single locus defines a strain distribution pattern (SDP) for that locus. This SDP can be compared with the SDP of any other segregating locus, whenever the latter information becomes available. If the respective SDP's reveal a significant excess of progenitor types, linkage may not be possible. The SDP of a particular locus identifies a chromosome region in which the locus resides. Once the RI strains have been characterized for numerous segregating loci scattered throughout the genome, newly discovered segregating loci can be mapped simply by typing each RI strain. Although matching SDP's indicate possible identity or close linkage of two loci, it should be kept in mind that two SDP's may match merely by chance $[p = (\frac{1}{2})^k$, where k is the number of RI strains$]$. As the linkage map becomes more complete, the procedure would establish ultimately the correct order of the genes, with the exception of closely linked factors.

In addition to detecting linkage, it is desirable to determine the linear order of the genes on a given chromosome. The facility with which multiple markers can be followed using RI strains lends itself to chromosome mapping. The study of such genes confined to a short segment of a chromosome is called fine structure analysis. The RI strains lend themselves quite easily to fine structure analysis inasmuch as discrete products of recombination events can be recovered as analyzed. Rather than deliberately attempting to uncover rare recombinants in specified regions, RI strains offer the opportunity for analysis of recombination events where they occur.

The power of the RI strains for fine structure analysis can be computed (Taylor, 1971, unpublished). RI strains derived by brother-sister mating have a mean of 0.04 of crossovers per centi-Morgan (cM) per line. In this respect, among 25 RI strains, one crossover would be expected to have occurred on an average in some line for each cM of chromosome (Taylor, 1971, unpublished). Expressing this another way, a chromosome 100 cM in length would be partioned into approximately 100 parts. If inbreeding were delayed a number of generations beyond the F_2 generation, the opportunity of crossing over is increased, making the derived RI strains less valuable for linkage detection, but more valuable for fine structure analysis. For each generation of random mating prior to inbreeding, the probability of crossing over increases by 0.005 per cM per line. Thus, 8 generations of random mating prior to inbreeding doubles the utility of these lines for fine structure analysis. This type of approach might be impractical unless an F_2 derived, large, random mating population, having been in existence for some time were available. It is important that population size remain large during the period of random mating, in order to minimize genetic drift and the attending complications (Taylor, 1971, unpublished).

CONGENIC LINES

In the ultimate analysis, the RI strains have been enhanced in their utility by the availability of additional lines of mice. This battery of mice is called congenic lines, and they are not to be confused with the RI strains. The congenic lines were developed independently from the initial cross of C57BL/6By to BALB/cBy by a regimen of skin-graft testing and backcrosses to B6 for at least 12 generations. This procedure resulted in congenic B6 lines, each of which differ from B6 itself by only an introduced chromosomal segment including a C-strain allele at a distinctive histocompatibility (H) locus. Each of these congenic lines has been tested against RI strains by means of skin-grafts to find which of the RI strains carry the C-strain allele and which the B6-allele at a particular H locus, thereby establishing their strain distribution patterns (SDP). A brief outline of the regimen followed for the development of the congenic lines is presented in Fig. 2.

Fig. 2. summarizes briefly Bailey's (1971) development of the congenic lines which he has used recently to good advantage in analyzing the complex murine histocompatibility system. In short, it should be emphasized that both the congenic lines and the RI strains are used for functional genetic analysis in order to establish linkage with the least amount of effort. A list of the various congenic lines developed is provided by Klein (1973).

In actual application of this system, when a given trait is analyzed, the SDP of the RI strains is considered and examined with SDP of other traits already available through research of other investigators. When an SDP matches that of the locus represented by an existing congenic line the latter line is then tested for that particular trait. In order for linkage to be detected, the congenic line which is tested usually must resemble the BALB/cBy progenitor strain in regard to the trait of concern. This is necessary because of the nature of the development of the congenic lines. When such correlation of a given trait between a congenic line and BALB/cBy occurs, it is concluded that a locus, at which differences in that trait are determined, is linked or is pleiotropic with the histocompatibility locus carried by the congenic line. If the histocompatibility locus, carried by the particular congenic line, has been mapped on a chromosome then the subsequent trait which an investigator examines is also determined. By comparing the position of the F_1 hybrids, one is also able to

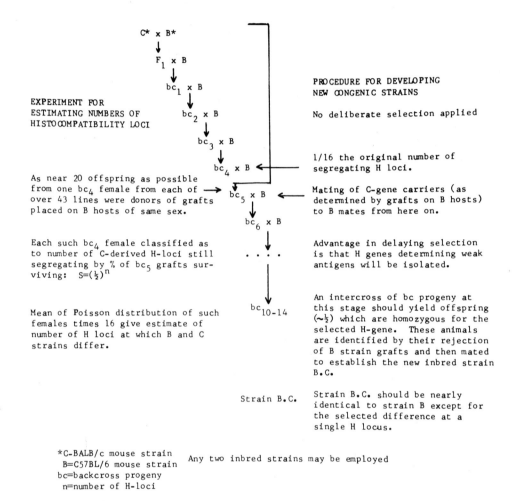

The diagram shows:

C* x B*
↓
F_1 x B
↓
bc_1 x B
↓
bc_2 x B
↓
bc_3 x B
↓
bc_4 x B ←——
↓
bc_5 x B ←——
↓
bc_6 x B
↓
. . . .
↓
bc_{10-14}
↓
Strain B.C.

EXPERIMENT FOR
ESTIMATING NUMBERS OF
HISTOCOMPATIBILITY LOCI

As near 20 offspring as possible
from one bc_4 female from each of ——→
over 43 lines were donors of grafts
placed on B hosts of same sex.

Each such bc_4 female classified as
to number of C-derived H-loci still
segregating by % of bc_5 grafts surviving: $S=(\frac{1}{2})^n$

Mean of Poisson distribution of such
females times 16 give estimate of
number of H loci at which B and C
strains differ.

PROCEDURE FOR DEVELOPING
NEW CONGENIC STRAINS

No deliberate selection applied

1/16 the original number of
segregating H loci.

Mating of C-gene carriers (as
determined by grafts on B hosts)
to B mates from here on.

Advantage in delaying selection
is that H genes determining weak
antigens will be isolated.

An intercross of bc progeny at
this stage should yield offspring
(~$\frac{1}{2}$) which are homozygous for the
selected H-gene. These animals
are identified by their rejection
of B strain grafts and then mated
to establish the new inbred strain
B.C.

Strain B.C. should be nearly
identical to strain B except for
the selected difference at a
single H locus.

*C-BALB/c mouse strain
B=C57BL/6 mouse strain   Any two inbred strains may be employed
bc=backcross progeny
n=number of H-loci

Fig. 2. Bailey's method for the development of new congenic lines
and for estimating numbers of histocompatibility (H) loci. Repro-
duced by personal consent of Dr. D. W. Bailey.

determine whether there is dominance for the high or the low aspects of a trait. Additionally, if the reciprocal F_1 hybrids do not exhibit any significant differences between each other, maternal effects are also eliminated. Conversely, if there is significant differences between the two reciprocal F_1's, maternal effects can be suspected.

APPLICATION OF THE METHOD

Advantages

The RI method of genetic analysis combined with a congenic line approach possesses a unique advantage in that one can determine quickly the probable location of a new gene by matching its pattern of distribution with those of other genes among a set of inbred strains that already have been developed. This is a great advantage over conventional approaches but derived from the replacement of the individual by the RI line as a unit of segregation. By the use of the RI method, one is able to identify genetic determinants in a short time, since the RI lines are already available and, in most instances, do not necessitate further crosses of various types as, for example, is the case with conventional Mendelian analysis. Additionally, the RI method has the advantage over conventional approaches in that (a) tissue from different individuals within an RI line may be pooled without introducing genetic heterogeneity; (b) once the RI strains are established, the time ideally required for production of the segregating generations can be avoided (c) the recessive characteristics of both progenitor strains are expressed in RI strains; (d) genetic differences tend to be maximized due to the elimination of heterozygotes; (e) genetic associations, due to either pleiotropy or linkage may be detected between traits expressed in utero, adult characteristics - male limited traits and female limited traits - and traits that require killing individuals at different stages or require different pretreatments, and (f) the F_1 hybrid of the progenitor lines accepts tissue or organ grafts from any of the RI strains.

Limitations

It should be noted that the RI method of genetic analysis, like most experimental tools, also has some limitations: (a) the method is applicable only to species of animals that are amenable to extensive inbreeding; (b) those species that have long generation times or exhibit inbreeding depression are poor candidates for

TABLE 1.

Summary of drugs, behaviors, and dosage levels in RI strain studies

DRUG	BEHAVIOR	CONTROL (Saline) Available (X)	DOSAGE LEVELS (mg/kg body weight) g/kg body weight)
Scopolamine	Toggle box activity	X	2.0mg 4.0mg 6.0mg
Amphetamine	Toggle box activity	X	0.5mg 1.0mg 2.0mg
Alcohol	Toggle box activity	X	0.5g 1.0g 1.5g 2.0g
Barbiturate	Toggle box activity	X	0.1mg[1] 1.0mg 10.0mg
		X	0.1mg[2] 1.0mg 10.0mg
Morphine	Toggle box activity	X	10.0mg 20.0mg
	Running activity	X	12.5mg 25.0mg 40.0mg
	Analgesia – latency to jump from hot plate	X	5.0mg[3] 10.0mg 20.0mg
	Analgesia – tail flick response		2.5mg 5.0mg 10.0mg
Chlorpromazine	Shuttle box avoidance		1.0mg 1.5mg 2.0mg 4.0mg

[1]Scores used represent all doses combined: single injections

[2]Scores used represent all doses combined: multiple injections

[3]Doses were repeated for multiple injections

the usual genetic analyses using RI strains; (c) the additional requirement for a number of known polymorphic markers necessarily
limits the application of the method to a better studied species;
(d) since only segregating loci can be analyzed using this system,
new mutations cannot be mapped using RI strains; (e) if a polymorphic locus of interest is not segregating in any extant of RI
strains, the RI method is not applicable.

Most laboratory species appear suitable for RI development and
study and among domestic animals, chickens, ducks and turkeys are
good possibilities for such development. Generally, the RI strains
can be used to study genes or gene combinations that are compatible
with survival and reproduction. The progenitor strains will be basically free of lethal genes, and gene combinations that are invia-
ble or sterile will be ultimately removed by natural selection.
The latter could be detected through the deficiency of certain unlinked marker gene combinations.

Although an extensive amount of time is required for developing new RI strains, another limitation of the method, a number of
already existing mouse RI strains are available. Thus, using these
RI strains, developed by Bailey (1971), Eleftheriou and co-workers
were able to detect and link a number of loci involved in behavioral responses and modification of certain behaviors dealing with
alcohol, chlorpromazine, amphetamine, scopolamine, morphine analgesia and tolerance, halothane anesthesia and barbiturate effects
(Oliverio and Eleftheriou, 1975a; Oliverio, Castellano and
Eleftheriou, 1975b; Shuster, Webster, Yu and Eleftheriou, 1975;
Castellano, Eleftheriou, Bailey and Oliverio, 1974; Oliverio,
Eleftheriou and Bailey, 1973; Elias and Eleftheriou, 1975).

Using these data we performed a major statistical analysis to
detect possible underlying common genetic-behavioral responses to
those pharmacologic agents.

STATISTICAL ANALYSES

Objectives

The data obtained from the various studies exploring drug-behavior relationships in the RI strains involved a number of different
measures of activity and analgesia. For most of the studies, a control (saline) condition was also available for the present analyses.
Table 1 summarizes the various drugs, dosage levels and control

groups which were used in our overall analyses. In addition, open
field activity (squares traversed) and emotionality (number of boli)
were included in two of the analyses, although these behaviors were
not tested under any drug conditions. All analyses consisted of
Pearson product-moment correlations among the strain distributions
for the RI strains, their two progenitor strains (C57BL/6By and
BALB/cBy) and the reciprocal F_1 hybrids. Scores entering the correlations were means for each strain (n = 11).

The major objectives of the analyses were to determine if significant strain (genotype) correlations existed among (1) the various dosage levels for each drug, (2) the behavioral measures, independent of drug administration, (3) the behavioral measures as they
were affected by different drugs at various dosage levels, and (4)
specific behaviors, measured independently of drug administration
and different, although possibly related behaviors, measured under
the various drugs and dosage levels.

All of the analyses must be considered essentially exploratory
in nature. The were designed only to provide indications of areas
for future research which could demonstrate whether or not a common
gene or set of genes affects two different phenomena. Caution must
be exercised in interpreting the RI strain correlations as we do
not have information regarding the within strain correlations. Consequently, we cannot determine the extent to which environmental
influences are contributing to the strain (genotype) correlations.
A conclusion that common genes are influencing two different phenotypic responses (e.g., activity and emotionality) can be made only
if high between strain correlations and low within strain correlations are found simultaneously (Roderick and Schlager, 1966). Thus,
the significant correlations obtained in the present analysis are
indicative of the importance of performing future studies in which
two or more measures are obtained on the same animals in order that
(1) both within and between strain correlations may be determined,
(2) strain distribution patterns (SDP's) may be compared under conditions of more complete environmental control, and (3) congenic
lines may be selected for testing. Environmental control is an
important aspect of any future studies as some of the past drug
studies were performed during various seasons and at different laboratories.

With these limitation in mind, the present correlational analyses provide indications as to the amount of prediction possible
from one strain distribution pattern to another using various drugs,

Pearson product-moment correlations for control (saline) conditions and open field behaviors

	Activity (Toggle Box) Scopolamine Control	Activity (Toggle Box) Alcohol Control	Activity (Toggle Box) Barbiturate Control	Activity (Toggle Box) Morphine Control	Activity (Running) Morphine Control	Activity (Open field)	Analgesia (Hot Plate) Morphine Control
Activity (Toggle Box) Alcohol Control	.95**						
Activity (Toggle Box) Barbiturate Control	-.05	-.12					
Activity (Toggle Box) Morphine Control	.89**	.96**	-.11				
Activity (Running) Morphine Control	.07	-.08	.57	-.06			
Activity (Open field)	.31	.24	.25	.21	.22		
Analgesia (Hot Plate) Morphine Control	-.23	-.34	-.26	-.35	.10	-.05	
Emotionality	-.23	-.17	-.48	-.08	-.43	-.79**	.06

* $p < .05$ ** $p < .01$

TABLE 3.

Pearson product-moment correlations between control and dosage levels

Scopolamine
(Mean number of toggle box crossings)

	Saline	2.0mg	4.0mg
2.0mg	.09		
4.0mg	-.73*	.66*	
6.0mg	-.76**	.65*	.99**

Amphetamine
(Mean number of toggle box crossings)

	Saline	0.5mg	1.0mg
0.5mg	.81**		
1.0mg	.63*	.96**	
2.0mg	.58	.93**	.96**

Chlorpromazine
(Difference scores before-after drug)
(Shuttle box avoidance)

	1.0mg	1.5mg	2.0mg
1.5mg	.79**		
2.0mg	.78**	.80**	
4.0mg	.65*	.98**	.76**

Alcohol
(Toggle box activity)

	Saline	0.5g	1.0g	1.5g
0.5g	.71*			
1.0g	.73*	.99**		
1.5g	.45	.85**	.89**	
2.0g	.27	.78**	.80**	.96**

Barbiturate
(Toggle box activity)

Saline minus average for all doses: Single injection .72*

Saline minus average for all doses: Multiple injection .62*

Morphine
(Analgesia - hot plate latency)
(single injection)

	Saline	5.0mg	10.0mg
5.0mg	.60*		
10.0mg	.58	.89**	
20.0mg	.57	.89**	.94**

Morphine
(Analgesia - hot plate latency)
(Multiple injections)

	Saline	5.0mg	10.0mg
5.0mg	-.57		
10.0mg	-.34	.82**	
20.0mg	-.45	.77**	.56

Morphine
(Analgesia - tail flick latency)

	2.5mg	5.0mg
5.0mg	.66*	
10.0mg	.41	.77**

Morphine
(Toggle box activity)

	Saline	10.0mg
10.0mg	-.25	
20.0mg	-.17	.97**

Morphine
(Running activity)

	Saline	12.5mg	25.0mg
12.5mg	-.57		
25.0mg	-.34	.82**	
40.0mg	-.45	.77**	.56

* p < 0.05   ** p < 0.01

dosage levels, and behavioral tasks. They also provide hypotheses
regarding the extent to which common genes affect different dosage
levels of the same drug, various behaviors under different drugs,
and, to some extent, similar and dissimilar behaviors as measured
by different laboratory tasks.

Results

Behaviors independent of drug effects. Table 2 presents the
Pearson product-moment correlations for behaviors under the control
(saline) conditions, open field activity and emotionality (defecation). Toggle box activity was measured in four different studies.
It might be expected that the correlations for this type of activity
would all be quite high because the various control conditions are
essentially experimental replications. It should be noted that a
single major gene effect was established for base-line toggle box
activity in the scopolamine study (Oliverio, Eleftheriou, and
Bailey, 1973). While the correlations for control toggle box activity are very high for the scopolamine, alcohol, and morphine
studies, this same activity measured in the barbiturate study does
not correlate significantly with any of the others. This discrep-
ancy for the barbiturate study is most likely a consequence of experimental variation. The scopolamine, alcohol, and morphine
studies were all performed during the months of July and August,
while the barbiturate study was carried out during January and
February. However, it appears likely that seasonal (or laboratory)
variation significantly affects the phenotypic expression of activity, even when the same genes are involved.

The only other significant correlation between behaviors measured independently of drug effects occurs for open field activity
and emotionality. It is particularly important to obtain the within
strain correlations for these variables in order to properly evaluate the extent to which strain correlations reflect common sets of
genes because open field activity and emotionality have been found
to be both positively and inversely related and, in some instances,
unrelated, depending upon the strain or strains chosen for study
(Elias and Elias, in press).

Several conclusions may be reached regarding the large number
of very low correlations among the various control behaviors. First,
there is no basis to assume a common genetic component for the response of jumping off a hot plate (analgesia), activity level, and/
or emotionality. Apparently, all of these behaviors have different

sources of genetic variation under control conditions. One question
of interest is whether correlations among control conditions will
be altered when drug conditions are introduced. Thus, it is extremely important to establish firmly genotype-behavior relationships
for the RI strain base-line behaviors prior to examining these relationships under drugs. Second, there is no basis to assume that
activity level will be determined by a common gene or set of genes
independent of a given laboratory task. Toggle box activity, running activity (in a small cage), and open field activity apparently
involve different genes. It is clear, however, that sources of
environmental variation cannot be completely ruled out even though
two of the studies of toggle box activity and the study of open
field activity were performed in the same laboratory at the same
time of year (July-August).

Control-dosage and dosage-dosage relationships. Table 3 presents the Pearson product-moment correlations for the control and
dosage levels for each drug. It is immediately apparent that the
dosage levels for most drugs, with a few exceptions, are significantly correlated. This finding might be expected in view of the
fact that the same pathways of drug action are involved, and thus,
some sets of common genes are affecting particular behaviors regardless of dosage level. However, it should not be concluded that
it is unimportant to determine drug-dose relationships, but rather
that it is encouraging to find that the strain distribution pattern
is not altered drastically from dosage to dosage. Furthermore, high
correlations between dosage levels are not found for all types of
drugs and behaviors. For example, the correlations for induction
and eduction times under various doses of halothane anesthesia
shown in Table 8 of the chapter by Elias and Pentz are considerably
lower than those in the present analysis. These low correlations
may reflect the diffuse effects of general anesthetics such as halothane. The few low correlations among dosages found in the present
analysis occur for analgesia and running activity under the highest
doses of morphine. It is possible that at very high doses of a
drug, genetic pathways, perhaps different from those at lower doses,
determine behavioral effects.

The control-dosage correlations in the present analysis are of
considerable interest. Very different relationships are observed
for different drugs. For example, the scopolamine, amphetamine and
alcohol studies all involved measures of toggle box activity; yet,
the patterns of their control-dosage correlations are quite different. For scopolamine, base-line toggle box activity appears to be

TABLE 4.

Pearson product-moment correlations for selected behaviors under various drugs.

	Scopolamine (Toggle Box)			Amphetamine (Toggle Box)			Morphine (Analgesia-Single inj.)			Morphine (Analgesic-Multiple inj.)			Barbiturate (Running)	
	2.0mg	4.0mg	6.0mg	0.5mg	1.0mg	2.0mg	5.0mg	10.0mg	20.0mg	5.0mg	10.0mg	20.0mg	SI[1]	MI[2]
Amphetamine (Toggle Box Activity)														
0.5mg	.11	-.42	-.44											
1.0mg	.25	-.18	-.21											
2.0mg	.18	-.22	-.24											
Morphine (Analgesia-Single injection)														
5.0mg	.64*	.76**	.75**	-.05	.11	.04								
10.0mg	.53	.51	.50	.18	.30	.21								
20.0mg	.51	.55	.53	.19	.34	.21								
Morphine (Analgesia-Multiple injection)														
5.0mg	.76**	.71*	.68*	.11	.26	.13	.91**	.78**	.79**					
10.0mg	.58	.55	.53	.12	.23	.10	.94**	.95**	.95**					
20.0mg	.60*	.59	.56	.15	.29	.17	.93**	.90**	.96**					
Barbiturate (Toggle Box Activity)														
SI	.06	-.09	-.08	.00	-.11	-.10	-.21	-.24	-.41	-.03	-.22	-.33		
MI	.15	-.03	-.02	-.01	-.14	-.06	.11	.05	-.18	.17	.07	-.06		
Morphine (Running Activity)														
12.5mg	-.16	.10	.09	.04	.17	.15	-.03	.03	.21	-.08	-.12	.12	-.76**	-.89**
25.0mg	-.06	.08	.07	.18	.33	.36	-.21	-.14	-.02	-.19	-.25	-.13	-.49	-.75**
40.0mg	-.14	.07	.05	-.03	.06	-.08	-.03	-.03	-.19	-.05	.02	.12	-.40	-.74**

[1]Scores represent saline minus average for all doses: single injection. [2]Scores represent saline minus average for all doses: multiple injections.

* p < .05 ** p < .01

unrelated to the toggle box activity at the lowest dosage level.
However, this relationship becomes inverse and significant at higher dosage levels. Opposite relationships are observed for amphetamine and alcohol. At low doses, baseline activity correlates positively with activity under the influence of these drugs and falls
off progressively at higher dosage levels. These relationships
may be contrasted with those for morphine where baseline toggle box
activity is unrelated to drug-influenced activity regardless of
dosage level. With a few exceptions, control conditions in most of
the morphine studies are unrelated to drug conditions.

Generally, the control-dosage correlations clearly indicate
that genotype-phenotype relationships for control behaviors must be
established independently of genotype-phenotype relationships for
behavior under drugs in order that the genotypic interactions for
behavior and drug effects may be clearly elucidated. It must be
emphasized that the biometric (correlational) approach only indicates possibilities as to where this search might begin. When the
RI strains are used as a genetic model, confirmation of specific
genetic determinants can only be made by establishing SDP's and testing the appropriate congenic lines. For example, loci for baseline
toggle box activity and its modification by scopolamine have been
identified through this method (Oliverio, Eleftheriou, and Bailey,
1973).

Relationships among behaviors under drug conditions. Table 4
presents the correlations for selected behaviors under various
drugs. Only three significant blocks of correlations were found.
Generally, it might not be expected that behaviors would correlate
highly when they are measured under the influence of different
drugs since many of the pathways of drug effects have been traced
and very likely involve many different genes.

Two of the blocks of significant correlations are of considerable interest in terms of hypothesis generation. The third block
of correlations most likely reflects the common genetic pathways
for multiple versus single injections for the analgesic response
to morphine when this response is measured in terms of latency to
jump from a hot plate. However, this same analgesic response is
also highly correlated with toggle box activity under scopolamine.
The relationship is positive, i.e., those strains high in toggle
box activity under scopolamine tend to have longer latencies in response to hot plate stimulation under morphine. Furthermore, the
data presented in Table 5 indicate that the correlations for base-

TABLE 5

Pearson product-moment correlations for various behaviors under morphine

		Habituation[1] Analgesia Hot Plate		Toggle Box Activity		Running Activity			Single inj.-Analgesia Hot Plate			Multiple inj.-Analgesia Hot Plate		
		10.0mg	20.0mg	10.0mg	20.0mg	12.5mg	25.0mg	40.0mg	5.0mg	10.0mg	20.0mg	5.0mg	10.0mg	20.0mg
Toggle Box Activity	10.0mg	-.75**												
	20.0mg	-.81**												
Running Activity	12.5mg	-.11		.33	.25									
	25.0mg	-.27		.59	.55									
	40.0mg	.12		.31	.19									
Single inj. Analgesia Hot Plate	5.0mg	.39		-.44	-.40	-.03	-.21	-.10						
	10.0mg	.19		-.25	-.15	.03	-.14	-.03						
	20.0mg	.30		-.22	-.17	.21	-.02	.19						
Multiple Analgesia Hot Plate	5.0mg	.69*		-.58	-.55	-.08	-.19	-.04						
	10.0mg	.45		-.46	-.40	-.02	-.27	.02		See Table 4				
	20.0mg	.53		-.41	-.41	.12	-.13	.12						
Analgesia Tail flick Response	2.5mg	.41		.58	.53	-.02	.15	-.12	-.25	-.18	-.13	-.38	-.27	-.23
	5.0mg	-.77*		.63*	.71*	-.03	-.14	-.20	-.15	.08	.02	-.38	-.14	-.22
	10.0mg	.46		.54	.62*	-.01	.36	-.20	.14	.21	.20	.05	.03	.02

[1]Difference scores for analgesic responses between single injections (prior to habituation) and multiple injections (habituation). Scores for 5.0, 10.0, 20.0 mg were pooled for each strain.

* p < .05

** p < .01

TABLE 6

Pearson product-moment correlations between activity and emotionality measures (no drug) and behaviors under various drugs. "X"
indicates those correlations between a control behavior and the
same behavior under drug conditions which are presented in Table 3.

		Toggle Box Activity (Scopolamine Study)	Toggle Box Activity (Barbiturate Study)	Running Activity	Open-field Activity	Emotion-ality
Scopolamine	2.0mg	X	-.05	.32	-.29	-.12
Toggle Box	4.0mg	X	.00	-.04	-.50	.18
Activity	6.0mg	X	.02	-.03	-.48	.16
Amphetamine	0.5mg	X	-.48	-.30	.15	-.08
Toggle Box	1.0mg	X	-.60*	-.38	.05	-.02
Activity	2.0mg	X	-.55	-.37	.19	-.18
Alcohol	0.5g	X	-.07	.31	-.17	.10
Toggle Box	1.0g	X	-.14	.24	-.19	.16
Activity	1.5g	X	-.21	.05	-.55	.48
	2.0g	X	-.06	.17	-.62*	.40
Barbiturate	SI[1]	.21	X	.40	.44	-.42
Toggle Box Activity	MI[2]	.22	X	.47	.27	-.40
Morphine	10.0mg	X	-.37	.01	.47	-.15
Toggle Box Activity	20.0mg	X	-.33	-.01	.46	-.15
Morphine						
Hot Plate Analge-	5.0mg	-.35	-.14	-.13	-.70*	.43
sia	10.0mg	-.11	-.26	-.13	-.67*	-.51
Single injection	20.0mg	-.17	-.47	-.31	-.72*	.65*
Morphine						
Hot Plate Analge-	5.0mg	-.14	-.09	-.06	-.69*	.36
sia	10.0mg	-.11	-.22	-.15	-.74**	.58
Multiple injection	20.0mg	-.14	-.36	-.21	-.78**	.60*
Morphine	2.5mg	.17	-.38	-.57	.65*	-.44
Tail flick response	5.0mg	.09	-.20	-.34	.54	-.28
Analgesia	10.0mg	-.05	-.23	-.45	.35	-.32
Morphine	12.5mg	-.28	-.74**	X	-.42	.48
Running Activity	25.0mg	-.18	-.62*	X	-.07	.07
	40.0mg	-.22	-.65*	X	-.39	.67*

[1]Saline minus average for all doses: single injection. [2]Saline minus average for all doses:
* p <0.05 ** p <0.01   multiple injections.

line toggle box activity and morphine analgesia are low and insignificant. As stated previously, there are separate loci controlling
baseline activity and activity under scopolamine. Although the basis for the scopolamine-morphine relationship is unknown, further
research utilizing within strain correlations, SDP's derived from
the same subjects, and tests of congenic lines may establish common
genetic influences. One note of caution must be made regarding
this particular analgesic response under morphine. It is significantly correlated with open field activity and emotionality, i.e.,
the strains that exhibit long latency analgesic responses tend to
be less active and more emotional in the open field situation
(Table 5). Thus, the predominant behavior tested in the morphine
analgesia study may involve an emotional response to pain which
includes freezing. A comprehensive study of scopolamine, morphine,
and several measures of activity and emotionality may be necessary
to clearly establish the genetic relationships affecting behavior
under these drugs.

The second block of significant correlations which is of interest in terms of hypothesis generation concerns the relationship of
toggle box activity under barbiturate and running activity under
morphine. The correlations for these two types of activity under
control conditions are relatively high (Table 2), but did not reach
significance. Further, they are positively correlated under control
conditions, but negatively correlated under drug conditions. The
drug scores in both cases were measures of the difference in activity between control and drug conditions. When these scores were
compared with their respective control conditions, the correlations
for the barbiturate study SDP's were high and positive, while correlations for the morphine study SDP's were relatively low and negative. Thus barbiturate affected toggle box activity similarly for
all strains and morphine reversed the strain distribution patterns.
Since the control behaviors appear to be unrelated, it may be hypothesized that the potential common genetic variance is attributable
to the gene-drug (morphine) and gene-behavior (toggle box activity)
pathways. This hypothesis receives further support as baseline
toggle box activity in the barbiturate study correlates significantly with running activity under morphine (Table 6). As with the
significant correlations discussed previously, an adequate test of
this hypothesis must include 1) within strain correlations, 2) the
matching of SDP's and 3) the testing of congenic lines.

Relationships among behaviors under a single drug (morphine).
Four separate morphine studies were conducted. Two involved

measures of analgesia. Thus, it is of interest to determine whether
a common gene might possibly affect these various behaviors. Table
5 presents the correlations for all behaviors under morphine. Several important relationships are observed. Contrary to expectations,
morphine does not produce similar SDP's for the two measures of activity or, with one exception, the two measures of analgesia.
Again, this would seem to suggest that different activity measures
and different analgesia measures are influenced by different genes.
Thus, it is impossible to conclude that morphine has a unitary effect on "activity" or "analgesic response"; rather the effect is
highly dependent upon the specific labortory task.

Again, contrary to expectations, the correlations for toggle
box activity and the analgesic tail flick response were high and
positive; i.e., the more active strains exhibited longer latencies
for the analgesic responses. Since the control data for tail flick
response were not available, it is not known if this relationship
is present under saline conditions. Finally, it may be noted from
the data in Table 5 that the habituation measure of the analgesic
(hot plate) response to morphine is the best predictor of toggle
box activity under morphine, although it is not strongly predictive
of the hot plate response. Further research of the type described
previously may clarify these relationships between analgesic effects
and activity under morphine.

Relationships among activity measures and drug behaviors. The
data in Table 2 suggested that various control activity measures
may be genetically independent. Thus, an attempt was made to search
out any significant relationships between specific types of activity
and drug behaviors. These data are presented in Table 6. Because
the control measures of toggle box activity were not significantly
correlated in the scopolamine and barbiturate studies, both were
included in this analysis. The open-field emotionality measure
(defecation) was also included.

It appears that the control toggle box activity measure in the
scopolamine study and the control running activity measure in the
morphine study are unrelated to any other behaviors under drugs.
However, the control toggle box activity measure in the barbiturate
study is predictive of running activity under morphine.

Apparently, the best predictors of drug behavior are open-
-field activity and emotionality measures. Open field activity is
significantly related to toggle box activity under high doses of

alcohol and both types of analgesic responses to morphine, although, for the tail flick response, only the correlation involving the lowest dosage level reaches significance. Emotionality in the open field situation is significantly related to morphine analgesic responses (hot plate) and running activity at the highest dosage levels. It would seem that open field behaviors may be important indicators of drug effects and it would be helpful if future studies involving drug modification of activity included these measures in order to assess potentially different gene-drug-activity relationships than those previously explored.

CONCLUSIONS

Some final notes of caution must be advanced regarding interpretation of the foregoing correlation analyses. An extremely large number of exploratory correlations were performed. It is thus possible that some of the significance levels may have been attained by chance. Consequently, further investigations of these relationships are necessary.

The correlations serve only to generate hypotheses and estimate the amount of possible prediction between SDP's involving different phenotypic responses. Thus, the correlational approach is not a substitute for the multivariate analyses and multiple contrasts designed to identify specific major loci for two or more biological and/or behavioral phenotypes. The latter objective includes a search for the matching of SDP's for the two or more phenotypes of interest and comparisons with the appropriate congenic lines which are subsequently compared with the progenitor strains.

Common genetic influences may occur through (a) pleiotropic effects of the same gene(s) (b) linked gene effects, or (c) two or more behavioral measurement techniques which measure essentially the same phenomena. Consequently, it is also important to establish the actual components of a behavior (e.g., activity) which a particular gene influences through variations in experimental tasks.

Certainly many drug effects, particularly drug effects on behavior, may be subject to polygenic influence. However, this does not preclude the possibilities that linked genes may be identified for drug-behavior relationships or that specific loci, some of which have been identified, may exert pleiotropic effects on related behaviors or the same behavior under different drugs.

REFERENCES

BAILEY, D. W., 1971. Recombinant-inbred strains: an aid to finding identity, linkage and function of histocompatibility and other genes. Transplantation 11:325.

CASTELLANO, C., ELEFTHERIOU, B. E., BAILEY, D. W., & OLIVERIO, A. 1974. Chlorpromazine and avoidance behavior: A genetic analysis. Psychopharmacologia 34:309.

DENENBERG, V. H. 1959. Learning differences in two separated livers of mice. Science 130:451.

ELIAS, M. F., & ELEFTHERIOU, B. E. 1975. A behavior genetic investigation of induction and eduction times for halothane anesthesia. Behav. Res. Methodol. Instr. (in press).

ELIAS, M. F., & ELIAS, P. K. Motivation and activity. In J. E. Birren and W. J. Schaie (Eds.) Handbook of the Psychology of Aging. New York: Van Nostrand Reinhold Company. (in press).

FULLER, J. L., & THOMPSON, W. R. 1960. Behavior Genetics. New York: Wiley.

GREEN, E. L. 1974. Some systems of mating useful in mouse genetics. Exp. Anim. 7:1.

KLEIN, J. 1973. List of congenic lines of mice. Transplantation 15:137.

LERNER, I. M. 1954. Genetic Homeostatis. New York: Wiley.

LEWONTIN, R. C., & HUBBY, J. L. 1966. A molecular approach to the study of genic heterozygosity in natural populations. II. Amount of variation and degree of heterozygosity in natural populations of Droxophila pseudobscura. Genetics 54:595.

McLAREN, A., & MICHIE, O. 1956. Variability of response in experimental animals. A comparison of the reactions of inbred F_1 hybrid, and random bred mice to a narcotic drug. J. Gent. 54:440.

MEIER, G. 1964. Differences in maze performances as a function of age and strain of house mice. J. Comp. Physiol. Psychol. 58:418.

MORDKOFF, A. M., & FULLER, J. L.   1959.   Heritability of activity
    within inbred and crossbred mice: A study in behavior genetics.
    J. Hered. 50:6.

OLIVERIO, A., ELEFTHERIOU, B. E., & BAILEY, D. W.   1973a.   Explora-
    tion activity: genetic analysis of its modification by scopo-
    lamine and amphetamine.   Physiol. & Behav. 10:893.

OLIVERIO, A., CASTELLANO, C., & ELEFTHERIOU, B. E.   1975b.   Morphine
    sensitivity and tolerance: A genetic investigation in the
    mouse.   Psychopharmacologia   (in press).

OLIVERIO, A., & ELEFTHERIOU, B. E.   1975a.   Motor activity and al-
    cohol: Genetic analysis in the mouse.   Pharm. Biochem. &
    Behav.   (in press).

RODERICK, T. H., RUDDLE, F. H., CHAPMAN, V. M., & SHOWS, T. B.
    1971.   Biochemical polymorphisms in feral and inbred mice.
    Biochem. Genet. 5:457.

RODERICK, T. H., & SCHLAGER, G.   1966.   Multiple factor inheritance.
    In E. L. Green (Ed.) Biology of the Laboratory Mouse.   New
    York: McGraw-Hill.

SNELL, G. D., & CHERRY, M.   1972.   Loci determining cell surface
    alloantigens.   In P. Emmelot and P. Bentvelzen (Eds.) RNA
    Viruses and Host Genome in Oncogenesis.   Amsterdam: North-
    Holland Publishing Co.   Pp. 221.

SPROTT, R. L., & ELEFTHERIOU, B. E.   1974.   Open-field behavior in
    aging inbred mice.   Gerontologia 20:155.

SHUSTER, L., WEBSTER, G. W., YU, G., & ELEFTHERIOU, B. E.   1975.   A
    genetic analysis of the response to morphine in mice: Anal-
    gesia and running.   Psychopharmacologia   (in press).

WRIGHT, S.   1923.   Mendelian analysis of pure breeds of livestock.
    I.   The measurement of inbreeding and relationship.   J. Hered.
    14:339.

GENETIC ANALYSIS OF MORPHINE EFFECTS: ACTIVITY, ANALGESIA,

TOLERANCE AND SENSITIZATION

Louis Shuster, Ph.D.

Department of Biochemistry and Pharmacology
Tufts University School of Medicine
Boston, Massachusetts   02111

CONTENTS

INTRODUCTION

The question of individual variability in response to narcotic drugs is of major importance in the clinical evaluation of
analgesic agents. Lasagna & Beecher (1954) found that 30 to 35%
of several groups of post-operative patients did not experience
any pain relief after the double blind administration of morphine
sulfate, 10 mg per 70 kg. Even when the dose was raised to 15 mg,
25% of the patients reported no analgesia.

There are also important differences in the response to
narcotic drugs among subjects who are not in pain. Lasagna,
Von Felsinger & Beecher (1955) injected volunteers with 4 mg
heroin or 15 mg morphine. About one-half of the subjects reported that the injections did not produce any euphoria, and
that they had no desire to repeat the experience.

It is obvious that subjective influences, such as the attitudes of the subjects towards pain and pleasure, are important
determinants of the way in which human subjects respond to narcotic drugs (Beecher, 1959). However, it is becoming clear from
recent experiments that the genetic background of an animal can
influence strongly its objective responses to narcotic drugs.

Analgesic Response

Strain differences in the analgesic response of two strains
of mice to morphine were reported by Gebhart & Mitchell (1973).
These workers used the hot plate method, and found that morphine
was 1.6 times more effective in producing analgesia in CF_1 mice
than in CFW mice. There was no difference in pre-injection latency or in the rate of development of analgesic tolerance.

Tilson & Rech (1974) found that Fischer rats were more reactive to footshock and showed less analgesia after morphine, as
determined by the flinch-jump method, than Sprague-Dawley rats.

Oliverio & Castellano (1974) compared the analgesic response
of three strains of mice to morphine, using the hot plate method
of Eddy & Leimbach (1953). They found that BALB/cJ and DBA/2J
mice were more sensitive than C57BL/6J mice to both morphine and
heroin.

These studies were extended in a subsequent paper by Oliverio,
Castellano & Eleftheriou (1974). These authors used BALB/cBy,
C57BL/6By, their reciprocal F_1 hybrids, and 7 recombinant inbred
(RI) strains. Dose response curves are illustrated in Fig. 1.
Strains BALB/cBy and CXBH showed the greatest analgesic response.

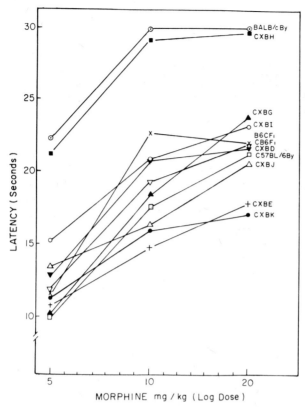

Fig. 1. Analgesic response of 11 strains of mice determined by
the hot plate method at 30 minutes following a single intraperitoneal injection of 5, 10 or 20 mg per kg of morphine sulfate.
Each point is the mean value obtained from 10 mice. [Data of
Oliverio et al. (1974); presented by permission].

Strains BALB/cBy and CXBH showed the greatest analgesic response.
The lowest analgesic response was exhibited by strains CXBE and
CXBK. Intermediate values were obtained for all the other strains.
Oliverio et al. (1974) concluded that their results suggest a
genetic model based on more than two loci.

Shuster et al. (1974) examined the analgesic response to
morphine of the same recombinant inbred strains, using the tail-
flick assay of D'Amour & Smith (1949). Their results were somewhat different from those of Oliverio et al. (1974).

There was a genetic difference in the baseline response, i.e.
latency to tail-flick between uninjected mice of different strains
(Table I). The difference between groups were statistically signif-

icant (p < 0.005). A tentative strain distribution pattern (SDP),
based on the statistical rank order of all the strains, indicated
a possible linkage of one locus for tail-flick. However, when
congenic lines B6.C-H-23 and B6.C-H-25c were tested, both resembled
progenitor strain C57BL/6By, and linkage could not be confirmed.
There was no correlation between the baseline response and the
analgesic response determined after the injection of morphine
sulfate.

The greatest analgesic response was exhibited by progenitor
strain C57BL/6By (Fig. 2). Even at the lowest dose of morphine
sulfate (2.5 mg/Kg),the mice of this strain showed a maximal analgesic response. The analgesic response of the other progenitor
strain, BALB/cBy, was significantly less (p < 0.05). The response
of both F_1 hybrids was similar, indicating a lack of sex-linkage
or maternal influence.

The area under each curve in Fig. 2 was calculated in minute-
seconds and used as a measure of the analgesic response to a
given dose of morphine sulfate. The values for all three doses
were combined and adjusted for body weight from analyses of covariance to give a mean value for each strain (Table II). The
various strains could be divided into three groups: very sensitive
(C57BL/6By); least sensitive (CXBG and CXBK); and intermediate
(all the remaining strains). The RI strains vary in coat color
from white to black, but there was no correlation between coat
color and latency of response to thermal pain. The statistical
grouping of the analgesic response of the RI lines did not provide
a distinctive strain distribution pattern that could be used to
arrive at the possible linkage of the two or more genes that seem
to determine the analgesic response to morphine.

There are some striking differences between the results of
Oliverio et al. (1974) and Shuster et al. (1974c) with respect to
the analgesic response of B6 and C mice, and the recombinant inbred strains derived from them. Thus, Shuster et al. (1974c) found
that the analgesic response of B6 mice was considerably greater
than that of C mice, while Oliverio et al. (1974) reported opposite findings. The most likely explanation for these differences
is the two different assay methods used. Vogt (1973) has pointed
out that the hot plate assay may give results that differ from
those obtained by other means because it can be affected by
changes in motor activity. If an analgesic test dose increases
the motor activity of a mouse, the analgesic activity determined
by the hot plate test may be lower than that found by other methods.
This difference could arise because the animal does not stay in
one place long enough to feel the pain as soon as a mouse that remains stationary. Miller (1948) has reviewed some of the problems
associated with the hot plate method.

Table I.

Baseline response (latency to tail-flick) to thermal pain
of two progenitor strains, BALB/cBy and C57BL/6By, their reciprocal F1 hybrids, B6CF$_1$ and CB6F$_1$, and seven of their derived recombinant inbred lines, CXBD, CXBE, CXBG, CXBH, CXBI, CXBJ, CXBK and congenic lines B6.C-H-23^c and B6.C-H-25^c, Means ± S.E.

Magnitude of Response*	Strains	N	Latency to tail flick in seconds ± S.E.
High	BALB/cBy	36	2.54 ± 0.09
	CXBG	34	2.61 ± 0.11
	CXBH	34	2.59 ± 0.06
	CXBI	27	2.49 ± 0.11
	CXBJ	36	2.42 ± 0.07
Intermediate	C57BL/6By	34	2.00 ± 0.15
	CXBD	32	2.11 ± 0.11
	CXBE	36	1.99 ± 0.09
	B6.C-H-23^c	5	2.30 ± 0.36
	B6.C-H-25^c	10	2.40 ± 0.36
Low	B6CF$_1$	33	1.55 ± 0.05
	CB6F$_1$	29	1.61 ± 0.05
	CXBK	35	1.54 ± 0.07

* A number of statistical tests were responsible for this grouping. However, for easy inspection, any value in this table that differs by 0.33 from any other value is statistically significant at $p < 0.005$.

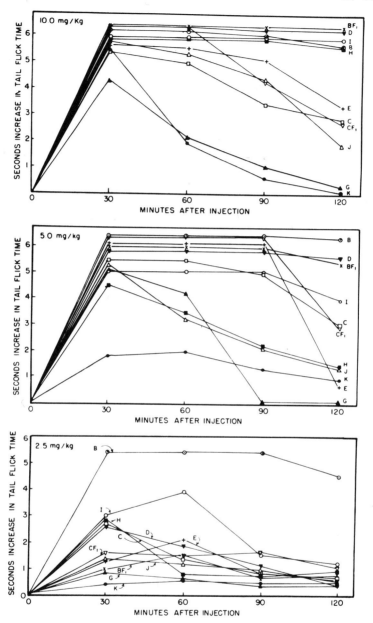

Fig. 2. Analgesic response of 11 strains of mice determined by
the tail-flick method following the injection of 2.5, 5.0 or 10.0
mg/Kg morphine sulfate. Each point represents the mean value obtained from 10-12 mice. The mouse strains are designated by the
following abbreviations: B (C57BL/6By); C (BALB/cBy), D (CXBD);
E (CXBE), BF$_1$ (B6CF$_1$), CF$_1$ (CB6F$_1$); G (CXBG); H (CXBH); I (CXBI);
J (CXBJ); K (CXBK).

Table II

Analgesic area under the curve for three different doses of morphine sulfate in progenitor strains BALB/cBy and C57BL/6By reciprocal F_1 hybrids, $B6CF_1$ and $CB6F_1$, and seven RI strains: CXBD, CXBE, CXBG, CXBH, CXBI, CXBJ, and CXBK. Class means are ranked from high to low, with vertically aligned asterisks indicating non-significant differences.

Magnitude of Response	Strains[a]	N	Mean Area under the curve $\pm$ S.E.				
Group 1[b]	K	35	149.09 $\pm$ 23.6 *				
	G	34	189.16 $\pm$ 25.2 *				
2	J	36	307.11 $\pm$ 29.4	*			
	H	34	309.18 $\pm$ 22.3	*			
3	C	36	370.83 $\pm$ 21.6		*		
	E	36	402.58 $\pm$ 21.4		* *		
	BF_1	33	431.96 $\pm$ 43.4			* *	
4	I	27	457.49 $\pm$ 32.3			*	
	D	32	463.83 $\pm$ 34.3			*	
	CF_1	29	468.35 $\pm$ 33.0			*	
5	B	34	617.33 $\pm$ 25.9				*

a Strain designations are the same as those indicated in Fig. 2.

b Based on one-way, two-way analyses of variance, Student-Newman-Keuls multiple range test, and Tukey's W estimate, groups with non-overlapping asterisks (vertical comparisons) are significantly different at least at the 0.05 level (d.f. = 332, Tukey's W = 68.49).

Both Oliverio & Castellano (1974) and Shuster et al. (1974c)
found that B6 mice show a considerably greater running response to
morphine than do C mice. Strain CXBH, which exhibited the same
high analgesic response in the hot plate test as C mice, also
showed a low running response to morphine. The opposite conclusion does not necessarily apply i.e., those strains that show a
low analgesic response in the hot plate test do not necessarily
exhibit greater motor activity. For example, strains CXBE and
CXBK showed both a low analgesic response and a low running response. The genetic determinants for the running response are
different from those for the analgesic response. One cannot
therefore, draw up any simple rules for relating the two responses
as determined by any tests.

Running Response

When mice are injected with morphine or related narcotic
drugs they exhibit a characteristic increase in motor activity.
Marked variability in the running response of both random-bred
Swiss-Webster mice and pure-bred C3H/HeJ mice was reported by
Goldstein & Sheehan (1969). In many of their experiments, these
investigators discarded two-thirds of the animals because of a
poor running response to levorphanol in a preliminary screening
test.

The running response of three inbred strains of mice to several doses of morphine was determined by Oliverio & Castellano (19-
74). They found that C57BL/6J mice were most sensitive, BALB/cJ
mice gave an intermediate response, and DBA/2J mice exhibited no
increase in motor activity after the injection of as much as 20
mg per kg morphine sulfate. Shuster et al. (1974a) found that
A/J mice show a poor running response to 25 mg per kg morphine
sulfate, C57BL/6J mice show a good response, and the response of
B6AF$_1$/J hybrids is intermediate between those of the parental
strains.

Some strains of mice appear to respond to narcotics like
rats--i.e. their motor activity is decreased. Thus, Hano et al.
(1963) reported that the injection of morphine into mice of the
ddo strain produced a decrease in motor activity. Miller & Cochin
(1974) made a similar observation with CD-1 mice. The motor activity of DBA/2J mice is decreased by the injection of methadone
(Santos et al., 1973). ICR mice do not run in response to morphine
(Eidelberg & Erspamer, 1974).

The running response to morphine of the Rl strains derived
from BALB/cBy and C57BL/6By was analyzed by Shuster et al. (19-
74c). Fig. 3 summarizes the response of the two progenitor strains,

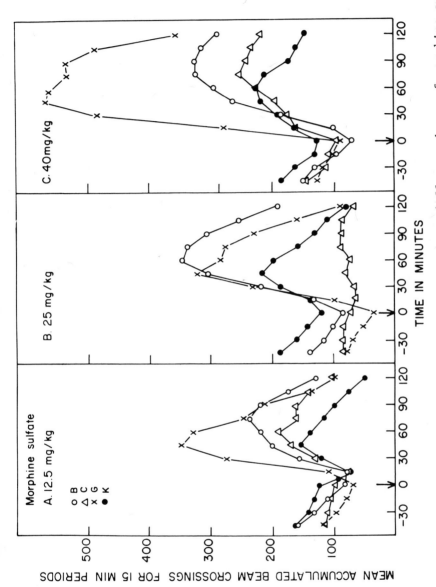

Fig. 3. Running response of four strains of mice to three different doses of morphine sulfate.
The value for each 15-minute period represents the mean value from 10-12 individual mice.
Data of Shuster et al. (1974c). Strain abbreviations as in Fig. 2.

their reciprocal F_1 hybrids, and seven RI strains to three different doses of morphine sulfate. C57BL/6By mice exhibited a
significantly greater response at each dose than did BALB/cBy
mice. The two F_1 hybrids gave similar values that were intermediate between those of the two progenitor strains. These results indicate a lack of sex linkage or maternal influence, and
also a lack of dominance.

There was no correlation between spontaneous activity prior
to injection and the subsequent response to morphine. Strain
CXBK, which displayed one of the lowest responses to morphine, had
the highest pre-injection activity.

In order to simplify genetic analysis, the mean values for
running activity were compared at 60 minutes after morphine injection. Statistical ranking of these values is presented in
Table III. The 11 strains could be divided into three major
groups: high (CXBG); low (BALB/cBy, CXBD, CXBK and CXBE); and
intermediate (all the other strains).

Table III

Combined means of activity scores 60 minutes after injection
of the three doses of morphine sulfate in the two progenitor
strains, BALB/cBy and C57BL/6By, their reciprocal F_1 hybrids and
their seven RI strains. Class means are ranked from high to low,
with vertically aligned asterisks indicating non-significant differences ($P = < 0.05$, d.f. = 345).

Strain	N	Class Means	S.E.	
G	34	409.23 ± 51.84	*	
J	36	344.97 ± 19.73	*	
I	34	343.05 ± 24.99	*	
BF_1	33	292.05 ± 26.54	*	
B	36	287.97 ± 32.56	*	
H	36	284.52 ± 28.96	*	
CF_1	30	265.06 ± 25.04	*	
D	32	204.40 ± 22.87		*
K	35	191.11 ± 19.47		*
C	36	163.02 ± 19.20		*
E	36	145.58 ± 25.55		*

Table IV

Hypothetical genetic model for combined means of 60-minute raw activity scores following injection of 3 different doses of morphine sulfate. Tentative designation of a given strain is based on statistical rank order (Table II). Strain distribution pattern (SDP) indicated as BALB/cBy-allele (C) or C57BL/6By-allele (B).

Strain	Locus 1		Locus 2	
C	$a_1 a_1$		$b_1 b_1$*	
B	$a_2 a_2$		$b_2 b_2$	
BCF_1 & CBF_1	$a_1 a_2$		$b_1 b_2$	
		SDP		SDP
D	$a_1 a_1$	C	$b_1 b_1$	C
E	$a_1 a_1$	C	$b_1 b_1$	C
G	$a_1 a_1$	C	$b_2 b_2$	B
H	$a_2 a_2$	B	$b_2 b_2$	B
I	$a_2 a_2$	B	$b_2 b_2$	B
J	$a_2 a_2$	B	$b_2 b_2$	B
K	$a_1 a_1$	C	$b_1 b_1$	C

* a_1 and a_2 or b_1 and b_2 are alleles at their respective loci. No dominance implied.

A hypothetical locus model based on this ranking is presented
in Table IV. The model postulates at least 2 loci with no dominance of alleles at either locus. An analysis of running scores at
75 minutes after injection was also carried out. Statistical
ranking yielded only two major groupings. A model to explain these
results (Table V) postulates a single locus with a strain distribution pattern identical to that of one of the loci in Table IV.
A number of congenic lines were examined in order to verify linkage postulated from the observed SDP, but no definitive linkage
could be determined.

Oliverio et al. (1974) have examined the exploratory activity
of the same RI strains in a toggle box (Fig. 4). These authors
also suggested that the running response to morphine is under the
control of two or more genetic determinants.

Narcotic Tolerance

The development of tolerance to the running response to
narcotics has been described by Shuster et al. (1963) in C57BL/6J
mice, and by Goldstein & Sheehan (1969) in Swiss-Webster mice.
Oliverio & Castellano (1974) found that tolerance to morphine
running developed more readily in C57BL/6J mice than in BALB/cJ
mice. These authors also observed differences between the same
strains in the rate of development of analgesic tolerance, as
determined by the hot plate test.

A more detailed analysis of tolerance was carried out with
the RI strains (Oliverio et al., 1974). Three or more loci seem
to be involved in the development of analgesic tolerance, and the
genetic picture is too complex to sort out at present.

Physical Dependence

Craving. One measure of physical dependence is the persis-
tence of drug-seeking behavior after withdrawal. Nichols & Hsiao
(1967) described genetic differences in the extent to which pretreated rats will choose to drink solutions or morphine in preference to plain water. Two distinct sublines were obtained by selective breeding.

Ericksson & Kiianmaa (1971) found a marked difference in the
consumption of morphine solutions by two strains of inbred mice
after they had received daily injections of morphine for three
weeks. C57BL/6J mice drank considerably more morphine than
CBA/Ca mice. These strains exhibit a similar difference in their
preference for solutions of ethanol instead of water. F_1 and F_2
generations were also tested, as well as backcrosses. Preference

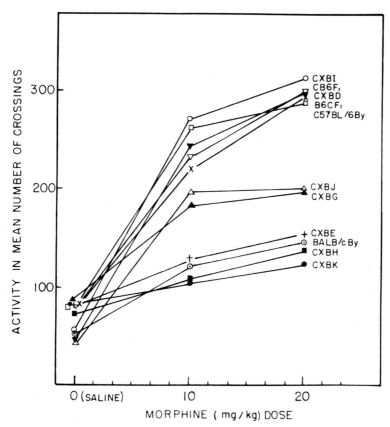

Fig. 4.   Exploratory activity of 11 strains of mice following intraperitoneal injection of saline or morphine sulfate (10 or 20
mg per kg).   Each point is the mean value for 10 mice.   [Data of
Oliverio et al. (1974), presented by permission].

Table V

Combined means of raw scores 75 minutes after injection of three doses of morphine sulfate in the two progenitor strains, BALB/cBy and C57BL/6By, their reciprocal F_1 hybrids and seven RI lines. Class means are ranked from high to low, with vertically aligned asterisks indicating non-significant difference. The SDP for the seven RI lines is also indicated.

Strain	N	Class Means ± S.E.	Strain Distribution Pattern of RI lines[a]	
G	34	357.26 ± 46.94 *		
J	36	347.81 ± 23.58 *	D	C^1
I	34	336.47 ± 27.34 *	E	C
BCF_1	33	323.12 ± 30.65 *	G	B^1
B	36	299.75 ± 22.84 *	H	B
H	36	295.64 ± 17.65 *	I	B
CBF_1	30	290.56 ± 44.67 *	J	B
D	32	217.75 ± 25.91 *	K	C
K	35	164.40 ± 16.98 *		
C	36	164.08 ± 21.94 *		
E	36	160.52 ± 25.33 *		

1. C indicates the BALB/cBy strain allele while B indicates the C57BL/6By allele.

a. Note that the SDP of this locus is identical to the second locus of Table IV.

for morphine was a dominant trait. Calculations showed that
about 90% of the variance in morphine consumption was due to
genetic factors. C57BL/6J and F_1 females showed a greater preference for both morphine and alcohol than did males.

Withdrawal. Naloxone jumping is a commonly-used measure of
physical dependence in mice. Addicted mice will jump in place
(Marshall & Weinstock, 1971) or off a platform (Maggiolo &
Huidoliro, 1961) when injected with small doses of the narcotic
antagonists such as naloxone or nalorphine. The injection of
nalorphine into narcotic-tolerant animals increased the spontaneous
activity of the Catholic University strain of Swiss-Webster mice
(Maggiolo & Huidobro, 1961) but decreased the spontaneous activity
of DBA mice (Maggiolo & Huidobro, 1961) and C57BL/6J mice (Shuster
et al., 1963). Way et al. (1969) found that naloxone produced
considerably less jumping in the Berkley-Pacific strain of Swiss-
Webster mice than in the Hooper Foundation strain. More recently,
it has been observed that morphine-dependent ICR (Horton) mice
jump much less in response to naloxone than do Simonsen Swiss mice
(Brase et al., 1974). It is of interest that treatment with
cholinergic antagonists decreased the incidence of jumping in
the high-jumping strain, but increased the jumping response in
the low-jumping strain.

                              Sensitization

     In some cases, the repeated administration of morphine to
mice leads to an increased running response to morphine, rather
than tolerance. This observation was first reported by Hano et
al. (1963) for mice of the ddo strain. Some of the features of
morphine sensitization have been described by Shuster et al.
(1974a; 1974b). Increases of up to four-fold in the running
response of B6AF$_1$/J hybrids have been observed. Sensitization
has the characteristic feat res of a specific narcotic response:
it is blocked by the narcotic antagonist naloxone; sensitization
can be produced by treating with levorphanol, but not with its
pharmacologically inactive enantiomer, dextrorphan.

     The genetic determinants for sensitization are different
from those for the running response. The extent of sensitization
in C57BL/6J and A/J mice is considerably less than that obtained
with the B6AF$_1$/J hybrid (Fig. 5).

     The RI lines derived from C57BL/6By and BALB/cBy were ex-
amined for sensitization. The most sensitive strain was BALB/cBy.
The injection of 25 mg/Kg morphine sulfate once a day for four
consecutive days produced a 7.5-fold increase in the running response of this strain (Table VI). The smallest response was ob-

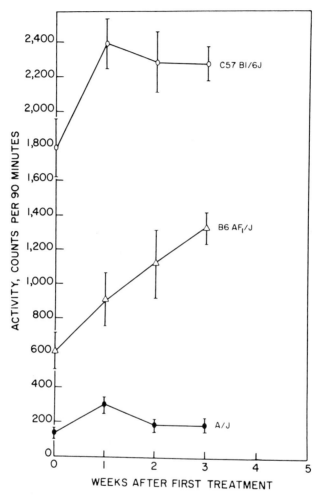

Fig. 5. Sensitization to the running response to morphine in mice
pretreated with morphine. Mice of three strains were injected
intraperitoneally with morphine sulfate, 25 mg per kg, once a
week. Running activity was determined after each injection.
Every point is the mean number of light beam interruptions during
the first 90 minutes after injections for 10 individual mice ±
S.E.M. [Reproduced from Shuster et al. (1974a); by permission].

Table VI

Sensitization to morphine of BALB/cBy and C57BL/6By mice, their reciprocal F_1 hybrids, and 7 derived recombinant inbred strains. The mice were injected once a day with 25 mg per kg morphine sulfate, i.p. Running activity was determined after the first injection (Day 0) and after the fifth injection (Day 4). Strain abbreviations as in Fig. 2.

Strain	n	Running activity after 25 mg/Kg morphine sulfate		Ratio, Day 4/ Day 0
		counts/90 min $\pm$ S.E.		
		Day 0	Day 4	
C	9	136 $\pm$ 62	1143 $\pm$ 270	8.40
H	8	843 $\pm$ 210	2749 $\pm$ 240	3.26
CF_1	9	307 $\pm$ 102	854 $\pm$ 160	2.78
E	9	458 $\pm$ 136	1126 $\pm$ 212	2.46
J	9	1225 $\pm$ 177	2785 $\pm$ 269	2.27
D	9	440 $\pm$ 94	959 $\pm$ 213	2.18
BF_1	9	640 $\pm$ 116	1331 $\pm$ 186	2.08
G	9	2471 $\pm$ 153	3893 $\pm$ 402	1.58
B	5	1678 $\pm$ 122	2476 $\pm$ 438	1.48
K	6	567 $\pm$ 46	766 $\pm$ 171	1.35
I	9	2431 $\pm$ 111	2904 $\pm$ 379	1.19

tained with strains CXBG, C57BL/6By, CXBK and CXBI.

Some of the small changes shown in Table VI may be attributed to the fact that the initial response was already so close to a maximal value that little sensitization could be demonstrated. However, Shuster et al. (1974a) showed that in the case of C57BL/ 6J mice the use of a test dose of 5 mg/Kg did not reveal greater sensitization than a dose of 25 mg/Kg morphine sulfate.

Morphine sensitization has also been reported in CD-1 mice by Miller & Cochin (1974). These authors also found (personal communication) a good correlation between increased running response and increased body temperature following the injection of morphine into sensitized mice. However, it is not clear whether the increase in temperature is a separate response or whether it results from the increased running activity.

SOME NEUROCHEMICAL CONSIDERATIONS

Neurohormones. Different strains of mice have been shown to differ in the amount of neurohormones contained within the whole brain or some of its regions (Maas, 1962, 1963; Schlesinger, et al., 1965; Karczmar & Schudder, 1967; Kempf,et al., 1974); in the activity of certain neurohormone-synthesizing and degrading enzymes (Kessler et al., 1970; Ebel et al., 1973); and in the rate of turnover of neurohormones in the central nervous system (Maruyama et al., 1971; Valzelli, 1973).

It is tempting to attribute genetic difference in the response to narcotic drugs to these neurochemical differences. So far it has not been possible to ascribe any of the acute or chronic responses to narcotic drugs to a change in either the content or metabolism of any known neurohormone within the brain. There are some indications that narcotic addiction may involve an increase in serotonin turnover (Way et al., 1973) but this theory remains controversial because of the appearance of several conflicting reports. Naloxone-induced withdrawal has been associated with changes in dopamine metabolism (Iwamoto et al., 1973). However, no one has yet established a clear-cut correlation between the genetic control of neurohormone metabolism and genetic determinants of the pharmacological response in the narcotic drugs.

Narcotic Receptors. Pert & Snyder (1973) and Lowney et al (1974) have demonstrated the presence in mammalian brain of specific receptors that combine reversibly with narcotics and narcotic antagonists. The concentration of such receptors in the brains of recombinant inbred strains of mice has been examined by Baran et al.

(1974). There were differences of as much as 70% in the amount
of receptor in different strains (Table VII). These differences
were due to a difference in the amount of receptors, rather than
affinity (Fig. 6). Mixing experiments ruled out any difference
that could be attributed to the presence of activators or inhibitors of binding.

Statistical separation of binding values into three classes,
together with the observation that both progenitor strains and the
reciprocal F_1 hybrids were within the same group suggests that
two or more genetic determinants may control narcotic binding.

In the case of the CXBK strain, low binding was accompanied
by a very low analgesic response to morphine (Table VII). However,
CXBH mice, with the highest amount of naloxone binding, did not
exhibit the greatest analgesic response. Regression analysis of
the data from all strains showed a positive, but not significant
correlation ($r = 0.48$, d.f. $= 9$) between the amount of narcotic
receptors and the analgesic response to morphine as determined
by the tail-flick assay. There was no correlation with the
analgesic response to morphine as determined by the hot plate
method (Oliverio et al., 1974).

Because the extent of binding is similar for both progenitor
strains, it is difficult to derive a strain distribution pattern.
Testing of appropriate backcrosses is now underway and may help
to reveal the genetic determinants of binding.

The normal role of narcotic-binding receptors in the brain
is still unknown. They do not appear to be related to either the
distribution or the metabolism of acetylcholine, nor-epinephrine
or serotonin (Kuhar et al., 1973).

STATUS SUMMARY

It is clear that all the responses to narcotic drugs that
have been examined are strongly influenced by genetic determinants.
Differences between pure-bred, and recombinant-inbred, strains of
mice are especially striking. These findings explain some of the
discrepancies in the results of similar experiments carried out in
different laboratories. Contradictory claims concerning the
possibility of producing tolerance or sensitization to the stimulant actions of narcotic drugs in mice can now be resolved by
taking into account the strains that were used. There still remain contradictory results derived from the use of different assay
techniques - as in the measurement of the analgesic response to
morphine. The choice of technique can also influence the genetic
analysis.

Table VII

Naloxone binding and analgesic response in the recombinant inbred strains, their progenitor strains and F_1 hybrid strains. Binding of naloxone to opiate receptors was assayed as described in the text, using 15 mice of each strain. The binding value of each brain extract was calculated from the results of triplicate incubations with 7 nM ^{3}H-naloxone, in the presence of 0.8 μM levorphanol or dextrorphan. The analgesic response is the area in minutes-seconds under the curve obtained by plotting increase in latency versus interval after intraperitoneal injection of morphine-sulfate (5 mg/kg). The numbers in brackets refer to the number of mice used for analgesic testing. Based on analyses of variance, Student-Newman-Keuls multiple range test, and Tukey's W estimate (12), groups with non-over-lapping asterisks (vertical comparison) are significantly different at least at the 0.05 level (d.f. = 154; Tukey's W = 123.38).

Magnitude of Grouping	Mouse Strain	Stereospecific naloxone binding (c.p.m./mg protein ± S.E.)		Analgesic response (min. x sec. ± S.E.)
High	CXBH	1044 ± 33*		326 ± 22 (12)
Inter-mediate	C57Bl/6By	968 ± 25	*	655 ± 7 (12)
	CXBJ	952 ± 27	*	326 ± 38 (12)
	BALB/cBy	948 ± 26	*	520 ± 24 (12)
	CXBI	940 ± 27	*	512 ± 10 (9)
	CXBE	934 ± 26	*	511 ± 25 (12)
	B6CF$_1$	923 ± 22	*	623 ± 10 (11)
	CB6F$_1$	915 ± 27	*	613 ± 7 (11)
	CXBD	893 ± 24	*	607 ± 12 (12)
	CXBG	884 ± 21	*	289 ± 12 (12)
Low	CXBK	609 ± 30	*	166 ± 37 (12)

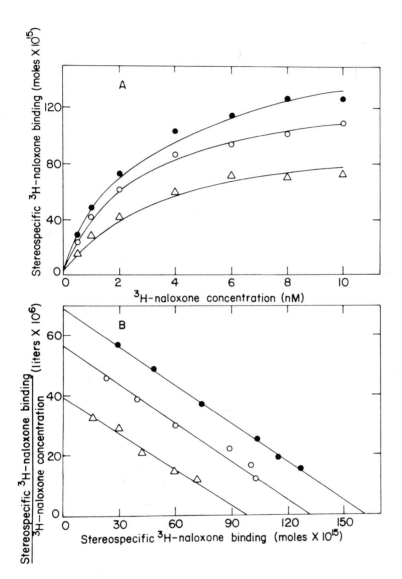

Fig. 6 (a). Effect of naloxone concentration on stereospecific
binding of ^{3}H naloxone to brain homogenates from different mouse
strains. (b) Scatchard plot of ^{3}H-naloxone binding to brain homogenates from different mouse strains. CXBH (●——●); CXBK (x——x);
all other strains (o——o). [Reproduced from Baran et al., (1974),
by permission].

While it has not yet been possible to define the exact number and location of the genetic determinants that control the response to narcotic drugs in mice, a good start has been made. The way is now clear for additional measurements with appropriate back-crosses and congenic lines. Even without complete genetic defin-ition we now have model strains that can be used to examine the neurochemical bases of narcotic tolerance and sensitization. A beginning has been made in relating the analgesic response to the number of narcotic receptors in the brain. Additional experiments should be carried out on genetic correlations of narcotic responses with the concentration and turnover of various neurohormones in the brain.

These studies are also important for the light they may shed upon individual variability in the response of human patients and addicts to narcotic drugs. For this purpose it would be helpful to establish genetic linkage between the response to narcotics and responses to other drugs, with the aim of being able to pre-dick analgesic refractoriness, addiction liability, or other clinically important variables.

REFERENCES

BARAN, A., SHUSTER, L., ELEFTHERIOU, B. E., & BAILEY, D. W., Opiate receptors and analgesic response in mice: basis for genetic difference. Brain Res. in press.

BEECHER, H. K., 1959, Measurement of subjective responses: Quanti-tative effects of drugs. Oxford University Press, New York.

BRASE, D. A., TSENG, L. F., LOH, H. H. & WAY, E. L., 1974, Choliner-gic modification of naloxone-induced jumping in morphine-dependent mice. Eur. J. Pharmacol. 26:1.

D'AMOUR, F. F. & SMITH, D. L., 1941, A method for determining loss of pain sensation. J. Pharmacol. Exp. Ther. 72:74.

EBEL, A., HERMETET, J. C. & MANDEL, P., 1973, Comparative study of acetylcholinesterase and choline-acetyltransferase activity in the brain of DBA and C57 mice. Nature New Biology 242:56.

EDDY, N. B. & LEIMBACH, D., 1953, Synthetic analgesics. II Dithienyl-butenyl- and dithienylbutylamines. J. Pharmacol. Exp. Ther. 107:385.

EIDELBERG, E. & ERSPAMER, R., 1974, Genetic factors modulating the actions of morphine in mice. Abstracts of the Fourth Annual

Meeting, Society for Neuroscience p. 199.

ERIKSSON, K. & KIIANMAA, K., 1971, Genetic analysis of susceptibil-
    ity to morphine addiction in inbred mice. Ann. Med. Exp.
    Biol. Fenn. 49:73.

GEBHART, G. F. & MITCHELL, C. L., 1973, Strain differences in the
    analgesic response to morphine as measured on the hot plate.
    Arch. Int. Pharmacodyn. Ther. 201:128.

GOLDSTEIN, A. & SHEEHAN, P., 1969, Tolerance to opiod narcotics.
    I. Tolerance to the running fit caused by levorphanol in the
    mouse. J. Pharmacol. Exp. Ther. 169:175.

HANO, K., KANETO, H., & KAKUNOGA, T., 1963, Pharmacological studies
    on analgesics. 5. Development of physical dependence in
    morphinized mice. Japanese J. Pharmacol. 13:207.

IWAMOTO, E. R., HOW, I. K. & WAY, E. L., 1973, Elevation of brain
    dopamine during naloxone-precipitated withdrawal in morphine
    dependent mice and rats. J. Pharmacol. Exp. Ther. 187:558.

KARCZMAR, A. G. & SCHUDDER, C. L., 1967, Behavioral responses to
    drugs and brain catecholamine levels in mice of different
    strains and genera. Fed. Proc. 26:1180.

KEMPF, E., GREILSAMER, J., MACK, G., & MANDEL, P., 1974, Corre-
    lation of behavioral difference in three strains of mice with
    differences in brain amines. Nature 247:483.

KESSLER, S., CIARANELLO, R. D., SHIRE, J. G. M. & BARCHAS, J. D.,
    Genetic variation in catecholamine-synthesizing enzyme activ-
    ities. Proc. Nat. Acad. Sci. (U.S.) 69:2448.

KUHAR, M. J., PERT, C. B. & SNYDER, S. H., 1973, Regional distribu-
    tion of opiate receptor binding in monkey and human brain.
    Nature (London) 245:447.

LASAGNA, L. & BEECHER, H. K., 1954, The optimal dose of morphine.
    J. Am. Med. Assoc. 156:230.

LASAGNA, L., VON FELSINGER, J. M., & BEECHER, H. K., 1955, Drug-
    induced mood changes in man. I. Observations on healthy sub-
    jects, chronically ill patients, and post-addicts. J. Am.
    Med. Assoc. 157:1006.

LOWNEY, L. I., SCHULTZ, K., LOWERY, P. J., & GOLDSTEIN, A., 1974,
    Partial purification of an opiate receptor from mouse brain.
    Science 183:749.

MAAS, J. W., 1962, Neurochemical differences between two strains
    of mice. Science 137:621.

MAAS, J. W., 1963, Neurochemical differences between two strains
    of mice. Nature 197:255.

MAGGIOLO, C. & HUIDOBRO, K., 1961, Administration of pellets of
    morphine to mice-abstinence syndrome. Acta Physiol. Latino-
    amer. 11:70.

MARSHALL, I. & WEINSTOCK, M., 1971, A quantitative method for
    assessing one symptom of the withdrawal syndrome in mice
    after chronic morphine administration. Nature 234:223.

MARUYAMA, Y., HAYASHI, G., SMITS, S. E., & TAKEMORI, A. E., 1971,
    Studies on the relationship between 5-hydroxytryptamine turn-
    over and brain tolerance and physical dependence in mice.
    J. Pharmacol. Exp. Ther. 718:20.

MILLER, L. C., 1948, A critique of analgesic testing methods.
    Ann. N. Y. Acad. Sci. 51:34.

MILLER, J. M. & COCHIN, J., 1974, The effect of continued morphine
    administration on motor activity in the mouse. The Pharmacolo-
    gist 16:248.

NICHOLS, J. R. & HSIAO, S., 1967, Addiction liability of albino
    rats: breeding for quantative differences in morphine
    drinking. Science 157:561.

OLIVERIO, A. & CASTELLANO, C., 1974, Genotype-dependent sensitivity
    and tolerance to morphine and heroine: dissociation between
    opiate-induced running and analgesia in the mouse. Psycho-
    pharmacologia 39:13.

OLIVERIO, A., CASTELLANO, C., & ELEFTHERIOU, B. E., 1974, Morphine
    sensitivity and tolerance: a genetic investigation in the
    mouse. Psychopharmacologia, in press.

PERT, C. B. & SNYDER, S. H., 1973, Opiate receptor: demonstration
    in nervous tissue. Science 179:1011.

SANTOS, C. H., III, MIDAUGH, L., BUCKHOLTZ, N. & ZEMP, J. W., 1973,
    Effects of methadone on activity and on brain monoamines in
    two mouse strains. Fed. Proc. 32:758.

SCHLESINGER, K., BOGGAN, W. O. & FREEDMAN, D. X., 1965, Genetics
    of audiogenic seizures: I. Relation to brain serotonin and
    norepinephrine in mice. Life Sci. 4:2345.

SHUSTER, L., HANNAM, R. V. & BOYLE, W. E., JR., 1963, A simple method for producing tolerance to dihydro-morphinone in mice. J. Pharmacol. Exp. Ther. 140:149.

SHUSTER, L., WEBSTER, G. W. & YU, G., 1974a, Increased running response to morphine in morphine-pretreated mice. J. Pharmacol. Exp. Ther., in press.

SHUSTER, L., WEBSTER, G. W. & YU, G., 1974b, Perinatal narcotic addiction in mice: sensitization to morphine stimulation. Internat. J. of Addictive Diseases, in press.

SHUSTER, L., WEBSTER, G. W., YU, G. & ELEFTHERIOU, B. E., 1974c, A genetic analysis of the response to morphine in mice analgesia and running. Psychopharmacologia, in press.

SUDAK, H. S. & MAAS, J. W., 1964, Central nervous system serotonin and norepinephrine localization in emotional and nonemotional strains in mice. Nature 203:1254.

TILSON, H. A. & RECH, R. H., 1974, The effects of p-chlorophenylanine on morphine analgesia, tolerance and dependence development in two strains of rats. Psychopharmacologia 35:45.

VALZELLI, L., 1973, Psychopharmacology--an introduction to experimental and clinical principles, p. 51 Spectrum Publications, Flushing, New York.

VOGT, M., 1973, Types of neurones involved in the analgesic effect of morphine. In Kosterlitz, H. W., Collier, H. O. J., & Villarael, J. E. (eds.). Agonist and antagonist actions of narcotic analgesic drugs. University Park Press, Baltimore, p. 139-141.

WAY, E. L., LOH, H. H. & SHEA, F. H., 1969, Simultaneous quantitative assessment of morphine tolerance and physical dependence. J. Pharmacol. Exp. Ther. 167:1.

WAY, E. L., HO, I. K. & LOH, H. H., 1973, Relation of brain serotonin to the inhibition and enhancement of morphine tolerance and physical dependence. In A. J. Mandell, (ed). New Concepts in Neurotransmitter Regulation. Plenum Press, N. Y. pp. 279-295.

EXPLORATORY ACTIVITY: GENETIC ANALYSIS OF ITS MODIFICATION

BY VARIOUS PHARMACOLOGIC AGENTS

Alberto Oliverio, M.D.

and

Claudio Castellano, M.D.
Laboratorio di Psiocobiologia e Psicofarmacologia
C. N. R.
Via Reno, 1
Rome, Italy

CONTENTS

INTRODUCTION

A number of biological differences between species or individuals is responsible for the difference in sensitivity or the variety of effects evident after the use of many psychopharmacological agents. Such is the case of lysergic acid diethylamide (Piala et al., 1959) or phenothiazines (Goldenberg & Fishman, 1961). While in some instances, as in the case of phenothiazines (Myrianthopoulos et al., 1962) or imipramine (Burnett et al., 1964) there is evidence for a clear-cut genetic control which may even rely on a major gene effect, in other instances more complex factors are involved. The study of psychopharmacogenetics represents the necessary approach to understand and account for the large individual variability in response to drugs evident in the clinical practice, and also to assess the nature of some individual differences at the level of the central nervous system.

In recent years, the existence of a large number of lines and inbred strains of laboratory mice has indicated that this species represents the choice material for behavioral genetics or pharmacogenetic analyses. While the first approach to the field of psychopharmacogenetics has been based on the use of inbred strains, a further step has been taken through the use of a new genetic device called the recombinant inbred strains (RI). The study of the effects of various psychotropic agents on the exploratory activity of inbred or recombinant inbred strains of mice has provided information on the type of mechanisms by which the individual genetic make-up modulates the reactivity of centrally acting drugs.

USE OF INBRED STRAINS IN PSYCHOPHARMACOGENETICS

A versatile possibility in psychopharmacogenetics relies on the use of inbred strains of mice. A large number of these strains is today available (Green, 1966; Medvedev, 1958; Staats, 1972), and proof of their genetic homozygosity results from a number of studies based on different immunological methods. Thirty-nine strains have also been characterized for their alleles, and as many as 16 polymorphic loci. The variability among these strains is, at least, as great as in any single feral or randombred population — a large group of inbred strains with unique alleles and no overlapping pedigrees being available as the best group to screen for a particu-

lar hoped for variant (Roderick et al., 1971). The existence of
a genetically homogeneous material and of well characterized
strains represents a very useful tool in the study of the mechanism of action of the centrally acting drugs upon the behavior,
and of the biochemical bases of individual differences or reactivity to drugs.

The first point to be considered in a psychopharmacological
approach is the existence of:

(a)   large behavioral differences among strains and within
strain behavioral homogeneity;

(b)   strain biochemical differences at various cerebral regions.

Within Strain Behavioral Homogeneity

This type of homogenity is clearly evident, for example, from
analysis of the avoidance behavior of different inbred strains of
mice trained in a shuttle box. If the performance of an inbred
strain is followed for a number of days (once the animals are
trained in the avoidance task), it is evident that the performance of the animals is very stable and does not fluctuate from
day to day. The genetic differences characterizing various inbred strains of mice result in clear behavioral differences, in
that various strains of inbred mice attain various avoidance levels.

By comparing the overall performance levels reached by 9
strains of mice, it was evident that three strains performed
very poorly (C57Bl/6J, C3H/HEJ and CBA), two (DBA/2J and C57Br/
CdJ) attained a very high level of performance, while the rest
of them showed intermediate values. The results of other learning tasks also showed that there was a positive correlation between active avoidance and maze learning, with the high avoiding
strains (DBA/2J, C57Br/cdJ and A/J) being also characterized by
high maze or Skinner box avoidance learning abilities (Bovet et
al., 1969; Renzi & Sansone, 1971).

Recently, our attention has been focused on three strains
of mice in order to conduct a genetic, biochemical and pharmacological analysis of behavior. A genetic analysis of avoidance,
maze learning, and wheel-running activity has been carried out
in mice belonging to three inbred strains and to their F_1, F_2,
and F_3 progenies. It has been demonstrated that while two
strains (SEC/1ReJ and DBA/2J) were characterized by high levels of avoidance and maze learning but by low levels of running

activity, a third strain (C57Bl/6J) attained poor avoidance and
maze levels, but was very active (Oliverio et al., 1972).

(1) The mode of inheritance in a given behavioral measure
was shown to depend on the crosses considered (Fig. 1). Crossing the C57Bl/6J strain with the high-avoiding low-running SEC/1
ReJ mice resulted in SEC/1ReJ-like progeny while crossing with the
high-avoiding low running DBA/2J mice yielded an offspring similar
to the C57Bl/6J phenotype. A similar dominance pattern was evident
for maze learning, the SEC/1ReJ strain being characterized by the
larger proportion of dominant genes in the three tests.

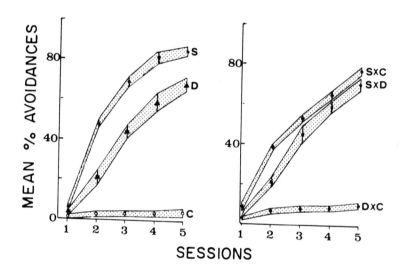

Fig. 1. Mean percentage avoidance (±95% confidence limits of the
mean during sessions 1-5 in three inbred strains of mice and their
F_1 offspring C = C57Bl/6J; S = SEC/1ReJ. (Oliverio et al., 1972.)

(2) Matherian analyses for segregation showed that the total
variance contained, in addition to an environmental component, a
significant genetic component.

(3) Estimates of heritability and genetic correlations were
assessed on F_3 mice and their F_2 parents. Estimates of heritability ($\underline{h}^2$) based on dam-offspring regressions or on sib correlations

were higher for avoidance and maze learning than for activity.
The estimates of the correlations between avoidance and activity were negative, and large enough to be ascribed to a pleiotropic effect. The positive genetic correlation evident between
avoidance and maze learning suggested also that these behaviors
were influenced by many of the same genes, though this effect
might also be ascribed to linkage effects. Thus, the two C57Bl/
6J x SEC1/ReJ and C57B1/6J x DBA/2J F_1 hybrid mice were very
similar for avoidance, maze and activity patterns to their SEC/1ReJ.
or C57B1/6J parents respectively. If these similarities do not
determine that the genetic differences affected learning ability
in the broader sense, an analogy between the brain mechanisms
characterizing each of these hybrids and its dominant parent
strain is somewhat conceivable.

The three inbred strains of mice used in the previous study
and their hybrids seem to be a very useful model for the study
of the genetic, biochemical, and pharmacogenetic aspects of behavior. A large number of results on the activity of DBA/2J and
C57B1/6J mice has already been reported indicating that the two
strains are characterized by low and high activity patterns,
respectively (van Abeelen, 1966; DeFries & Hegman, 1970; McClearn
et al., 1970). In support of our findings, Sprott (1974) has recently reported that DBA/2J and C57B1/6J mice are respectively
characterized by high and low passive avoidance learning and that
the F_1 hybrids are like their C57B1/6J parents. The two strains
were also found to differ in visual discrimination tasks, DBA/2J
mice requiring fewer trials to learn the task (Elias, 1970).
Thus, it seems that the strain differences observed with the active avoidance task are also observable with other paradigms such
as maze learning or passive avoidance.

In general, the two C57B1/6J x SEC1/ReJ and C57B1/6J x DBA/2J
hybrid mice are very similar for avoidance, maze, and activity patterns to therir SEC/1ReJ or C57B1/6J parents, respectively.

Strain Biochemical Differences

In regard the second point, e.g. evidence for biochemical
differences among strains, the results of different biochemical
estimates indicating clear differences between the brain chemistry
of the above cited strains and of their hybrids, suggest that
these lines and their crosses are an interesting model for correlations between individual differences in behavioral patterns
and brain biochemistry.

A number of findings indicate that these strains differ both
in behavior and also in brain chemistry. Measures of brain acetyl-

Table 1

Acetylcholinesterase Activity in Different Brain Regions
of Two Strains of Inbred Mice and Their F_1 Hybrids*
(mmol/g/h)

Frontal	2.15±0.37	1.94±0.39	2.20±0.30
Temporal	3.98±0.62+	2.26±0.49	3.62±0.66
Limbic	3.76±0.40	2.93±0.51	3.21±1.01
Occipital	2.23±0.31	1.87±0.24	1.55±0.15
Parietal	2.05±0.55	1.88±0.37	1.75±0.12
Overall	2.83±0.45	2.17±0.40	2.46±0.44

*From Ebel et al. (1973)

+Significantly different from the C57Bl/6J value (p<0.001)

cholinesterase (ACh-ase) activity have been carried out by Pryor
et al. (1966) in five strains of mice. These authors found large
differences between the strains, which become even more pronounced
if a regional analysis is performed. It is particularly interesting to note that the two strains characterized by high avoidance
levels (A and DBA/2J) also show a higher ACh-ase activity than the
two low-avoiding strains (C3H and C57Bl/6J). A more detailed analysis carried out by Ebel et al. (1973) and Mandel et al. in DBA/2J
and C57Bl/6J and their F_1 hybrids, revealed that DBA/2J mice have
higher ACh-ase (Table 1) and choline acetyltransferase (ChA) activities in the temporal lobe than C57Bl/6J mice. All these findings
indicate that behavioral differences must reflect some biochemical
differences at the brain level.

The adrenergic system. Eleftheriou (1971) has demonstrated
that clear differences exist between the regional brain noradrenaline
turnover of C57Bl/6J and DBA/2J mice. The experiments conducted
by Kempf et al. (1974) on the noradrenaline levels in various brain
areas of the three strains of mice C57Bl/6J, DBA/2J, SEC/1Re and
their F_1 hybrids have demonstrated the existence of clear correlations between neurochemical and behavioral data. It has been
demonstrated in particular that the two high-avoiding strains,
SEC/1ReJ and DBA/2J which are also characterized by low levels of
activity, exhibit higher levels of noradrenaline in the hypothalamus than C57Bl/6J mice. On the contrary, lower levels of noradrenaline are found in the first two strains when the pons and the
medulla oblongata are considered. It is very interesting to note
moreover that the hybrids are similar to their dominant parents

for both behavioral patterns and levels of regional brain noradrenaline (Fig. 2). For example, when wheel running is considered, the
F_1 offspring of C57B1/6J and DBA/2J mice is C57B1/6J-like while the
offspring of C57B1/6J and SEC/1ReJ mice is SEC/1ReJ-like. This is
also evident when the levels of noradrenaline in the pons and medulla oblongata are considered. Similarly, the dominance order
observed for maze learning is similar to that observed for cortical
noradrenaline. When the hypothalamic levels of noradrenaline are
considered, the behavioral-biochemical relationships are evident
in the offspring of C57B1/6J x DBA/2J mice while there is no correlation between the avoidance behavior of the C57B1/6J, SEC/1ReJ,
and C57B1/6J x SEC/1ReJ mice and their hypothalamic noradrenaline
levels.

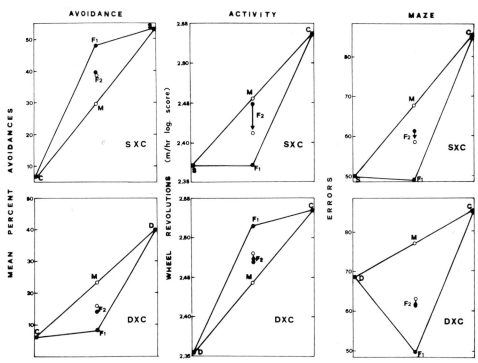

Fig. 2. Genetic triangles representing the observed and expected
population means in three strains of inbred mice (C, D, and S) and
their F1 and F2 progeny. The mean values for the nonsegregating
population forms the corner points of a triangle which is inscribed
in a square. The mean measurement for F_1 lies on the vertical line
which bisects the square, at a distance d above the midparent (M).
The expected means for F_2 (open circles) are at a distance d/2
above the midparent. The observed F_2 value are shown in filled-
in circles and an arrow points from the observed to the expected
means. The S strain is dominant over the C strain, while D mice
are recessive in relation to the C line. (Oliverio et al., 1972).

In general, these results indicate that a promising genetic approach is open to the study of the behavioral individuality and its biochemical bases; they also show that there are clear strain correlations between the levels of motor activity and the amounts of noradrenaline in the pons and medulla, or between those of cortical noradrenaline and those of avoidance or maze learning ability. Thus, the existence of these behavioral differences and of their possible biochemical correlates suggests that these strain dependent brain differences may represent the gound for the observed differences in sensitivity, or opposite types of responding to various centrally acting drugs. In fact, a number of pharmacogenetic experiments have demonstrated that the genetic factors modulate the individual reactivity to different psychotropic agents (Bovet & Oliverio, 1973).

Pharmacologic effects. The effects of different drugs on the behavior of the three strains considered above and their F_1 hybrids have been extensively investigated. Previous findings by Schlesinger & Griek (1970) indicate that DBA/2J mice have lower electroconvulsive shock (ECS) and metrazol seizure threshold than either C57Bl/6J mice or F_1 hybrid mice. Our data agree with these findings and show that DBA/2J and SEC/1ReJ have a lower metrazol sensitivity than C57Bl/6J animals. Here, too, the C57Bl/6J x SEC/1ReJ hybrids resembled the SEC/1ReJ phenotype, and the C57Bl/6J x DBA/2J mice resembled the C57Bl/6J inbred strain, thus confirming the dominance order observed for behavioral phenotypes such as avoidances activity or maze learning (Oliverio & Castellano, 1973).

In a second experiment, the effects of an adrenergic and two cholinergic agents were assessed on the exploratory activity of the different strains. The number of crossings occurring in a tilt-box was measured for 30 minutes. In undrugged mice, the exploratory activity clearly differed in the three strains, which agrees with previous findings (van Abeelen, 1966). Actually, the number of crossings was twice as high in the C57Bl/6J strain than in the other two lines: C57Bl/6J = 122.9±10.1; SEC/1ReJ = 56.9±4.1; DBA/2J = 65.0±3.9. Again, the offspring of the active C57Bl/6J mice show a low or a high exploratory activity depending on whether they come from a cross with SEC/1ReJ or with DBA/2J (C57Bl/6J x SEC/1ReJ = 60.2±6.1; C57Bl/6J x DBA/2J = 115.0±11.2). Differences in responses to amphetamine and to scopolamine were also found. Rather, surprisingly, both drugs reduced the activity in the C57Bl/6J strain, while they increased the number of crossings in SEC/1ReJ and DBA/2J (Fig. 3). The responses of the C57Bl/6J x SEC/1ReJ hybrids to amphetamine and scopolamine were essentially similar to those of the SEC/1ReJ mice. However, when examining the C57Bl/6J x DBA/2J hybrids, the usual pattern of dominance was absent. In fact, amphetamine decreased the number of crossings (like it did in the C57Bl/6J strain), while scopolamine enhanced the activity of

the C57Bl/6J x DBA/2J mice, as was observed in the DBA/2J strain.
The latter findings seem to indicate that the C57Bl/6J genotype
is dominant over the DBA/2J genotype as far as the response to amphetamine is concerned, but that it is recessive to the DBA/2J
genotype with regard to the effects of scopolamine. Physostigmine
diminished exploratory behavior in all strains. (Oliverio & Castellano, 1973).

These results are consistent with other evidence showing
that C57Bl/6J and DBA/2J mice differ in activity and may respond
to the same centrally active drugs in opposite directions (van
Abeelen et al., 1971). In addition it is evident that, although
amphetamine or scopolamine produce opposite effects depending on
the strain considered, a second cholinergic agent physostigmine,
exerts a depressing effect in all genotypes. Since the levels of
adrenergic and cholinergic mediators differ in the brains of mice
of these strains, it is possible that their different reactivities
to various adrenergic and cholinergic agents is related to this
neurochemical diversity.

The morphine-induced modifications of exploratory activity
and analgesia are particularly interesting in the study of the
role of cholinergic mechanisms since many of the effects of the
opiate have been ascribed to modifications of the cholinergic
synapses (Jhamandas et al., 1973). A number of findings indicate
that the effects of morphine on locomotor behavior are strain dependent. Thus, by using three strains of inbred mice C57Bl/6J,
BALB/cJ and DBA/2J which were previously tested for their behavioral and biochemical differences, it was shown that these strains
were clearly different when the morphine "running fit" is considered. (Fig. 4).

In fact, a threefold average increase was evident in the
C57Bl/6J strain, while a twofold increment appeared in the BALB/cJ
strain. Conversely, none of the doses employed suceeded in inducing the running fit in the DBA/2J mice.

In regard to analgesia (Fig. 5) as measured by the hot plate
method (Eddy & Leimbach, 1953), as modified by Goldstein and Sheehan (1969), it was clearly evident that the behavior of the three
strains was completely opposite to that observed for morphine-induced running. In fact, the analgesic effect was less evident in
the C57Bl/6J strain which was very sensitive to the stimulating
properties of the drug on activity. On the contrary, DBA/2J mice
were very sensitive to the analgesic effect of the opiate though
the same doses of morphine were unable to produce any effect on
the locomotor activity of this strain (Oliverio & Castellano, 1974).
These data clearly demonstrated that:

(1) The effects of opioid narcotics on both analgesia and

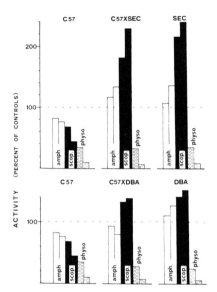

Fig. 3. Modification of exploratory activity (expressed as percent of control level) in three strains of mice and two F_1 hybrids. Amphetamine sulphate (o.5 and 1.0 mg/kg, i.p.), scopolamine hydrobromide (2.5 and 5.0 mg/kg, i.p.), and physostigmine sulfate (0.15 and 0.30 mg/kg), i.p., were injected 30 min. before the test. The lower and the higher dose of each drug are represented by the left and right columns, respectively. Each column represents the mean of crossings in a tilt-box for 15 mice. (Oliverio & Castellano, 1973).

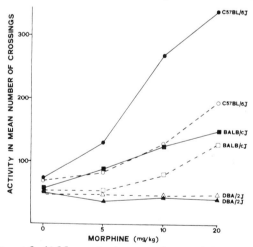

Fig. 4. Effects of different doses of morphine on the running activity of normal (solid lines) and tolerant (broken lines) mice. Each group consisted of 10 mice tested 30 min. after the injection of morphine (Oliverio & Castellano, 1974).

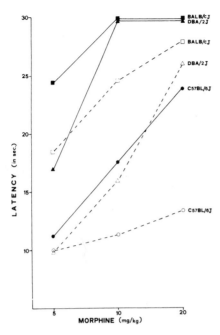

Fig. 5. Morphine-induced analgesia in normal (solid lines) and tolerant (broken lines) mice. The animals were tested 30 min. after the injection with different doses of opiate, (Oliverio & Castellano, 1974).

motor activity are strain dependent;(2) the effects of opiates on running activity and on analgesia are likely to imply two diferent sites of action in that are clearly dissociated; a negative correlation between the degree of running and analgesic responses caused by morphine being clearly evident in the strains considered.

These findings also show that the effects of morphine on the "running fit" and on analgesia are likely to involve two different neurophysiological systems since they are not a unitary phenomenon. It has been suggested that the neuronal and biochemical models which may account for the opiate-induced running activity do not explain opiate analgesia. The mechanism responsible for the "running fit" syndrome in mice seems to be associated with catecholamine depletion and to be faciliated by decreased serotonin levels (Cheney & Goldstein, 1971; Hollinger, 1969; Rethy et al., 1971). However, this model does not explain opiate analgesia and abstinence which seem to be regulated by cholinergic factors (Cheney & Goldstein, 1971; Domino & Wilson, 1973; Jhamandas & Dickinson, 1973). The clear dissociation observed between motor and analgesic effects of morphine further supports the hypothesis that the same neuronal and biochemical model cannot explain the two effects.

Since findings obtained by several investigators (Ebel et al., 19-
73; Mandel et al., 1973; Mack et al., 1973; Kempf et al., 1973)
have shown that these strains are clearly different for their regional brain levels of cholinergic and adrenergic transmitters, it
may be suggested that these biochemical differences might be responsible for the strain-dependent effects of opiates, and for the
dissociation between the effects of morphine on running and analgesia behavior.

When the genetic analysis of the effects of morphine on running activity and analgesia is extended to the F_1 hybrids of the
three strains considered (C57B1/6J, DBA/2J and BALB/cJ) it clearly
appears that the performance of C57B1/6J x BALB/cJ or C57B1/6J x
DBA/2J hybrid mice is similar to that of the C57B1/6J strain, thus
showing a dominance of this strain on the other two. In addition
the inheritance of morphine analgesia seems to be regulated by incomplete dominance, in that the performance of C57B1/6J x BALB/cJ
and C57B1/6J x DBA/2J hybrid mice resulted very similar to that of
the C57B1/6J strain. Due to large estimates of environmental variance it was impossible to show that the backcross population
[(C57B1/6J x BALB/cJ) x C57B1/6J and (C57B1/6J x BALB/cJ) x BALB/cJ
or (C57B1/6J x DBA/2J) x C57B1/6J and (C57B1/6J x DBA/2J) x DBA/2J]
contained a significant genetic component. Since the backcross
mice tested for morphine-induced analgesia were those that were
also tested 30 minutes earlier for morphine-induced "running fit",
correlations between analgesia and locomotor activity were also
calculated. (Castellano & Oliverio, 1974).

The genetic correlations between analgesia and locomotor behavior were negative and large enough to suggest that both behaviors were influenced by many of the same genes. As will be pointed
out by Shuster, in another section of this volume, the findings reported above do not clarify whether the mechanisms responsible for
these behavioral measures involve two different neurophysiological
systems or the same neuronal and biochemical models.

An initial repsonse to this question has been given by studying the relationships between septal lesions and morphine-induced
"running fit" and analgesia in DBA/2J and C57B1/6J mice. While no
change in morphine-induced "running fit" was evident in mice with
septal lesions, it was possible to antagonize morphine analgesia in
both strains (Castellano et al., 1974). In the same experiment, it
was shown that after inhibition of the synthesis of noradrenaline,
by pretreating the mice with α-methyl-p-tyrosine, the effects of
morphine on locomotor behavior were markedly reduced in C57B1/6J
and DBA/2J mice. On the contrary, pretreatment with α-methyl-p-
tyrosine (AMT) did not modify the analgesic effects of morphine.
Since considerable amount of data indicates that lesions of the
septum result in a decreased cholinergic input to other regions of

the limbic system (Kuhar et al., 1973; Srebo et al., 1973), the
data reported above suggest that when the morphine-induced analgesia
is considered, a reduction of the cholinergic activity in the limbic
system due to septal lesions interferes with the effects of morphine
on the analgesic behavior. On the contrary, the locomotor effects
of morphine activity are not modified by a reduction of the septal
function. The fact that septal lesions decreased morphine-induced
analgesia but not the "running fit", while AMT antagonized the effects of morphine on locomotor activity, but did not affect analgesia, it may be assumed that the same biochemical and neurophysiological model cannot explain the effects of opiates on running
and on analgesic behaviors and that, at lease in the mouse, the
limbic system modulates morphine-induced analgesia, but not the
effects of the opiates on locomotor activity. These findings support a number of data which indicate that the septal area is critical for eliciting analgesia (Wey et al., 1973), and that morphine-
binding activity is high in the limbic system (Kuhar et al., 1973;
Pert & Snyder, 1973).

     EEG and brain lesion studies. A further demonstration of the
difference existing between these strains, in respect to their reactivity to morphine, derives from the study of the EEG responses
to morphine in C57Bl/6J and DBA/2J mice (Oliverio, 1974) (Fig. 6).

     Recordings of the EEG activity in both strains during waking
were substantially similar, and the normal baseline sleep EEG generally showed larger spindles in the DBA/2J than in C57Bl/6J mice.
After a single injection of morphine, the EEG patterns were drastically altered in the C57Bl/6J strain which also exhibited a "running
Fit". This change occurred 3 to 10 minutes after the injection and
lasted as long as 45-60 min. Tracings from normally sleeping C57Bl/
6J mice looked almost idential to recording from the same subject
after morphine administration, with a clear increase in voltage and
the appearance of slow waves and spindles. Morphine, on the contrary, did not affect the EEG pattern or the locomotor behavior of
DBA/2J mice.

     Septal lesions resulted in a reduction of the analgesic ef-
fects of morphine in both strains, but did not modify the running
response and EEG correlates. In conclusion, the administration of
morphine, which was shown to stimulate the locomotor activity of
C57Bl/6J mice, is followed in this strain by an EEG pattern similar
to that evident in normally sleeping mice, while the injection of
the opiate was not followed by the appearance of higher levels of
locomotor behavior nor by any observable EEG modification in the
DBA/2J strain. Thus, it would seem that in the mouse, or at least
in these strains of mice, morphine-induced behavioral activation is
correlated to a sleep-like EEG pattern, a dissociation between EEG
and behavior similar to that described for some anticholinergic

112 A. OLIVERIO & C. CASTELLANO

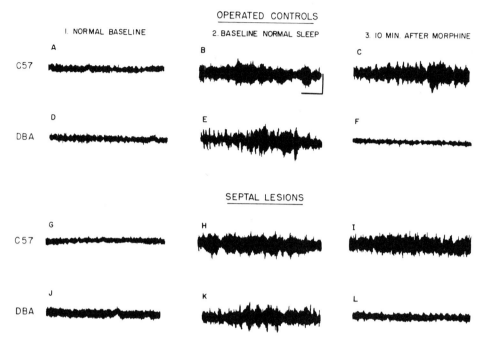

Fig. 6. Effects of a single injection of morphine on the EEG tracing recorded from the cortex in normal mice (operated controls) and
in mice with lesions of the septum. Samples of polygraphic recordings during waking (1., normal baseline), slow wave sleep (2., baseline normal sleep) and after the injection of morphine (20 mg/kg)
in C57Bl/6J and DBA/2J mice. The normal sleep EEG (B) and that after morphine injection (C) are similar in the C57Bl/6J strain. On
the contrary, the waking EEG (D), and that after morphine injection
(F) are similar in DBA mice. Septal lesions do not produce any major modification of the effects of morphine on the EEG patterns.
(Oliveriod, 1974).

agents. The fact that morphine did not increase the locomotor activ-
ivty of DBA/2J mice further supports also the possibility that the
lack of effect on EEG patterns may be ascribed to common neurophysiological mechanisms.

The fact that septal lesions antagonize morphine-induced analgesia but not the "running fit" or the sleep-like EEG activity seems
to confirm the hypothesis that locomotor or other excitatory patterns rather than the analgesic effects of morphine, are possibly
correlated to the EEG responses to the opiate.

USE OF RECOMBINANT INBRED (RI) STRAINS
IN PSYCHOPHARMACOGENETICS

Exploratory Activity

A useful tool in psychopharmacogenetics is represented by the recombinant inbred strains (RI). The RI strains are derived from a cross of two unrelated by highly inbred progenitor strains having then been maintained independently from the F_2 generation with strict inbreeding. This procedure fixes genetically the chance recombination of genes that occurred, although in ever-decreasing amounts, in each succeeding generation after the F_1. The resulting battery of strains can be looked upon, in a sense, as a replicable recombinant population (Bailey, 1971). Through this genetic analysis, it is possible to determine quickly the probable location of a new gene by matching the strain distribution pattern (SDP) with those of other genes among a set of inbred strains. The SDP method, therefore, is useful in searching for gene identity, since identical or similar SDP's of any pair of traits indicate possible pleiotropism or linkage of controlling genes. The advantage of this genetic analytic device is stressed elsewhere in this same volume.

Scopolamine and amphetamine. By applying this procedure to behavior, it has been possible (Oliverio et al., 1973) to conduct a genetic analysis of exploratory activity of mice and its modification by scopolamine and amphetamine (Fig. 7).

For this purpose seven recombinant inbred strains were used = CXBD, CXBE, CXBG, CXBH, CXBI, CXBJ and CXBK. These were derived from an initial cross of BALB/cBy (C) and C57Bl/6By (B6), followed by over 40 generations of full sib matings. In addition, a battery of congenic lines was developed independently from an initial cross of B6 to C by a regimen of skin-graft testing, and backcrossed to B6 for at least 12 generations. This procedure resulted in congenic B6 lines, each of which differ from B6 itself by only an introduced chromosomal segment including a C-strain allele at a distinctive histocompatibility (H) locus. Each of these congenic lines has been tested against RI strains by means of skin-grafts to find which of the RI strains carry the C-strain allele and which the B6-allele at a particular H locus, thereby establishing their (SDP) strain distribion patterns.

The pattern in which the RI strains exhibited low of high activity, and its modification by scopolamine was compared to the strain distribution patterns (SDPs) already determined for the H-loci. Matching SDP's indicate possible identity or close linkage of two genes. On the other hand, two SDP's may match merely by chance.

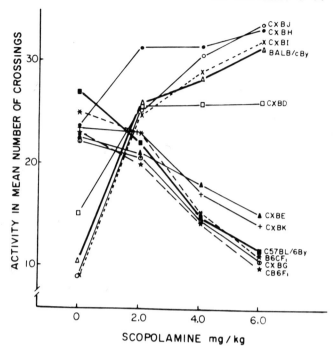

Fig. 7. Mean activity exhibited by BALB/cBy, C57Bl/6By, their reciprocal F₁ hybrids, B6CF₁ and CB6F₁ and the seven recombinant inbred strains after injection of saline or scopolamine at 2, 4, or
6 mg/kg of body weight. (Oliverio *et al*., 1973).

    The data obtained in the testing of all strains indicated
that, for basal exploratory activity, these strains were distinctly
grouped in two major categories. Thus, strains CXBD, CXBI, CXBJ,
and the progenitor strain BALB/cBy exhibited low basal exploratory
activity, while all the RI strains, and the two reciprocal F₁ hybrids were high in basal exploratory activity, and similar to the
other progenitor strain, C57Bl/6By.

    For the purpose of classifying all strains in their explora-
tory activity after injection of the drug, two major response categories were considered. The first category grouped all strains
according to a significant increase or decrease of activity following the lowest (2 mg/kg) scopolamine dose. It appeared that strains
CXBI, CXBJ, CXBD, CXBH, and progenitor strain BALB/cBy exhibited
a trend toward increase of basal exploratory activity, while all
other strains exhibited a trend toward decline in exploratory
activity.

    The second classification grouped all strains according to
their overall responses after the injection of scopolamine. Thus,

consideration was made whether a particular strain maintained an increasing or decreasing trend in exploratory activity during all three doses of scopolamine. Strains CXBE, CXBG, and CXBK, both reciprocal hybrids (B6CF$_1$ and CB6F$_1$), and progenitor strain C57Bl/6By maintained a persistent decline in exploratory activity with increasing levels of scopolamine. Strains CXBI, CXBJ, and progenitor strain BALB/cBy maintained a persistent increase in exploratory activity after drug injection. However, strains CXBD and CXBH exhibited no significant changes in exploratory activity following increasing levels of scopolamine. In short, these two strains exhibited their optimum scopolamine-induced modification of exploratory activity with the lowest dose of drug, and thereafter maintained a plateau in this response.

Several aspects of the statistical grouping of strains and crosses permitted the derivation of a genetic model of basal exploratory activity on the following rationale: (1) RI strains were distributed either high or low along with each of the progenitor strains, C57Bl/6By and BALB/cBy, with absence of intermediate groups; (2) the reciprocal F$_1$ hybrids, B6CF$_1$ and CB6F$_1$ were alike and identical in activity to the C57Bl/6By progenitor strain indicating dominance of the allele for high activiity or the C57Bl/6By genotype; (3) no evidence of maternal effects based on similarity of activity in the reciprocal F$_1$ hybrids; (4) confirmation that the controlling gene is in chromosome 4 since the congenic line H(w26) was BALB/cBy-like for exploratory activity; (5) data from backcross B6CF$_1$ x BALB/cBy consisting of two distinct groupings. This is in agreement with previous results demonstrating dominance of the C57Bl/6J strain over BALB/cJ strain for still other measures of activity (de Fries & Hegman, 1970; Oliverio & Messeri, 1973).

The genetic model which best explained the data obtained in the sustained scopolamine response postulated the existence of a second locus at which one allele controls dose-response related activity changes by this drug. These conclusions were primarily based on (1) the esistence of the plateau effect in strains CXBD and CXBH, although both of these strains exhibited quite dissimilar basal exploratory activity; (2) lack of pharmacologic "ceiling effect" in CBD strain; (3) the confirmation by the use of congenic lines H(w19) and H(w41) indicating that this effect is not a pleiotropic effect of the H-2 locus, although it is probably closely linked to it.

The symbol Exa was suggested to designate the locus, linked to H(w26) in chromosome 4 (LG VIII), for basal short-term exploratory activity, with Exa^h to designate the allele determining high level, and Exa^1 the allele determining low level of activity. The symbol Sco was additionally proposed to designate the second locus,

linked to H-2 in chromosome 17 (LG IX), one allele at which controls the sustained reactivity to scopolamine once the initial response has occurred, the other allele permitting reversal of exploratory activity determined at Exa. It was suggested that Sco^a
be used to designate the allele determining absence of dose-response
related activity changes by scopolamine, and Sco^P to designate the
allele with presence of dose-response related changes (Oliverio et
al., 1973).

In regards to the effects of amphetamine, this drug influenced
the RI basal activity in a manner opposite to that of scopolamine.
Generally, the results indicated a highly varied response of the RI
strains after amphetamine injection. This was evidenced by segregation of these strains into six major groupings which were significantly different from one another. Thus, based on the statistical
analyses it was concluded that the modification of basal activity
by d-amphetamine was due to a polygenic effect which is highly complex to analyze genetically. For this reason, no further genetic
testing was pursued for this effect.

Ethanol. Another centrally acting agent whose effects have
been investigated in a number of studies is ethanol. The RI technique has proved to be a very useful device to assess the role of
the genetic make-up in modulating the effects of alcohol upon behavior. While a number of previous studies have concentrated in
assessing the role of genetic factors in long term preference for
ethanol drinking (Rodgers & McClearn, 1962; Eriksson & Kiianmaa,
1971), our study was devolved to determine the acute effects of
alcohol on behavior.

Thus, the effects of alcohol on locomotor activity were tested on the RI strains by using a procedure similar to that described
for scopolamine. It was observed that alcohol induced a proges-
sive and persistent decline in motor activity, in all of the 11
strains (Fig. 8). However, when the effects of alcohol were represented in terms of percent variation in relation to previous control (saline injected) level, strains CXBD, CXBE and the progenitor
strain C57Bl/6By showed the highest decline of performance following ethanol administration, while all other strains were characterized by the lowest decline of performance.

In order to arrive at a testable genetic model for ethanol
modification of basal activity different congenic lines which
closely matched the RI lines SDP were tested. In all these con
genic lines, with the exception of line B6.C-H(w13K), alcohol at
the dose of 2 g/kg induced a decrement of performance similar to
that evident in C57Bl/6By mice. Congenic line B6.C-H(w13K) was
identical to BALB/cBy and different from C57Bl/6By in performance
in relation to alcohol-induced decrement of activity. This indi-

cated that although its SDP matched that for alcohol for all strains, with the exception of strain CXBD which is B6-like and CXBI and CXBK which are C-like, the gene exerting a major effect on alcohol-induced decrement of performance is linked to, or possibly identical with, the gene H(wl3K).

In addition, when the performance of the backcross BALB x B6CF$_1$ mice injected with 2 g/kg of alcohol is considered, two different and statistically separate groups were evident. This latter observation further supports the conclusion that the effects of ethanol on exploratory activity are controlled by at least one locus exerting an effect on this behavior.

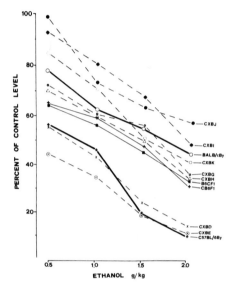

Fig. 8. Activity in mean number of crossings in the toggle box, for the 11 strains examined after saline (sal.) injection or different doses of ethanol (g/kg). (Oliverio & Eleftheriou, 1974).

From these findings it was clearly evident that the allele for the low decline in performance following ethanol administration is dominant, and that the locus exerting the major effect is in chromosome 4 (LG VIII). It was suggested the symbol Eam (ethanol activity modifier) be used to designate the locus, linked to H(wl3K) in chromosome 4 (LG VIII), for ethanol effects on motor activity, with Eam[h] to designate the allele determining a high or C57Bl/6By-like decline in activity by ethanol, and Eam[l] the allele determining a low or BALB/cBy-like decline in activity.

It must be stressed that recently, Fuller & Collins (1972)

have shown by means of Mendelian analyses, that two loci or two independent blocks of closely linked genes, control the major amount
of variance in ethanol intake and preference. In the study referred
to above, it was possible to demonstrate linkage for a gene modulating the effects of alcohol upon motor behavior, a trait different
from ethanol consumption, but which might possibly be related to it.

The studies reported until now demonstrate the utility of the
RI method in identifying the genes responsible for some drug effects.
However, this method does not always lead to clear cut results; in
fact, the RI technique is mainly useful when the parental strains
are different for the phenotype considered and when the number of
genes responsible for the trait under study is relatively low.

An example of the difficulty for arriving at linkage when a
more complex genetic model is represented are the effects of morphine on running and analgesia (Castellano & Oliverio, 1974). In
this case, the RI method was not as successful as for scopolamine
or alcohol, indicating a genetic model based on three or more genes,
as evident from the findings obtained by Shuster et al. (1974).
These findings will be reported in this volume elsewhere.

In general, the advantage of using a genetic approach in the
study of psychotropic drugs is mainly represented by the possibility of obtaining a genetic model for the action of a given agent,
and to eventually identify and link the gene(s) responsible for
its action. The genetic approach is also useful in that it offers
the possibility of arriving at the identification of strains or congenic lines available for further studies on the biochemical bases
of drug action. In addition to that, it has been demonstrated
that the same genes exert comparable biochemical effects in different animal species. (Kalmus, 1971). Thus, it is possible that
the same gene is responsible for the same pharmacological effects
in animals or in man, and that the study of biochemical genetics
in mice might prove to be useful also for man. Thus, psychopharmacogenetics represents a useful approach for understanding the function of the brain and also offers the possibility to study the biochemical action of genes which exert similar effects in different
species.

ENVIRONMENTAL FACTORS

Until now, we have considered a number of examples in which
the genetic make-up of the individual modulates the effect of
drugs upon behavior. However, it should also be remembered that
the environment may affect the action of different pharmacological
agents and in particular of the drugs acting upon the behavior.

It is known that, in man, the mechanisms responsible for individual differences in the reactivity to different psychotropic
agents such as tranquilizers or hallucinogens are modulated by
genetic differences (Vesell, 1972; Kalow, 1966). However, environmental factors may modify the effects of many psychotropic agents
such as psychodelic drugs or opiates.

Steinberg and her associates have clearly demonstrated that,
in a maze situation, past experience can have a great effect or
abolish the increase in activity following the administration of
different drugs and drug mixtures to the rat. Recently, it has
also been demonstrated that environmental factors also play an
important role in determining the stimulating effects of morphine
and that the genetic mechanisms are not the sole source of variation when the individual reactivity to opiates is considered.
(Oliverio & Castellano, 1974). It has been previously shown that
a single morphine injection is followed by a threefold increase
in activity of C57Bl/6 mice. To test the effects of past experience on the action of morphine, another group of mice was previously adapted to the testing apparatus and immediately after the
end of this session the same mice were injected with morphine
and tested again in the same set up. No stimulating effect was
evident under these conditions in relation to the control group,
showing that past experience modifies the effects of morphine.

In another schedule of experience, the animals were adapted
to the apparatus in absence of drug. Six hours later the mice
were subjected to a second 25 min. test and at the end of this
session they were injected with saline or morphine and immediately
retested during a third 25 min. long session. (Fig. 9). Under
these conditions, the experience of the animals was more consolidated than under the previous schedule, and the injection of morphine resulted in a complete block of their activity. However,
when, at the end of the session, the animals were removed and returned to their home cages, they exhibited extremely high levels
of locomotor behavior. Thus, after a few minutes, they were tested again in the apparatus and a high level of activity was evident
under these conditions. Therefore, it was concluded that exploration of a different environment was followed by the "running fit"
in the same xperienced animals in which the injection of morphine
previously resulted in a block of their activity.

Similarly, it was possible to reduce the running fit in experienced animals in which morphine resulted in a block of their
locomotor activity by arousing them either by switching off the 40
W lamp normally lighted in the cabin 1 meter above the toggle-
floor boxes, or by spraying a solution of eugenol inside the cabin
at the end of the morphine session.

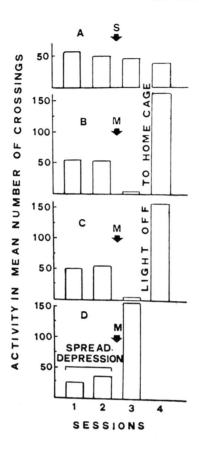

Fig. 9. Effects of past experience on the morphine-induced "running fit". Groups A and D were subjected to two 25 mm. long sessions (1 and 2) spaced by six hours. Animals of group D were subjected to cortical spreading depression during these two sessions. Immediately after session two the mice were injected with saline (S) or morphine (M) (20 mg/kg) and tested again for 25 minutes (session 3). At the end of this session the mice were either returned to their home cage for 2-3 minutes and then tested again for 25 minutes (session 4) or they were subjected to an additional session in total darkness. The performance of groups A and B during the third and fourth sessions was significantly different (t = 13.1, P < .001; t = 17.0, P < .001). Similarly, the performance of group C during session four was different from that of a control group (not shown) injected with saline and subjected to a similar schedule (t = 14.9, P < .001). In the mice tested under spreading depression during sessions 1 and 2 morphine significantly enhanced the performance in relation to that of another group of animals injected with saline (t = 17.9, P < .001). (Oliverio & Castellano, 1974).

To show that experience of the environment results in a clear change of the behavioral effects of morphine, a group of mice was subjected to functional decortication during the experience of the apparatus. In these mice, the injection of morphine was followed by clear excitatory effects, showing the importance of sensory inputs and experience in modulating the effects of the opiate.

These experiments stress the importance of the environment in influencing the action of centrally acting drugs. Study of these factors in animals might provide a useful tool for analysing the type of effects of morphine and of a number of "social drugs" in man depending on his social environment.

In summary the exploratory activity of mice measured by a simple and reliable test, such as the tilt-floor box, represents a useful behavioral pattern in the study of the genetic and environmental factors which modulate the reactivity to different psychotropic agents. The analysis of the genetic determinants of drug effects on behavior has not only important clinical implications but may also represent an important tool in a multidisciplinary approach to brain research.

REFERENCES

ABEELEN VAN, J. H. F., 1966, Effects of genotype on mouse behavior Anim. Behav. 14:218.

ABEELEN VAN, J. H. F., SMITS, A. J. M., RAAIJMAKERS, W. G. M., 1971, Central location of genotype-dependent cholinergic mechanism controlling exploratory behaviour in mice. Psychopармacologia, 19:324.

BAILEY, D. W., 1971, Recombinant inbred strains. Transplantation 11:325.

BOVET, D., BOVET-NITTI, F. & OLIVERIO, A., 1969, Genetic aspects of learning and memory in mice. Science 163:139.

BOVET, D. & OLIVERIO, A., 1973, Pharmacogenetic aspects of learning and memory. In G. Acheson et al. (eds.). Proceedings of the 5th International Congress on Pharmacology. Karger, Basel.

BURNETT, C. H., DEUT, C. R., HARPER, C. & WARLAND, B. J., 1964, Amer. J. Med. 36:222.

CASTELLANO, C., ESPINET LLOVERA, B. & OLIVERIO, A., 1974, Morphine reduced running and analgesia in two strains of mice following septal lesions or modification of brain amines. Arch. Pharmacol. (In press)

CASTELLANO, C. & OLIVERIO, A., 1974, A genetic analysis of morphine induced running and analgesia in the mouse. In press in Psychopharmacologia.

CHENEY, D. L. & GOLDSTEIN, A., 1971, The effect of p-Chlorophenyl-alanine on opiate-induced running, analgesia, tolerance and physical dependence in mice. J. Pharmac. Exp. Ther. 177:309.

DE FRIES, J. C. & HEGMAN, J. P., 1970, Genetic analysis of open-field behavior. In G. Lindsay & D. D. Thiessen (Eds.) Contribution to behavior-genetic analysis. The mouse as a prototype. New York, Appleton-Century-Crofts, p. 23.

DOMINO, E. F., & WILSON, A., 1973, Effects of narcotic analgesic agonists and antagonists on rat brain acetylcholine. J. Pharmac. Exp. Ther. 184:18.

EBEL, A., HERMETET, J. C. & MANDEL, P., 1973, Comparative study of acetylcholinesterase and choline-acetyltransferase enzyme activity in brain of DBA and C57 mice. Nature New Biology, 242:56.

EDDY, N. B., & LEIMBACK, D., 1953, Synthetic analgesics. II. Dithie-
    nylbutenyl-and dithienylbutylamines. J. Pharmacol. Exp. Ther.
    107:385.

ELEFTHERIOU, B. E., 1971, Regional brain norepinephrine turnover
    rates in four strains of mice. Neuroendocrinology 7:329.

ELIAS, M. F., 1970, Differences in reversal learning between two
    inbred mouse strains. Psychon. Sci. 20:179.

ERIKSSON, K., KIIANMAA, K., 1971, Genetic analysis of susceptibility
    to morphine addiction in inbred mice. Amer. Med. Exp. Biol.
    Fenn. 49:73.

FULLER, J. L., COLLINS, R. L., 1972, Ethanol consumption and prefe-
    rence in mice: a genetic analysis. Ann. N. Y. Acad. Sci.,
    197:42.

GOLDENBERG, H. & FISHMAN, V., 1961, Species dependence of chlor-
    promazine. Proc. Soc. Exper. Biol. & Med. 108:178.

GOLDSTEIN, A. & SHEEHAN, P., 1969, Tolerance to opioid narcotics.
    I. Tolerance to the "running fit" caused by Levorphanol in
    the mouse. J. Pharmac. Exp. Ther. 169:175.

GREEN, M. C., 1972, (For the Committee on Standardized Genetic
    Nomenclature for Mice). Standard Karyotype of the mouse,
    Mus musculus. J. Hered. 63:69.

HOLLINGER, M., 1969, Effects of reserpine, α-methyl-p-tyrosine,
    p-chlorophenylalanine, and pargyline on levorphanol induced
    running activity in mice. Arch. Int. Pharmacodyn Ther. 179:
    419.

JHAMANDAS, K. & DICKINSON, G., 1973, Modification of precipitated
    morphine and Methadone abstinence by acetylcholine antagonists.
    Nature New Biology, 245:219.

JHAMANDAS, K., PINSKY, C. & PHILLIS, J. W., 1970, Effects of mor-
    phine and its antagonists on release of cerebral cortical
    acetylcholine. Nature 228:176.

KALMUS, H., 1971, Comparative primate genetics and human heredity
    in Comparative Genetics in Monkeys, Apes and Man (A. B.
    Chiarelli, ed.) New York Press, London.

KALOW, K., 1966, Genetic aspects of drug safety. Appl. Ther., 8:
    44.

KEMPF, E., GREILSHAMER, J., MACK, G., & MANDEL, P., 1974, Corre-
    lation of behavioral differences in three strains of mice
    with differences in brain amines. Nature 247:483.

KUHAR, M. J., PERT, B. C. & SNYDER, S. H., 1973, Regional distri-
    bution of opiate receptor binding in monkey and human brain.
    Nature 245:447.

KUHAR, M. J., SETHY, V. H., ROTH, R. H. & AGAJANIAN, G. K., 1973,
    Choline: Selective accumulation by central cholinergic
    neurons. J. Neurochem. 20:581.

MACK, C., GREILSAMER, J., KEMPF, E. & MANDEL, P., 1973, Neuro-
    chemical correlates of genetically observed differences in
    performance levels in mice. Abstract IV Int. Meeting of the
    International Society of Neurochemistry, Tokio.

MANDEL, P., EBEL, A., HERMETET, J. C., BOVET, D. & OLIVERIO, A.
    1973, Etudes des enzymes du systeme cholinergique shez les
    hybrides F1 de Souris se distinguant par leur aptitude au
    conditionnement. C. R. Acad. Sci. (Paris) 276:395.

MCCLEARN, G. E., WILSON, J. R.,& MEREDITH, W., 1970, The use of
    isogenic and heterogenic mouse stocks in behavioral re-
    search. In G. Lindzey & D. D. Thiessen (Eds.), Contribu-
    tions to behavior-genetic analysis: the mouse as a prototype.
    New York, Appleton-Century-Crofts.

MCCLEARY, R. A., 1961, Response specificity in the behavioral
    effects of limbic system lesions in the cat. J. Comp. Physiol.
    Psychol. 54:605.

MEDVEDEV, N. N., 1958, On the breeding of the laboratory strain
    mice. Biulletini Moskoskogo Obestva. Ispitateki Prirodvi
    63:117.

MYRIANTHOPOULOS, N. C., KURLAND, A. A. & KURLAND, L. T., 1962,
    Hereditary predisposition in drug-induced parkinsonism.
    Arch. Neurol. 6:5.

OLIVERIO, A., 1974, Genotype dependent electroencephalografic be-
    havioral and analgesic correlates of morphine: an analysis
    in normal mice and in mice with septal lesions. Brain Res.
    82:101.

OLIVERIO, A. & CASTELLANO, C., 1973, In D. Bovet & A. Oliverio,
    Pharmacogenetic aspects of learning and memory. In G. Acheson
    et al. (Eds.) Proceedings of the 5th International Congress
    on Pharmacology, Karger, Basel.

OLIVERIO, A. & CASTELLANO, C., 1974, Experience modifies morphine-
    induced behavioral excitation of mice. Nature (In press).

OLIVERIO, A., CASTELLANO, C. & MESSERI, P., 1972, A genetic analy-
    sis of avoidance, maze and wheel running behavior in the mouse.
    J. Comp. Physiol. Psychol. 79:459.

OLIVERIO, A., CASTELLANO, C. & MESSERI, P., 1973, Genotype dependent
    effects of septal lesions on different types of learning in
    the mouse. J. Comp. Physiol. Psychol. 82:240.

OLIVERIO, A., ELEFTHERIOU, B. E. & BAILEY, D. W., 1973, Exploratory
    activity, genetic analysis of its modification by scopolamine
    and amphetamine. Physiol. Behav. 10:893.

OLIVERIO, A. & MESSERI, P., 1973, An analysis of single-gene ef-
    fects on avoidance, maze, wheel-running and exploratory be-
    havior in the mouse. Behav. Biol.

PERT, C. B., & SNYDER, S. H., 1973, Opiate receptor: demonstration
    in nervous tissue. Science 179:1011.

PIALA, J. J., HIGH, J. P., HASSERT, G. L., BURKE, J. C. & CRAVER,
    B. N., 1959, Pharmacological and acute toxicological compari-
    sons of triflupromazine and chlorpromazine. J. Pharmacol.
    & Exper. Therap. 127:55.

PRYOR, G. T., SCHLESINGER, K. & CALHOUN, W. H., 1966, Differences
    in brain enzymes among five inbred strains of mice. Life Sci.
    5:2105.

RENZI, P. & SANSONE, M., 1971, Discrininated lever-press avoidance
    in mice. Communs. Behav. Biol. 6:315.

RETHY, C. R., SMITH, C. B., & VILLARREAL, J. E., 1971, Effects of
    narcotic analgesics upon the locomotor activity and brain
    catecholamine content of the mouse. J. Pharmac. Exp. Ther.
    176:472.

RODERICK, T. H., RUDDLE, F. H., CHAPMAN, V. M. & SHOWS, T. B., 1971,
    Biochemical polymorphisms in feral and inbred mice (Mus mus-
    culus). Biochem. Geneti. 5:457.

RODGERS, D. A., MCCLEARN, G. E., 1962, Mouse strain differences in
    preference for various concentrations of alcohol. Quart. J.
    Stud. Alcohol 23:26.

SCHLESINGER, K. & GRIEK, B. J., 1970, The genetics and biochemistry
    of audiogenic seizures. In G. Lindzey & D. D. Thiessen (Eds.)

Contributions to Behavior-genetic analysis. The mouse as a prototype. (New York, Appleton-Century-Crofts).

SHUSTER, L., WEBSTER, G. W., YU, G., ELEFTHERIOU, B. E., 1974, A genetic analysis of the response to analgesia and running after morphine in mice. Submitted to Psychopharmacologia.

SPROTT, R. L., 1974, Passive-avoidance performance in mice: Evidence for single-locus inheritance. Behav. Biol. 11:231.

SREBRO, B., ODERFELD-NOVAK, B., KLODOS, I., DABOWSKA, J. & NARKIE-WICZ, O., 1973, Changes in acetylcholinesterase activity in hippocampus produced by septal lesions in the rat. Life Sci. 12:261.

STAATS, J. L., 1972, Standard nomenclatura for inbred strains of mice: Fifth listing. Cancer Res. 32:1609.

STEINBERG, H., RUSHTON, R., & TINSON, C., 1961, Nature 192:533.

VESELL, E., 1972, Introduction: genetic and environmental factors affecting drug response in man. Fed. Proc. 31:1253.

WEY, B., LOH, H. H. & WAY, E. L., 1973, Brain sites of precipitated abstinence in morphine-dependent rats. J. Pharmacol. Exp. Ther. 185:108.

ALCOHOL IMBIBITION AND BEHAVIOR: A COMPARATIVE GENETIC
APPROACH

Kalervo Eriksson, Ph.D.

Research Laboratories
State Alcohol Monopoly
Alko, Box 350
SF-00101 Helsinki 10
Finland

CONTENTS

INTRODUCTION

Alcoholism is a major and difficult problem in many countries.
In those countries from which at least relatively valid statistical figures are available, i.e., the northern and western European
countries, Britain, the USA, Canada and Australia, one can estimate that approximately 4-6% of the men and 0.1-1.5% of the women
suffer from alcoholism or problems caused by excessive drinking.
It is impossible to estimate the exact number of alcoholics, because the occurrence and frequency figures are totally dependent
upon how one defines alcoholism.

Most definitions of alcoholism are based on general drinking
behaviors, such as the frequency and amounts consumed at one time.
It is very difficult to obtain valid information about behaviors
of this type with the use of simple interviews or questionnaires.
Also, included in some definitions of alcoholism are the social
consequences that are often seen as a result of excessive drinking. One of the most important definitions of alcoholism is that
made by Jellinek (1960), the leading authority in this area. He
expounded the disease concept of alcoholism and showed that the
disease is manifested in various ways. On this basis, he devised
five major categories for alcoholics, designated as alpha, bets,
gamma, delta or epsilon. His classification system takes into
consideration the periodicity of the drinking, the amounts consumed,
the signs of severe or mild intoxication, signs of physical de-

pendence and withdrawal, and difficulties in human relationships.
Alcoholism as described by Jellinek is, therefore, a very complicated and complex "disease," which is manifested as many different
syndromes.

Although producing a single definition of alcoholism that is
both uniform and valid appears to be nearly an impossible task,
several operational definitions have been used successfully, despite
their defects, for mapping the occurrence of the problem and its
social consequences. Finding a definition suitable for use in
psychogenetic studies is, however, even more difficult and is
very much dependent upon the aim of the experiment. On the basis
of Jellinek's criteria, one can assume that alcoholism is not a
uniform and clearcut disease. No matter what definition one uses,
there is always the dange of obtaining erratic interpretations due
to a biased weighting of the environmental, behavioral and physiological factors underlying the definition. For instance, definitions
emphasizing the social consequences of alcoholism have little value
when trying to measure the basic metabolically-determined behavior
involved with alcoholism.

The role of genetic factors in the etiology of alcoholism is
a very old and controversial question, and has been the cause of
much heated debate. A very common popular misconception is that
if the existence of genetically-determined metabolic and behavioral
factors in the etiology of alcoholism is accepted, the environmental
part, i.e., social and psychiatric causes, must be ruled out. This
is seldom true with any phenomena, and certainly is not with ones
such as alcoholism. One of the fundamental rules in genetics is
that the inherited genotype together with environmental factors
makes the phenotype. There are actually only a few physical properties in man or animals which, like eye color, are completely determined by inherited factors without any environmental influence.
Most of the phenotypic traits, especially those regulated by many
loci or genes, are strongly dependent upon the environment.

Since 1947, when Williams presented his genetotrophic theory
of alcoholism, there has been much argument concerning the importance
of "nature vs. nurture" in the production of alcoholism. Unfortunately, almost all of the argument has been generated by this misconception. When this nature vs. nurture controversy started,
many scientists felt that it was necessary to choose sides, which
further polarized the discussion. McClearn (1973) has crystallized
these attitudes and statements very well in his recent review, and
I can simply agree with him:

"The dichotomous view that a trait must be due either to
heredity or to environment has also permitted the development of a curious prejudice with respect to theories of

the etiology of alcoholism. The burden of proof seems
to fall on the proponent of the hereditary role. Environmental factors are assumed to be relevant unless demonstrated
not to be; genetic factors are assumed a priori to be irrelevant, and can be admitted only after rigorous demonstration. For example, in reports of the incidence of alcoholism within families, one frequently finds a statement
to the effect that, because there is no positive proof for
the direct inheritance of a tendency towards alcoholism,
the statistics must be interpreted as revealing the adverse
effects of family environment. Another aspect of this same
type of bias is the willingness of many investigators to
conclude that the demonstration of some particular environmental factor confirms the importance of environmental factors as a class, and negates the influence of genetic variables as a class."

Many of those who eschewed any genetic influence in alcoholism,
also criticized the use of animal models as a tool in alcohol
research. Although they were readily willing to accept the results of experimental surgery, cancer surveys and biomedical research in general, all of which are based on animal experimentation,
they completely rejected the possibility that animal models have
any value in such a typically human behavioral disturbance as alcoholism.

One may ask if it really is useful to do research on the role
of genetic factors in this field, because we have no way to effect
or alter them at present, nor are we likely in the near future.
This is true, but there are several other reasons for conducting
research on this question. In order to arrive at an appropriate
understanding of alcoholism, it will be necessary to clarify the
basic genetically-determined metabolic and behavioral factors which
may be involved in the tiology of the disease. During the past
two decades, massive amounts of new information about the metabolism
of alcohol in the liver and in the brain, and its effects on behavior, have been accumulated. Since the majority of the individual metabolic processes in general are under genetic control, it is
obviously important to determine the significance of genetic factors in the metabolism of alcohol and the extent to which these
factors are thereby able to influence behavior. Finally, because
the genotype and the environment do interact in the formation of
the phenotype, we may be able to manipulate the environment of the
known genotype in such a way that the phenotype is altered.

The study of inherited drinking behavior and the metabolic
and behavioral traits correlated with it, can only be approached
with an understanding of the basic nature of polygenic inheritance,
the problems of valid estimation of the phenotype, the main path-

ways of alcohol metabolism in the body, the possibilities and
limitations of animal models, and the basic methods used in the
estimation of heritability. The aim of this review is to examine
the fundamental questions and evaluate new data in the field of
the psychopharmacogenetics of alcoholism in the light of the
background presented above.

THE CONCEPT OF QUANTITATIVE INHERITANCE

Many important characteristics in both man and animals are
inherited through a polygenic system. This means that the characteristic is produced by a quantitatively variable phenotype which
is dependent upon the interaction of numerous genes. For example,
intelligence, many behavior traits, height and skin color are all
determined by polygenes. As will be discussed later, there appear
to be genetic factors which contribute to individual differences
in alcohol drinking, the metabolism of alcohol and its metabolites
in the body and behaviors related to alcohol consumption and intoxication; it is very likely that these factors are also under
polygenic control and are regulated by many genes and their alleles.

The general nature of polygenic inheritance and the biometric
methods suitable for estimating the heritability are thoroughly
discussed by Falconer (1960) and Mather & Jinks (1971). During
the last decade, new information has been obtained with the use
of computer-assisted new statistical assays, which have made it
possible to classify, transform and analyze the massive amounts
of new data collected and reanalyze old material.

Man has 23 chromosome pairs in which thousands of genes are
located. Some of them are called "major genes" because they affect obvious qualitative differences or characteristics in an
individual. Genes which regulate the quantitative differences
in traits are called polygenes or "minor genes." The different
units of a polygenic system can be located on different chromosomes. The transfer of these polygenes from parents to offspring
follows Mendelian laws and exhbits phenomena such as segregation,
recombination, dominance, epistasis, sex linkage and autosomal
linkage. The polygenes affecting a certain characteristic constitute a system, in which each particular unit has a small,
quantitatively, almost equal additive influence. A system can
occupy two or more loci where the genes or their alleles are
situated.

The typical feature of quantitative and polygenically determined traits is that the characteristic varies between individuals across a wide range, in such a way that the intermediate types
are more abundant in the population and the extreme types relative-

ly rare. Such characteristics usually follow a normal distribution; consequently, their occurrence and frequency, and inter- and intraclass correlations can be analyzed with statistical methods suitable for normal distributions.

The basic assumption in the studies on the genetics of alcohol consumption cited and criticized in this review is that the genetic factors influencing drinking are under polygenic control. This assumption has been validated in work with animals; there is not enough information with humans, but it seems likely that such factors in man would also be polygenically inherited. Once this assumption is made, it becomes possible to evaluate statistically the probability that such factors do exist and the degree to which they affect alcohol intake.

If it is assumed that the genotype and the environment are not correlated, that individuals of one genotype are no more likely to be born and reared in a particular environment than are those of any other genotype, then the total phenotypic variance, V_p, in the population can be expressed as the sum of the genetic variance, V_G, and the environmental variance, V_E:

$$V_p = V_G + V_E$$

In this formula, the environmental contribution, V_E, is broadly conceived to include all nongenetic influences ranging from cytoplasmic factors of the egg cell, through intrauterine conditions and nutritional status, to the effects of the family surroundings and the social group.

Many assumptions must be made concerning the nature of the genetic variance component, V_G, in polygenic systems, although we have actually rather little solid evidence about it. Nevertheless, the biometric models applied to the polygenic traits of plants and animals have fit the observed results very well, and we have no reason to believe they would not be equally successful with polygenic traits in man. In simple models, the influence of each gene in the polygenic system is assumed to be only additive with that of all other genes, and, consequently:

$$V_p = V_A \text{ (additive effect)} + V_E$$

If we take into consideration such phenomena as dominance and gene interaction, the mode of polygenic inheritance becomes more complicated. The basic genetic component can be split into three parts:

$$V_G = V_A \text{ (additive effect)} + V_D \text{ (dominance effect)} + V_I \text{ (interaction)}$$

and the final phenotypic variance can be expressed as:

$$V_p = V_A + V_D + V_I + V_E$$

The relative part of the total phenotypic variance of the population contributed by the genetic variance is called the heritability (h^2). This theoretical value, h^2, can be presented as a "narrow sense heritability" based on the simple model for which only the additive component, V_A, of the genetic variance is calculated. Or it can be presented as a "broad sense heritability" in which dominance effects and interactions are also taken into consideration.

All the basic literature concerning the methods for analyzing and estimating heritability cannot be reviewed in detail here, but the interested reader will find reviews of the behavioral genetic analyses made in experimental animals in Hirsch (1967), and the classical analysis methods on the genetics of human behavior in Partanen et al. (1966) and in Jinks & Fulker (1970).

PROBLEMS IN DETERMINING ALCOHOLIC PHENOTYPE

One of the most important factors in all genetic analyses made in either humans or animals is the question of valid measurement of the phenotype. Very much attention must be placed on evaluating the actual nature and validity of the measure used. Usually all measures used in biometric analyses of a behavioral trait actually sample a complex group of many psychological and physiological properties. Some of these properties will be unrelated to the trait under study. Without proper and careful analysis of the nature of the measure used, it is possible that these unrelated properties will produce erroneous conclusions.

Measuring the drinking behavior of experimental animals

Most genetic analyses of voluntary alcohol intake by experimental animals are based on self-selection experiments in which the subjects have free access to a weak ethanol solution [usually 5-15% (v/v)], tap water and standard laboratory food.

Basically, three different measures have been used in such studies. The most frequently seen is the alcohol preference score: i.e., the amount of ethanol solution consumed as a percentage of the total fluid consumption, often abbreviated as E/T. This measure or phenotypic score is greatly dependent upon the total fluid requirement of the subject. This does not present a problem if environmental aspects such as temperature, humidity, water content of the food and composition of the diet remain unchanged. However, one must still questions whether it is reasonable to relate alcohol consumption to the fluid intake. Another difficulty with preference scores is that when alcohol solutions of different concentrations are used, the scores change, which makes it very difficult to compare results obtained by different experimenters. Finally, the alcohol preference score is a relative value which must be subjected to an arc-sine transformation before it can be properly used in biometrical genetic analyses, or other statistical treatments based on the variance ratio. Such transformations have not usually been done (Brewster, 1968).

Another widely used measure is the amount of alcohol consumed per unit of body weight. The figures are often presented as the ml absolute alcohol/100 or 1000 g body weight or the grams ethanol/ 1000 g per day. The amount of alcohol consumed per unit of body weight seems reasonable when one is trying to interpret the results from a pharmacological point of view, since it probably reflects well the pharmacological and physiological effects of alcohol. It can, however, sometimes give a misleading picture. For example, in most small rodents there is a great size difference between the sexes so that the males are heavier than the females. With this measure one often observes a sex difference in alcohol intake (Eriksson & Malmström, 1967; Eriksson, 1972) which can be partly an artifact produced by difference in the rates of metabolism relative to body size in the sexes. When this measure is used to determine phenotype in selective breeding studies (Mardones, 1960; Eriksson, 1968, 1969, 1972), it must be remembered that this measure includes the body weight as a factor. On the other hand, this measure will produce relatively comparable results when used with different concentrations of alcohol. Eriksson (1969) has experimentally demonstrated that genetically different rat strains tend to drink roughly constant amounts of alcohol per unit of body weight over a range of concentrations from 5 to 10% (v/v). The amount of alcohol consumed by the individual rats is, to a large extent, determined by the strain and not by the concentration of alcohol offered. The same feature may be found in the material presented by Thomas (1969), who tested the alcohol consumption of inbred mice strains (C57BL and DBA) and the derived offspring generations.

The third measure, actually used rather seldom in genetic studies (Eriksson, 1972), is the percentage of the total energy requirement obtained from alcohol. This measure can be calculated if the ethanol intake, the food intake and the joule content of the food and alcohol are recorded. This measure is probably very useful when trying to correlate drinking behavior with nutritional factors and energy metabolism. It is not, however, limited to this, since in practive in free-choice situations when environment, ethanol concentration and diet are not changed, it give almost identical results to those obtained with the other measurements.

The correlation between these three phenotypic measures is approximately +0.96. The preference for alcohol joules (or calories)
does not, however, reflect any artifact from the body size, which
can be seen in the data presented by Eriksson (1972). Furthermore,
it shows well the metabolic role of ethanol in relation to the
total energy intake, independent of the concentration used: even
the results from different animal species can be compared with
certain limitations. This measure, as well as the other two, has,
however, little ability to reflect addiction to, dependence on or
motivation for alcohol, which will be discussed in more detail
later in this review.

     The statements presented above show that even in such an ap-
parently simple situation as that used in self-selection experiments, the determination of phenotype can be difficult. According to some authors, the importance of the concentration offered
must also be considered. Rodgers & McClearn (1962) and Kakihana
& McClearn (1963) have stated that, in genetic experiments, several
different concentrations should be used for determining the subjects'
behavior towards alcohol. Fuller (1964) studied the preference
for alcohol in mice when six different concentrations were offered
simultaneously and demonstrated that the inbred strains differed
as to the concentrations as which their preference scores reached
50%. According to him, the preference figures obtained with the
six different concentrations can be used for calculating the "alcohol score", which can serve as a measure of the phenotype of
spontaneous alcohol drinking.

     Cicero & Myers (1968) have presented experimental results
showing that a single test solution can be employed as a measure
of an animal's alcohol consumption. The animals are presented
with a series of concentrations increasing daily. The concentration just higher than the one at which alcohol solution still constitutes over one-half of the animal's total fluid intake is then
taken as the representative measure of alcohol drinking behavior.

     The above procedures are based on the assumption that the
point at which alcohol solution intake equals water intake, i.e.,
when the preference score is 50%, has some particular significance.
There is, however, no evidence that this point has any significance
for the animals. Within the range of about 5-15% (v/v) animals
tend to drink a relatively constant amount of alcohol, regardless
of whether the concentration is so low that they consume more solution than water, or so ghigh that relatively little solution
needs to be drunk. If we wish to determine if there are genetic
factors influencing alcohol consumption, we should use a measure
of phenotype which is as free as possible from artifacts. Any
concentration in the middle of this range appears to be equally
good for producing such measures, and there is no _a priori_ reason

for insisting upon the concentration which produces a preference score of 50%. This range of concentrations also has the advantage of probably being physiologically active and is comparable to the concentrations most commonly imbibed by man. As pointed out by Cicero & Hill (1970), the alcohol solutions should be made from distilled ethanol only, rather than chemically purified alcohol.

Other environmental factors must also be well controlled. The ambient temperature, consistency and composition of the diet, special dietary factors, lighting, handling procedures, etc., are all factors which can strongly affect the phenotypic value observed in alcohol drinking experiments. The general standardization of environmental factors and measuring techniques from the point of view of genetic studies on alcohol consumption is broadly discussed by Eriksson (1969).

The alcoholic phenotype in human samples

Finding a qualitatively and quantitatively reliable measure of the phenotype of human behavior towards alcohol is even more difficult than in animals. In general, the determination and measurement of the phenotype has been based on interviews or questionnaires presented to the people collected for a family or twin study.

In the largest and most exhaustive twin studies for examining the inheritance of drinking behavior, Patanen et al. (1966) presented their subjects with 183 multiple-choice questions, 40 dealing with alcohol drinking. Most of the questions concerned personal information and social and psychological matters. Those questions concerning alcohol drinking behavior included: (1) When did you most recently drink any alcoholic beverage? (2) What types of beverages did you drink? (3) How long did the drinking last? (4) Did you get intoxicated? (5) How much money did you spend the last time you were drinking? (6) Did you have a hangover? (7) If so, how long did it last? (8) Did you drink anything for the hangover? (9) How much do you usually consume? (10) How long does a drinking bout usually last? (11) Have you ever neglected your work because of drinking? (12) Have you ever been arrested because of drinking? Questions of a similar nature have also been used by Loehlin (1972) in his large National Merit Twin study.

There are many sources of error in such questionnaires. However, it is probably not possible to obtain much more valid information by developing better and more suitable questions. Another approach has been attempted in some population studies in which the social consequences of excessive drinking were used as the criteria for the phenotype. Only subjects who had suffered such consequences as hospitalization for alcohol problems, being arrested for excessive intoxication, or the need for psychiatric treatment because of drinking, were included. One advantage to these studies is that the "phenotype" is determined independently from the study situation, while a disadvantage is that the sample is highly selected, not randomized and that the study cannot give information about people with normal drinking habits or abstainers. In theory, information about the latter two groups is just as important for determining the genetic influence on drinking as is information about heavy drinkers. The use of such social criteria or of more precise questions in questionnaires is not, however, likely to improve the validity of their estimates of heritability, because the basic criticisms against these studies are not primarily against the accuracy of their phenotypic measures, as will be discussed later in this review.

GENETIC ASPECTS OF ALCOHOL DRINKING
IN HUMAN POPULATIONS

Twin studies

About the only way to get relatively valid quantitative data on the heritability of some behavioral and physiological traits in humans is the classical twin study. The basic idea is that monozygous twins (MZ) have the same chromosomal material. Consequently, any differences with the pairs must, for all practical purposes, be caused only by environmental factors. Normal dizygous (DZ) fraternal twins, however, have on the average only one-half of their genes in common; therefore, genetic variability will contribute to their phenotypic variance.

If the zygosity of the twins is validly diagnosed, the following formula can be used for quantitatively estimating heritability:

$$\text{Heritability } (h^2) = \frac{\text{Variance DZ} - \text{Variance MZ}}{\text{Variance DZ}}$$

More precise estimates for the environmental source of variance can be made by comparing data from twins reared together with that from twins reared together with that from twins brought up separately. The mathematical approach and methods for twin studies is comprehensively presented by Partanen et al. (1966) and described in a more general form by Jinks & Fulker (1970).

It is now possible to make a very accurate diagnosis of zygosity in twin studies on the basis of 20-50 blood group markers. However, it is also possible to determine zygosity by questioning about the similarities and differences of various characteristics, such as hair color and eye color, and how often one twin is mistaken for the other. It has been shown that the latter procedure produces results in agreement with the blood group diagnosis technique 93-98% of the time (Loehlin, 1972; Myrhed, 1974). Therefore, if large enough samples are used, this method should give acceptable results.

The very first twin study of alcohol-related behavior was conducted by Kaij (1960) in Sweden. His data came from 48 MZ pairs of twins and 126 DZ pairs. He determined the presence of chronic alcohol drinking on the basis of three criteria: (1) a pathological desire for alcohol, (2) a physical dependence on alcohol and (3) the occurrence of blackouts during intoxication. The concordance of the MZ twins on these phenotypic traits was greater than that of the DZ twins. With some reservations, the author stated that the results supported the assumption that drinking habits are influenced by genetic factors and that such factors play an important role in the appearance of chronic alcoholism.

Partanen et al. (1966) made a large study of the drinking behavior of all the male twins born in Finland between 1928-37: a total of 902 pairs, of which 172 were accurately diagnosed as monozygotic and 557 as dizygotic. On the basis of their exhaustive questionnaire they could formulate three criteris measuring drinking behaviors: (1) Density, (2) Amount and (3) Lack of Control. "Density" was calculated by the linear combination of all of the questions concerning the frequency with which alcohol is imbibed; "Amount" was calculated from those questions dealing with the quantity of alcohol used during one drinking occasion; and "Lack of Control" combined the questions about the ability to regulate the amount consumed and the duration of a drinking bout. The results showed that there are genetic factors strongly influencing whether a person abstains, drinks normally or drinks excessively, "Density" showed a heritability of 0.40. "Amount" had a value of 0.27. Both of these values are highly significant statistically. All of the other traits including "Lack of Control", and characteristics involved with the social consequences of drinking failed to show evidence of significant heritability.

Jonsson & Nilsson (1868) collected a very large body of data about the drinking behavior of approximately 7500 pairs of twins in Sweden. Rather valid zygosity diagnoses were known from 1500 pairs. The authors distributed large questionnaires to the subjects and found that variations in alcohol drinking behavior could be explained mainly by social-environmental factors. A genetic influence was seen, however, in the determination of the quantity of alcohol consumed, which agrees nicely with the results of Partanen et al. study.

Rather recently, Loehlin (1972) collected a massive amount of data from 850 like-sexed twins in the USA in the National Merit Twin study. The higher heritability values (h^2) were produced in response to questions about whether the subjects had a hangover ($h^2 = 0.62$), if they had never done any heavy drinking (0.54), if they had used alcohol excessively (0.36), if they had gone on the wagon ever (0.36), and if they had ever had a drink before breakfast or instead of breakfast (0.36). These results are all in nice agreement with the previous studies. The measures showing the most genetic influences are those which might be explained in part by physiological or metabolic factors, such as the ability to drink a certain amount at one time and the sensitivity to alcohol.

Family studies: brother-sister comparisons

Another way to get information about the inherited background of alcoholism is to check the frequency of the disease in the families of alcoholics as compared to the frequency in control families. Åmark (1951) conducted an extensive family study in Sweden, using 349 brothers, 265 sisters, 265 fathers and 200 mothers of 203 male alcoholics. His results showed that the morbidity risk was 21% in brothers, 26% in fathers, 2% in sisters and 0.9% in mothers. In male children who had one alcoholic parent the morbidity risk was 33%; the figure for the sons of non-alcoholic parents was only 17%. Åmark points out that alcoholism is a family disease, which often is involved with psycho-pathological and depressive illnesses, but he also states that environmental factors in alcoholic families are often worse than in normal families, which could cause the higher alcoholism rate in these families.

Winokur et al. (1970) also conducted an extensive study on 259 male alcoholic patients and their immediate relatives. The authors tried to check the occurence of psychic illnesses in the relatives of the alcoholics, the existence of heritability for alcoholism, and if there actually are many different diseases present in these families. Their results showed that the morbidity risk of alcoholism was 30-50% in the male relatives of alcoholics and only 4% in female relatives. They also studied relatives of the alcoholics who were adopted into or fostered in non-alcoholic families. In those people with one biological parent who was an alcoholic, the morbidity risk was twice as high as in people whose parents were not alcoholics, despite the fact that the former subjects were not reared by their alcoholic parent. The authors concluded that alcoholism is a family disease, partly caused by an inherited basis; this genetic factor was thought to produce a higher rate of mental and emotional disorders in all relatives, and, in male relatives, a higher rate of alcoholism.

In many family studies (Åmark, 1951; Winokur & Clayton, 1968; Winokur et al., 1970), it has been shown that the frequency of alcoholism is much higher in men than in women. Similar statistics can be obtained from most industrialized countries, in which the disease is found in 4 to 6% of the men, but only 0.1 to 1.5% of the women. Obviously, there are many social and environmental reasons why the frequency might be different in men and women. If it were true, however, that the rate was higher in men for reasons other than the social factors, or if the disease which appears in men as alcoholism is often manifested in women as e-motional disorders, then we could assume that alcoholism has a gen-etic sex-linked basis, with material on the X-chromosome. The evidence for this is, however, so weak that we should take a very careful attitude towards this hypothesis, as Winokur et al. (1970) point out. The relative increase in alcoholism among women in recent years can be seen as further evidence against this hypothe-sis.

Half-sibling and adoption studies

The major criticism directed at the conventional family studies is that one usually cannot tell whether the higher frequency of alcoholism in the relatives of alcoholics is caused by shared genetic material within the family, or by the environmental in-fluences from living in an alcoholic family. In experiments with half-siblings or adopted children, it is possible, to a large ex-tent to eliminate the confounding by these environmental factors.

Schuckit (1972) conducted an extensive study with 98 half-siblings of 41 alcoholic probands, using severe consequences of alcohol abuse as the criterion of alcoholism. It was found that alcoholism occurred in only 10% of the cases stepparent was an alcoholic and their biological parent was not, but in 40% of the cases in which the real parent was an alcoholic and the stepparent was a non-alcoholic. The rate was 64% in those subjects who had an alcoholic as their biological parent, but were brought up in a non-alcoholic household. Schuckit's data is from too few subjects to allow for a comprehensive statistical analysis of heritability, but the results are in agreement with the hypothesis that poly-genic inheritance is involved in alcoholism.

One of the earliest adoption studies was made by Roe in 1944. This experiment is particularly important to examine because it is very often cited as an argument against the hypothesis of inherited susceptibility to alcoholism; even as recently as 1971, it was quoted in a special report to the U.S. Congress, edited by Keller & Rosenberg.

Roe's data came from 61 adopted children; 36 had a biological father who was an alcoholic, while neither of the biological parents of the remaining 25 were alcoholics. At the time of the study, the mean age of the alcoholic-parentage group was 32 years, and that of the control group was 28 years. In the former group, 21 of the subjects were males, while only 11 of the subjects in the control group were men. The use of alcohol in the group with alcoholic parentage was reported to be as follows: 7% regular, but not necessarily heavy, use; 63% occasional use; 30% abstinence The respective figures for the control group were 9%, 55% and 36%. On the basis of these data, Roe stated that since there were no statistically significant differences between the groups, environmental rather than hereditary factors appear to be the determining influence on alcohol drinking behavior.

It seems that the results of Roe's study have been completely misunderstood, and that some later authors have misinterpreted tham on purpose. First of all, at the time of this study, in the early 1940s, heavy drinking started at a later age than it does now. In Åmark's (1951) study, the modal age for the emergence of alcoholism was 37-38 years. Thus, Roe's subjects probably had not yet developed what would be their eventual behavior towards alcohol. Second, in her alcoholic parentage group, the number of abstainers was smaller than in the control group, while the number of occasional drinkers was higher, which actually shows a tendency, although not significant, for the alcoholic parentage group to be more attracted to alcohol drinking. Third, the phenotype upon which the experiment was based initially, excessive drinking by the fathers of the experimental group subjects, is statistically a rather rare behavior. The number of subjects in Roe's study was so low that it would have been almost impossible to find a statistically significant difference in the frequency of this phenotype in the offspring groups. Since less than 1.5% of women in general show this phenotype, there would be very little chance that even one would have been seen in the 14 women in the control group. If the rate is twice as high in the children of alcoholics, as suggested by the data of Winokur et al. (1970), it is also unlikely that any would have been found among the 15 women in the experimental group. Among the men, the expected frequency would be 0.55 in the control group and 2.10 for the alcoholic parentage group. These numbers are so low that statistical analyses are inappropriate. Nevertheless, if the figures for the men were analyzed, the expected x^2 would be only 0.24, which is far from significant. With such few subjects, the rate of alcoholism would have to be more than ten times higher than normal in the sons of alcoholics in order to produce a significant ($p < 0.01$ difference between the groups.

Recently, Goodwin et al. (1973) have done a well-controlled

adoption study in Denmark. The purpose of the study was to determine whether men raised apart from their biological parents
were more likely to have drinking problems or other psychiatric
difficulties if one of their biological parents was an alcoholic.
The sample consisted to 55 male adoptees with a parent who had
been hospitalized at least once for alcoholism, and 78 control
adoptees without known alcoholic biological parents. The psychi-
atrist who made the interviews had no knowledge about the parentage of the subjects until the end of the study. The results showed
that the alcohol proband groups had more than twice the number
of alcohol problems shown by the controls; this difference was
statistically significant.

Only in a fraction of the adoption cases is the child of
an alcoholic parent placed in a socially healthy family immediately after birth. Usually, the children are transferred to their
foster homes at a varying early age, but, nevertheless, not before having spent some time with their biological parents. Consequently, the effect of the original home environment can almost
never be completely excluded. On these grounds, it is always
possible to criticize adoption studies and deny their importance.

GENETIC MARKERS AND ALCOHOLISM

An old topic for discussion on the etiology of alcoholism is
the association of alcoholism to some special type of genome or
genetic marker. At present, there are only a few possibilities
for determining genetic linkage groups in humans. The most commonly used marker genes are the blood group markers, especially
those of the ABO system, plus color blindness factors, and the
ability to taste phenylthiocarbamide (PTC). On the basis of
prior knowledge about the frequency and distribution of alcoholism,
it seems unlikely that any of these markers should be correlated
with it. For example, color blindness defects have quite a different frequency than alcoholism or excessive drinking. On the other
hand, a special type of alcohol dehydrogenase enzyme (ADH) is
present in the retina of the eye, which could, at least in theory,
provide a weak basis for this hypothesis. The distribution of ABO
blood groups is different in many nations which nevertheless have
rather similar frequencies of alcoholism. The rate of alcoholism
is quite different in men and women, although they have similar
blood group distributions. Nevertheless, there are great differences in alcohol consumption rates and drinking behaviors, as
well as blood groups, between different races and ethnic groups,
which again offers some possibilities for the hypothesis that
there is some association between the blood groups and alcohol
drinking.

Alcoholism and blood group markers

Achté (1958) was the first to execute a large correlational analysis about the ABO blood group distributions in alcoholic and control populations. His sample was racially uniform, but otherwise randomized, which increases the value of the study. He studied the distribution of blood groups in 212 alcoholics and 1383 controls in Finland, and could not find any difference between the groups. Later Nordmo (1959) presented data from 939 alcoholics in Colorado, which seemed to show that alcoholism is more common in people having blood group A. Similar results were also obtained by Billington (1956) and Speiser (1958), who studied the ABO blood group distribution in patients with liver cirrhosis.

Later, Camp & Dodd (1967) and Camp et al. (1969) obtained results from much larger studies which did not support the assumption of an association between alcoholism and blood group A. The frequency of blood group A was no higher in the alcoholics in their experiment than in the controls. They did find, however, that the frequency of blood group A was higher in those alcoholics who did not secrete the salivary ABH blood groups substances, or stated in another way, fewer blood group A alcoholics secreted the salivary substances. The results were seen as indicating that something interfered with this excretion mechanism in blood group A alcoholics, probably as a result of excessive alcohol consumption.

Swinson & Madden (1973) have also conducted a study on how the ABO blood groups and the excretion of the ABH blood groups substances were distributed among 448 alcoholic patients. They could only confirm that in blood group A, alcoholics there were significantly more non-secretors of the ABH substances. They also pointed out that correlations between blood groups and alcoholism need not be caused by a genetic association, since there are such great ethnic differences in the frequency of blood grouping. Such correlations could be produced in at least four different ways: (1) technical faults caused by the sampling of ethnic groups with different drinking habits, (2) the pleiotropic gene effect, (3) coincidental associations and (4) alterations in the frequency of the trait as a consequence of the illness.

Alcoholism and color vision defects

The discussion about the association between alcoholism and color blindness started when Cruz-Coke (1965) reported an exceptionally high frequency of the defects in patients with liver cirrhosis. Later, Cruz-Coke & Varela (1966) reported evidence that the tendency

towards excessive drinking was correlated with color blindness.
In addition they assumed that color vision tests were sensitive
enough to show heterozygotic color vision defects in women and
reported marked sex differences in the color discrimination ability of the children of alcoholics, with the defects of the daugh-
ters correlating strongly with the defects of their alcoholic
fathers. On this basis, the authors concluded that women are the
carriers of both color vision defects and alcoholism, both traits
being linked on the X-chromosome.

This hypothesis has been strongly criticized by many authors.
Fialkow et al. (1966) tested male alcoholics with liver cirrhosis
before and after treatment. They found a high frequency of color
blindness defects, especially in those having severe cirrhosis,
before the tratements; but when the same patients were tested
after treatment, they produced normal results. The authors also
stated that the color vision defect frequency observed was so
high in female patients that it could not be attributed to X-
linked inheritance.

Winokur (1967) and Jacoby (1967) also criticized the hypothesis relating color blindness and alcoholism, because they could
not confirm the results in their family studies, particularly with
regard to women. Gorell & Thuline (1967) studied 81 cirrhosis
patients, 55 of whom were known to be alcoholics, but they could
only find 5 subjects with color vision defects: this gives a
lower frequency than the 7.7% which is typical in normal populations. Thuline (1972) reported that no correlation was found between alcoholism and color blindness when studied in healthy
North American men.

Varela et al. (1969) conducted a new experiment using more
sensitive testing methods and reported that male alcoholics had
more blue-yellow color vision defects than non-alcoholic male
controls. They also stated that female relatives of alcoholics
showed less ability to discriminate colors than did female controls.
Sassoon et al. (1970) reported preliminary information that blue-
yellow color vision defects are more common in alcoholics, and the
frequency of the defect seems to be higher in families where there
is alcoholism. Nevertheless, they also pointed out that non-alcoholic families have not been studied as thoroughly.

If blue-yellow color vision defects were connected with alcoholism, it would not support the hypothesis of X-chromosome linked
inheritance, since this defect is autosomally located (Wald, 1968).
Finally, Smith (1972) tried to repeat Fialkow et al.'s study, by
checking carefully the color vision defects of 172 male cirrhotic
alcoholics and 33 female alcoholics. He studied them both before
and after treatment, and concluded that the defects were acquired

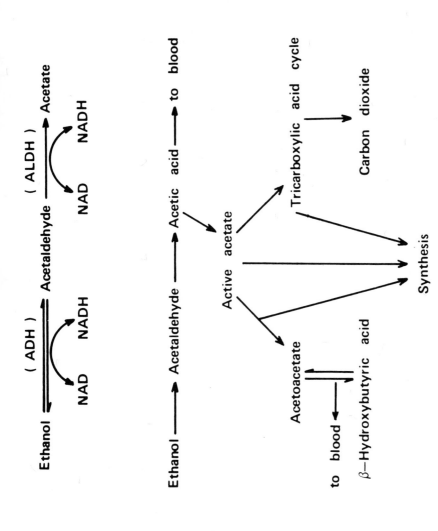

Fig. 1. Schematic diagram for the primary pathway of ethanol oxidation: ADH = alcohol dehydrogenase; ALDH = aldehyde dehydrogenase. Relationships to the general metabolic pathways also indicated.

as a result of excessive drinking since they could no longer be
found after treatment.

Mardones (1972) tried to explain these contradictory results
through the hypothesis that at least some types of alcoholism
could be controlled by a polygenic system including an X-linked
major gene. The present author, however, agrees with Thuline
(1972) who states that the hypothesis of acquired color vision
defects as a result of alcohol abuse rests on better experimental
ground than does the hypothesis of an X-linked inheritance of
alcoholism.

INDIVIDUAL AND ETHNIC DIFFERENCES
IN ETHANOL METABOLISM

It will only be possible to present a brief schematic picture
of ethanol metabolism here, for the purpose of clarifying the
genetic control of it and its possible role in drinking behavior.
The major portion (95-99%) of ethanol is metabolized in the liver
with only a small remnant being oxidized in other tissues. Ethanol
is oxidized to acetaldehyde primarily by alcohol dehydrogenase
(ADH); the acetaldehyde is then oxidized to acetic acid by aldehyde dehydrogenase (ALDH). The first reaction is reversible and
requires the presence of nicotinic acid diamide (NAD-NADH) as a
hydrogen acceptor (Fig. 1). The acetaldehyde produced from ethanol
is physiologically a very active substance. It is poisonous in
small quantities. It is also the substance which accumulates when
an alcoholic who is taking disulfiram ("Antabus") drinks alcohol,
and is the probable cause for the nauseous feelings produced. Recently, there has been much speculation on the importance of acetaldehyde in controlling the consumption of alcohol and the addiction to it (Seixas & Eggleston, 1973). For the present discussion,
however, the most important point is that the formation and metabolism of acetaldehyde are influenced genetically through variations
in enzymes such as ADH and ALDH and also in the NAD system.

It is in some way surprising to find that only a few studies
have been done in the field of genetic factors in the metabolism
of alcohol in humans. Vesell et al. (1971) and Vesell (1972)
have done a genetic-environmental analysis of the elimination
rate of ethanol, in 14 pairs of twins and six prisoners living in
a common environment. The subjects were given 1 ml/kg of 95%
ethanol solution orally in a standardized situation; the ethanol
elimination rate was then followed by taking blood samples for
four hours. They found that the heritability value for ethanol
elimination rate was 0.98: i.e., the rate was almost totally controlled by genetic factors. This heritability value is probably
too high, and their estimates of elimination rates were somewhat

confounded by variations in absorption rates. Nevertheless, their finding seems real. Quite recently, Forsander & Eriksson (1974) have reported preliminary data obtained from 6 MZ and 8 DZ male twin pairs in Finland. A heritability value of approximately 80% was found for ethanol elimination rates, and a heritability value of 60-80% for the acetaldehyde levels in the peripheral blood. Both studies cited here were done with too few subjects to allow for further speculation and more research is needed to answer this question.

One way to get indirect evidence about genetic differences in alcohol metabolism is through ethnic comparisons. Fenna et al. (1971) studied the alcohol elimination rate in North American Caucasians, Eskimos and Indians. The authors showed that the rate is faster in Caucasians (approximately 0.14 per mille per h) than in Indians (0.10 per mille per h) or Eskimos (0.11 per mille per h). Later, Wolff (1972, 1973) studied facial flushing in Caucasians, Japanese, Taiwanese and Koreans. He found that Mongolians tended to become flushed after only small oral doses of alcohol, while Caucasians generally showed no sign of flushing even with greater doses of ethanol. The authors assumed that the differences found were caused by variations in the reaction responses of the autonomic nervous system to alcohol, and that these variations are under genetic control.

It is is true that genetic factors cause differences in alcohol elimination rate or acetaldehyde levels in the blood, the question remains as to what kind of genetically-controlled mechanisms are responsible.

Alcohol dehydrogenase (ADH) in the liver is the most important enzyme for ethanol elimination in humans as well as animals (Wartburg & Papenberg, 1966). The microsomal enzyme system of the liver (MEOS) is also believed to metabolize alcohol, but its importance has been very controversial (Lieber & DeCarli, 1968). It has been found that ADH is present in various forms or isoenzymes. Murray & Motulsky (1971) have reported in addition that the liver ADH isoenzymes present are different in various phases of ontogeny, the enzymes of the fetus or young child being different from those of the adult. Wartburg et al. (1965) reported the discovery of an "atypical" ADH isoenzyme, the kinetics of which are different and more active than the "normal" ADH type. In a later study, Wartburg & Schürch (1968) stated that this "atypical" ADH was present in about 20% of the people in Switzerland and 4% of those in London. A similar study made in Japan (Ogata & Mizohata, 1972) gave quite different results. The "normal" type of ADH was extremely rare in the Japanese and the frequency of this "atypical" ADH was high.

Probably, the differences in ethanol elimination rates cannot

be explained by the different types of ADH. In both human and
animal studies, the presence of more active ADH isoenzymes have
not been found to have much effect on the ethanol elimination
rate. On the other hand, variations in ADH and possibly also
genetically caused variations in the enxymes oxidizing acetaldehyde may effect the levels of acetaldehyde found in the blood
after drinking ethanol.

CHROMOSOMAL ABNORMALITIES AND ALCOHOLISM

If we accept the hypothesis that some basic inherited metabolic system can have an influence on an individual's alcohol
metabolism, and perhaps even the susceptibility to ethanol dependence, we can assume that the genetic material controlling
these systems could be found in the chromatin or cytoplasm. Consequently, it is not reasonable to simply exclude the possibility
that certain chromosomal aberrations can be one cause for alcoholism. Conversely, it might be possible for excessive drinking of
ethanol to cause genetic changes in the reproductive cells, which
are passed on to the offspring rendering them more susceptible to
alcohol abuse.

DeTorok (1972) has presented data which seem to show that
chromosomal aberrations are more common in alcoholics than in a
control population. He found a higher frequency of either mono-
somal or polysomal chromosomes in three areas of the caryotypes
of alcoholics. His subjects consisted of 100 transient alcoholics, 20 dry alcoholics, 100 alcoholics with organic brain syndromes
and 60 controls. They were rather heterogeneous with respect to
sex, race and age. In the case of age, the alcoholics and controls
were not matched: only 17% of the controls were in the oldest
age bracket, 60-69 years, while 34% of the alcoholics were in this
category. Since there is some evidence that age can be one factor
producing a higher frequency of chromosomal defects, some doubts
are cast on the conclusion that excessive use of alcohol alone
produces more chromosomal abnormalities. At most, deTorok's data
would appear to show that alcohol abuse raises the frequency of
these abnormalities through an interaction with aging. For instance, the life style of alcoholics and the health problems related to alcohol abuse could be more conducive to the development
of viral infections which could, over several years, produce a
sizeable amount of cumulative chromosomal damage.

It is probably not possible to collect valid data about the
innate chromosomal defects of alcoholics in comparison to non-
alcoholics, in order to determine if any differences found are
the cause or the result of drinking. Recently, Cadotte et al.
(1973) studied the effects of ethanol on chromosomes in vitro.

They cultured human lymphocytes in different ethanol concentrations
and found that the number of chromosomal breaks, aneuploidy and
other fatal chromosomal changes did not differ from the respective
figures for the control cultures. Similarly, Kohila et al. (unpublished data) recently studied goniomitosis, i.e., the number
of chromatid breaks and gaps in metaphase, in rats subjected to
prolonged obligatory consumption of alcohol. They did not find
any increase in aberrative changes in comparison to the control
group.

These findings do not mean that ethanol has no effect on reproductive cells and no teratogenic effects on the fetus. Van
Thiel et al. (1974) have shown that ethanol inhibits vitamin A
metabolism in the testes. Alcohol dehydrogenase is required for
the conversion of retinol (vitamin A) to the bioactive retinal
which is essential for normal spermatogenesis in the testes.
Ethanol was found to inhibit this reaction in testicular homogenates, which could explain the sterility often observed after
chronic prolonged ethanol drinking in male alcoholics. Quite
recently, Badr & Badr (1975) have reported the induction of higher
frequencies of dominant lethal mutations in male mice intubated
with doses of 40% (v/v) ethanol solution. In this study, the
question remains open as to whether the results were caused by
a direct effect of ethanol in the system, or as an indirect consequence of the stress and health damage produced by such a high
alcohol concentration.

ANIMAL EXPERIMENTATION

Formerly, a popular misconception was that voluntary alcohol
drinking was, in some way, a unique type of behavior existing only
in human beings. During the last decade, masses of experiments
have been done with experimental animals such as guinea pigs,
hamster, mice, rats and monkeys. These experiments have rather
consistently shown that in a normal free choice situation, in which
the subject has ad libitum access to tap water, standard food and
a weak ethanol solution (5-20% v/v), most animal species and most
individuals willingly drink the alcohol solutions and often prefer them to water. Typically, the consumption of alcohol increases
during the first few weeks to an asymptotic level and then changes
very little, provided that the situation remains constant (Lester,
1966; Eriksson, 1969; Wallgren & Barry, 1970).

Although it is now generally accepted that animals will drink
alcohol voluntarily, there is still much debate as to whether their
consumption is for the same reasons as that of humans, and the degree to which it can be used as a model suitable for studying the
etiology of alcoholism. Part of the problem has come from the

previously-encountered difficulty in defining alcoholism. An
operational approach is to use the characteristics generally accepted as being typical signs of alcoholism as a set of criteria:
(1) The subject quite frequently drinks voluntarily an intoxicating
amount of alcohol.
(2) The subject chronically drinks alcohol to the detriment of his
health, and develops problems such as liver cirrhosis.
(3) Alcohol is imbibed for its pharmacological effects.
(4) The voluntary drinking leads to physical dependence.
(5) The subject shows a strong motivation to drink alcohol.
Although there are drawbacks to this approach, these criteria do
present a means for evaluating the usefulness of animal experimentation in this field, and the degree to which the results can probably
be generalized to humans.

At present, most of these criteria have been satisfied in
animal studies. The AA strain of rats developed by selective outbreeding for high alcohol consumption (as will be discussed later
in this review) show in general a high preference for 10% (v/v)
alcohol solution in a free choice situation, and drink large amounts
of the solution every day. Since alcohol consumption by rats tends
to occur in peaks during the night, the rate of alcohol intake is
much higher at these times; high enough that many of the AA rats
reach blood alcohol levels (over 1 per mille) which have independently been shown to produce clear signs of intoxication (Eriksson,
1972). From the consistency of the daily intakes of alcohol, it
can be concluded that these rats repeat this behavior, i.e., drinking to intoxication, nearly every night for as long as alcohol is
available.

Since these rats have ad libitum access to an adequate diet
and to water at all times, the simplest explanation for their behavior appears to be that they are drinking for the pharmacological
effects of alcohol. The fact that rats and monkeys will volunari-
ly self-inject rather large amounts of alcohol also suggests that
the pharmacological effects of alcohol are reinforcing for animals.
A recent finding that morphine injections suppress voluntary alcohol consumption by rats (Sinclair, 1974 b,c), while drinking of
water and saccharin solution is not reduced and food consumption
returns to normal several days before alcohol drinking does, can
be seen as evidence that the rats are drinking alcohol for its
pharmacological effects.

All of the physiological consequences of chronic or acute
alcohol intake seen in man, such as intoxication, liver cirrhosis,
tolerance and dependence, have also been demonstrated in animals.
Freund (1969, 1973) produced dependence, as evidenced by withdrawal symptoms, in mice using a liquid diet containing alcohol as the
only source of water and energy. Goldstein (1972, 1973) showed

clear withdrawal symptoms in mice housed in an inhalation chamber
containing ethanol in the air. Similarly, Ellis & Pick (1969)
produced withdrawal symptoms in monkeys after 10-18 days of continuous dosage with alcohol.

The above studies have used measures such as tremor and convulsions upon withdrawal of alcohol as their evidence for dependence. There is, however, no a priori basis for deciding what behaviors should constitute a withdrawal symptom: our only definition
for a withdrawal symptom, and thus for dependence, is that the behavior should be present only after experience with alcohol has
been abruptly terminated, and not present either in naive animals
or in animals that still have alcohol available. According to this
definition, the "alcohol-deprivation effect" (Sinclair & Senter,
1968; Sinclair et al., 1973) would qualify as a withdrawal symptom,
and thus as evidence that dependence can be induced with voluntary
access to alcohol. This effect is a temporary increase in alcohol
consumption by rats or monkeys after several days in which alcohol
is withheld. It is not seen in aive animals but only in ones
that have had prolonged prior experience with drinking alcohol. It
then develops as a function of how long the animals are deprived of
alcohol.

Although voluntary consumption of ethanol solution rather than
water in a free choice situation could be seen as an indication of
motivation for alcohol, such findings have not been convincing for
some authors who have claimed that the drinking somehow may have
occurred by chance, i.e., without motivation. Recently, however,
Sinclair (1974a) has shown that rats selected for having high preferences for a 10% (v/v) alcohol solution in a free choice situation,
readily learn to work for it when housed in an operant-conditioning
chamber with free access to food and water. Rats were also willing
to continue working for alcohol when weights totalling about one-
third of the animal's body weights were attached to the back of the
alcohol lever so as to increase the effort needed to press it. This
result appears to satisfy Cicero & Smithloff's (1973) definition of
psychological dependence on alcohol: i.e., the willingness to perform work or overcome an imposed barrier in order to obtain it.

It could be argued that since these criteria were satisfied
in different experiments, the results cannot be used for determing
the extent to which drinking behavior in animals constitutes a
model for alcoholism. It should be remembered, however, that according to Jellinek, alcoholism is mainifested in various ways.
The alcoholic types also are not permanent: successive retyping
has shown that roughly one-half of the alcoholics will drift from
one type of alcoholism to another within two or three years. Consequently, it is probably unreasonable to expect one animal to ful-
fill all of the criteria in a single experiment, since we would not

expect any single alcoholic to show all the characteristics of
alcoholism at one time.

Genetic analyses made in inbred animals

One method for obtaining evidence about genetically-determined
behavior towards ethanol is through the study of the differences
between inbred lines produced by special brother-sister matings.
After 20 generations of inbreeding, the strains are practically
homozygous, which means that roughly 99% of the loci are homozygous
in all individuals. On this basis, one can assume that variations
between individuals within one strain are caused solely by the
environment; the phenotypic variance component, V_p, within the
strain is then equal to the environmental variance, V_E. When
crossing pure parental lines, one produces heterozygous F_1 hybrids,
which are again individually similar, but have a different genotype than either of the parents. The F_2 hybrids then receive all
the genetic variation present in the parental lines, and their
total variance includes both genetic and environmental components.
Consequently, if the behavioral trait studied is genetically determined, the total variation within the F_2 hybrids should be greater than in the F_1 hybrids.

One of the first inbred strain studies was made by McClearn
& Rodgers (1959) in which they checked the self-selection behavior
towards 10% ethanol solution of C57BL/Crgl and A/Crgl inbred mice
and their F_1 and F_2 hybrid and backcross populations. They demonstrated that C57BL mice prefer the ethanol solution while the A
strain avoids it. Later, Rodgers (1966) demonstrated that voluntary ethanol intake is very different in inbred mice strains, with
the preference scores forming a continuous series ranging from a
minimum of less than 5% in the DBA/2J strain to about 90% in C57BL
mice.

Fuller (1964) conducted a six-bottle choice study in inbred
mice using different alcohol concentrations. He also observed the
very high alcohol preference of C57BL mice, the rather low preference of the A and C3H mice and the very strong avoidance of the
DBA mice. Brewster (1968) did a biometrical reanalysis of Fuller's
and McClearn & Rodger's (1962) earlier published data, and was
able to show that approximately 80% of the total variance in voluntary drinking behavior of these mice was under genetic control. In
addition, he could demonstrate that this genetic control had an
additive polygenic nature. The same author also presented his own
data on the alcohol consumption of Maudsley Reactive (MR) and
Maudsley Non-reactive (MNR) rat strains in which the heritability
was 0.72. He concluded that genetic influences on the alcohol
drinking behavior of rats and mice are very strong.

The experiments cited above, in different laboratories, using different alcohol concentrations and different standard foods, have conclusively proved that normal self-selection of alcohol in inbred mice is under genetic control. The results are in surprisingly good agreement with one another, and the basically very small differences found in the estimates of heritability are easily explained by difference in environmental factors and procedures.

One very important control for determining if the phenotype measuring technique used had an effect on the results of the analyses and if the drinking is indeed under genetic control, is to see if it is possible to change the alcohol intake so much with variations in the experimental procedure that the genetic effect disappears. For this purpose, Eriksson (1971) conducted a genetic crossbreeding experiment using C57BL inbred mice with high alcohol preference scores and CBA/Ca mice with low scores. Their drinking behavior was first determined using 10% (v/v) ethanol solution in a normal free choice situation. In the second experimental phase, the animals were motivated to drink more alcohol by adding saccharin (0.003%) to the ethanol solution and quinine (0.002%) to the water. A complete biometric genetic analysis was made using the data from both experimental phases. Alcohol consumption (as ml/100 g body weight) gave heritability values ranging from 0.54 to 0.93 depending upon the estimation equation used, the sex of the animals, and the choice situation such as this, some inherited metabolic function limited the ethanol intake; the strain difference persisted despite the change in procedure and the estimates of heritability were similar in both situations. In addition, the author was able to show a clear dominance in the non-drinking direction.

Results reached by selective breeding

Inbred strains can be used as a model in quantitative estimation of the heritability of most biological, metabolic or behavioral traits. However, the standard inbred strains have been selected by a non-directional process for characteristics other than alcohol drinking behavior. Consequently, if we wish to discover and study the metabolic and behavioral correlates of alcohol drinking, the use of inbred strains presents severe problems. The differences in alcohol intake between the inbred lines are real; so are the differences in many other traits. There is, however, no a priori reason for suspecting that connections between these other traits and alcohol consumption are not merely coincidental. Strains differing in alcohol intake also differ on many other variables, but since the strains were not developed by selecting for alcohol drinking, these other differences need not have any real connection to the drinking behavior. A more useful approach is to use strains

specifically selected for drinking or avoiding alcohol, and then
observing the metabolic and behavior correlates of consumption.

This very useful and far-reaching idea was first presented
by Mardones (1960), who started two inbred rat strains from one
pair with high alcohol preferences and from a low-drinking pair.
He produced inbred rat strains which differ clearly on voluntary
alcohol intake. In this study, however, there is very little
genetic variation, and there is a strong possibility that any
strain differences, in addition to alcohol drinking behaviors,
are merely coincidental or are dependent, for instance, on only
one unusual strong metabolic factor.

More valid data can be obtained using heterogeneous outbred
populations with directional selection in every generation for
producing strictly separate lines. With this procedure, any
traits accidentally selected along with alcohol drinking behavior
in one generation would probably not be selected in the next;
therefore, any metabolic or behavioral characteristics still found
to be correlated with alcohol drinking after many generations
probably have a real connection to the drinking behavior. For
several years, this kind of selection has been carried out by
Eriksson (1968, 1969, 1971b, 1972). Through selective outbreeding,
the author has produced rat strains differing greatly in their
voluntary alcohol drinking (Fig. 2). The AA (Alko, Alcohol) rats
rats voluntarily drink 5-10 g ethanol per kg per day, taking an
average of 25-40% of their energy needs from the alcohol (Fig. 3).
The ANA (Alko, Non-Alcohol) strain almost completely avoids the
alcohol solution in a normal free choice situation, taking on the
average less than one g ethanol per kg per day and less than 10%
of their energy needs as alcohol.

Recently, Goldstein (1973) has succeeded in raising by selective outbreeding two mouse strains which show highly significant
differences in their susceptibility to alcohol withdrawal after
exposure to alcohol in a vapor chamber. It was concluded that
the susceptibility to seizures on withdrawal of alcohol can be inherited.

The animal strains described above can present many future
possibilities for searching for physiological inherited factors
correlated with alcohol drinking or with susceptibility to withdrawal. Such factors found with selectively outbred animals are
not likely to be correlated only by chance, but rather have some
real connection to the bases for differences in alcohol consumption
or withdrawal susceptibility.

A

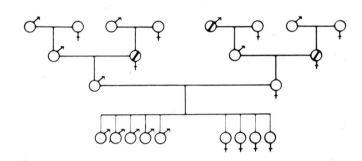

B

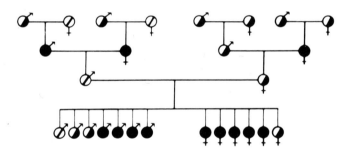

Fig. 2. Effect of genetic selection for low (A) and high (B)
voluntary alcohol consumption on the eventual drinking behavior of
the offspring. The percentage of black in each circle represents
the percentage of total fluid imbibed as alcohol solution.

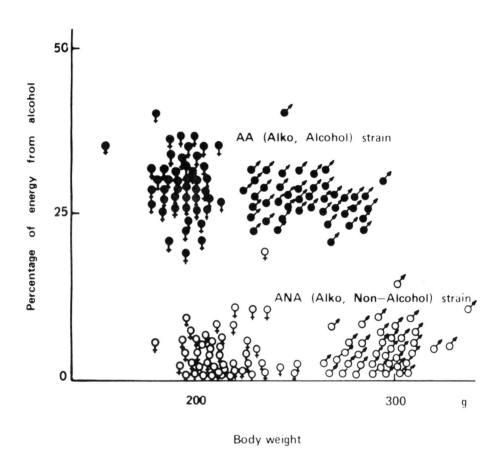

Fig. 3. Distribution of individuals from two rat strains selectively outbred for high (AA) and low (ANA) voluntary alcohol consumption.

INHERITED METABOLIC AND BEHAVIORAL
CORRELATES OF ALCOHOL INTAKE

If we accept the assumption that some inherited physiological factors can make a subject more susceptible to excessive alcohol drinking, more susceptible to physical dependence on alcohol, or in some other way determine the behavior towards ethanol, then it is a very important goal of biomedical research to find these factors.

In population studies, twin studies and family studies, attempts have been made to determine personality, emotional or psychic disorders involved with pathological alcohol drinking. All of these studies are valuable as a way for attempting to describe the alcoholic syndrome. So far, however, they have been of little use for determining the etiology of alcoholism, partly because of difficulties in collecting valid data about pre-alcoholic personality traits.

There is good evidence that some metabolic functions, such as the ethanol elimination rate and the levels of acetaldehyde accumulating in the blood when ethanol is consumed, are apparently inherited in humans as well as animals, but the question is still open as to how much these factors can affect drinking behavior.

As stated above, the specially selected animal strains can, in the future, have much value for mapping the physiological correlates of drinking and susceptibility to dependence. A large amount of multidisciplinary research is now being done with Goldstein's mice and Eriksson's rats, but unfortunately only relatively little data are currently available.

There has been much speculation in this field concerning the differences in liver ADH and ALDH. Numerous studies have shown that mouse strains with higher preferences for alcohol have higher levels of ADH activity (Bennet & Hebert, 1960; Eriksson & Pikkarainen, 1968; Schlesinger et al., 1966; Sheppard et al., 1966). It would be tempting to conclude that these animals drink more alcohol simply because the higher ADH activities allow them to eliminate it more rapidly. However, it has been found that the alcohol elimination rate in the heavy drinking C57BL mice strain is only very slightly higher than that in non-drinking strains, apparently because the ADH activity per se is not the rate-limiting factor in ethanol elimination. A similar but more likely hypothesis is based on the finding that the drinker strains also have higher levels of ALDH activity (Schlesinger et al., 1966; Sheppard et al., 1968). If alcohol consumption in mice is limited by the acetaldehyde levels produced, the higher ALDH activity might allow the drinker strains to consume more alcohol.

Deitrich (1972) has shown that different rat strains have different types of ALDH as a result of variations in at least two genetic loci. C. O. P. Eriksson (1973) has demonstrated that the AA rats and ANA rats do not in general differ significantly in their ethanol elimination rates. However, in the non-drinking ANA strain the acetaldehyde level in the blood and liver after intraperitoneal injection of ethanol is significantly higher than in the AA animals. Similarly, the different metabolic responses to ethanol can also be seen in the liver 3-hydroxybuturate/acetoacetate ratio, which was significantly decreased only in the ANA strain after ethanol administration.

Presently, there is much discussion concerning the interactions of acetaldehyde and the metabolism of brain amines, especially norepinephrine, dopamine and serotonin, and the possible role of these amines in alcohol drinking. Little research has been done so far with specially selected animal strains on this topic. Ahtee & Eriksson (1972) reported that brain 5-hydroxytryptamine (5HT) and 5-hydroxyindolylacetic acid (5HIAA) content is approximately 15-20% higher in the alcohol-preferring AA rats than in the ANA rats. In addition, Ahtee & Eriksson (1973) showed difference in the 5HT distribution in the brain: the serotonin content 34% higher in the hypothalamus, 24% higher in the midbrain thalamus, and 24% higher in the cortex of the AA rats than in the ANA animals. Recently, the same authors (1975) have presented a preliminary report in which they showed that brain dopamine content was 15-25% higher in the AA rats than in the ANA animals, but they chould not find any difference in norepinephrine content of the brains of these strains. The significance of these findings is still unclear, and much additional information is needed for explaining the relationship between amine metabolism in the brain and alcohol drinking.

Much data have been collected also concerning the behavioral differences in laboratory animal strains having different alcohol drinking behaviors. As stated earlier in this paper, studies made in inbred mice can be misleading because of coincidental correlations, unless the complete data are present for a large number of animals including all parental populations, offspring populations and backcross populations. Whitney (1972) conducted such a large study and found interesting connections between temperament and alcohol intake. He pointed out that increasing the level of environmental stimulation during testing appeared to decrease the alcohol consumption and increase the emotionality of both strains used. He also found that the correlation between alcohol preference and the defecation scores in an open field situation was -0.68. Eriksson (1972) also reported some preliminary data which seem to indicate that ANA rats have higher ambulation scores in an open field than do AA animals, but the strains did not differ in the amount of defecation or rearing.

It seems reasonable to believe that even in specially selected animals, such as Goldstein's mice or the AA and ANA rats, the comparative behavioral studies are useful only as a tool for mapping the metabolic connections to general behavior. They probably have only little value, for instance, when trying to determine personality or emotional characteristics directly involved with excessive drinking. If such connections are found, it is more likely that the personality trait and the drinking behavior are both influenced by some common metabolic factor. For instance, it is known that biogenic amines are important in the behavior of animals, affecting such traits as susceptibility to convulsions, stress behavior, aggression, open-field activity and general arousal. If they also influence alcohol drinking, they chould be responsible for correlations between behavioral traits and ethanol consumption.

CONCLUSIONS

(1) Because of the various ways in which alcoholism is manifested, it is very difficult to produce a simple, valid and inclusive definition of the disease.

(2) Finding such a defintion of alcoholism that can be used in genetic studies as a measure of phenotype is even more difficult.

(3) For the purpose of deciding the role that inheritance plays in determining alcohol drinking behaviors, information about abstainers and normal drinkers is just as important as information about alcoholics. Most human studies, however, have tended to emphasize only excessive drinking.

(4) A common misconception has been that the cause of alcoholism must be either genetic or environmental; that if genetic influences were accepted, then environmental ones would have to be eliminated. Actually, in phenomena such as alcoholism, the phenotype is determined through interactions between the genotype and the environment.
(5) It has been shown in animals that the metabolism of alcohol and alcohol drinking behavior are controled by polygenic systems: i.e., the inheritance is quantitatively influenced by the additive influences of many genes and their alleles. Traits controlled by such systems tend to follow a normal distribution.

(6) Even in animals, measuring the phenotype of drinking behavior in a simple self-selection situation is very difficult: various measures can be used, each with its own advantages and limitations.

(7) With humans, there are even more problems in determining the phenotype. The most common methods have utilized questionnaires, or the selection of subjects who have suffered certain social conse-

quences of excessive drinking, such as hospitalization. Although
the phenotypic measurement procedures are not perfect, they are
not the major criticism against most human studies. This is the
inherent difficulty in separating genetic from environmental influences. Twin studies may be in error because individuals with
similar appearances are often treated similarly by other people;
thus, monozygous twins would have more similar environmental influences that could lead to more similar drinking behaviors. A-
doption studies suffer from the fact that the children of alcoholic
parents who are adopted, or fostered into other families usually
have spent some time with their biological parents. In family
studies, it is even more difficult to separate the genetic and
environmental influences. Nevertheless, the general conclusion
from all of these experiments is that inherited factors do play a
role in determining drinking behaviors and can account for 20-40%
of the variance. In addition, half-sibling studies show that the
environmental influences of living in an alcoholic household are
much less important than had previously been thought.

(8) Attempts have been made to find genetic markers for alcoholism
with the ABO blood group types and with color vision defects, but
at present there appears to be no valid evidence that such traits
are linked genetically with excessive drinking.

(9) Genetic factors have been found to play a very strong role in
determining variation in ethanol elimination rates and the levels
of acetaldehyde that accumulate in the blood after alcohol consumption, in both animals and man. Ethnic differences in elimination rates are also thought to be genetically determined. Genetically determined differences in the types of alcohol dehydrogenase have also been discovered, but these are probably not responsible for the differences in elimination rate.

(10) It has been reported that alcohol abuse leads to an increase
in chromosomal abberations, but interactions with ageing appear
to be an alternative explanation for the results. Recent evidence
also suggests that alcohol may affect spermatogenesis.

(11) Research with animals has shown that they will reproduce most
of the characteristics usually associated with human alcoholism,
such as drinking to intoxication voluntarily, showing dependence
upon alcohol and demonstrating a willingness to work for alcohol
and a strong motivation to get it.

(12) Genetic factors have been found to explain over one-half of
the differences in alcohol consumption among inbred strains of mice
and rats.

(13) Strains of rats have been raised by selective outbreeding for

both high and low voluntary alcohol consumption, and strains of
mice for their susceptibility to withdrawal symptoms after prolonged ethanol inhalation. Physiological differences have been
found in these rats strains in their ability to metabolize acetaldehyde and in their levels of certain amines, such as serotonin
and dopamine, in the brain.

ACKNOWLEDGEMENTS

I would like to acknowledge my appreciation for the criticism
and helpful suggestions on this review provided by Dr. David
Sinclair and Dr. Olof Forsander.

REFERENCES

ACHTÉ, K., 1958, Korreloituvatko ABO-veriryhmät ja alkoholismi.
(In finnish, with german summary). Duodecim. 74:20.

AHTEE, L. & ERIKSSON, K., 1972, 5-hydroxytryptamine and 5-hydroxy-
indolylacetic acid content in brain of rat strains selected
for their alcohol intake. Physiol. Behav. 8:123.

AHTEE, L. & ERIKSSON, K., 1973, Regional distribution of brain 5-
hydroxytryptamine in rat strains selected for their alcohol
intake. Ann. N. Y. Acad. Sci. 215:126.

AHTEE, L. & ERIKSSON, K., 1975, Dopamine and noradrenaline content
in the brain of rat strains selected for their alcohol intake.
Acta Physiol. Scand. (in press)

ÅMARK, C., 1951, A study in alcoholism. Acta Psychiat. Neurol.
Scand. Suppl. 70:256.

BADR, F. M. & BADR, R. S., 1975, Induction of dominant lethal
mutation in male mice by ethyl alcohol. Nature (London)
253:134.

BENNET, E. L. & HEBERT, M., 1960, Investigation of possible biochemical differences correlatedwith ethanol preference in
mice. Univ. Calif. Radiation Lab. Quart. Report No. 3208.

BILLINGTON, B. F., 1956, Note on distribution of bloodgroups in
bronchiectasis and portal cirrhosis. Australas. Ann. Med.
5:20.

BREWSTER, D. J., 1968, Genetic analysis of ethanol preference in
rats selected for emotional reactivity. J. Hered. 59:283.

CADOTTE, M., ALLARD, S. & VERDY, M., 1973, Lack of ethanol in
vitro on human chromosomes. Ann. Gent. 16:55.

CAMPS, F. E. & DODD, B. E., 1967, Increase in the incidence of
non-secretors of ABH blood group substances among alcoholic
patients. Brit. Med. J. 1:30.

CAMPS, F. E., DODD, B. E. & LINCOLN, P. J., 1969, Frequencies of
secretors and non-secretors of ABH blood group substances
among 1000 alcoholic patients. Brit. Med. J. 4:457.

CICERO, T. J. & HILL, S. Y., 1970, Ethanol self-selection in rats:
A distinction between absolute and 95 per cent ethanol.
Physiol. Behav. 5:689.

CICERO, T. J. & MYERS, R. D., 1968, Selection of single ethanol
test solution in free-choice studies with animals. Quart.
J. Stud. Alc. 29:446.

CICERO, T. J. & SMITHLOFF, B. R., 1973, Alcohol oral self-administration in rats: Attempts to elicit excessive intake and
dependence. In: Alcohol Intoxication and Withdrawal. Experimental Studies. Ed. by M. M. Gross, Plenum Press, New
York-London. Advan. Exp. Med. Biol. 35:213.

CRUZ-COKE, R., 1965, Color-blindness and cirrhosis of the liver.
Lancet 1:1131.

CRUZ-COKE, R. & VARELA, A., 1965, Color-blindness and alcohol
addiction. Lancet 2:1348.

DEITRICH, R. A., 1972, Genetic basis of phenobarbital-induced
increase in aldehyde dehydrogenase: Implications for
alcohol research. Ann. N. Y. Acad. Sci. 167:73.

ELLIS, F. W. & PICK, J. R., 1969, Ethanol-induced withdrawal reactions in Rhesus-monkeys. Pharmacologist 11:256.

ERIKSSON, C. J. P., 1973, Ethanol and acetaldehyde metabolism in
rat strains genetcially selected for their ethanol preference
Biochem. Pharmacol. 22:2283.

ERIKSSON, K., 1968, Genetic selection for voluntary alcohol consumption in the albino rat. Science 159:739.

ERIKSSON, K., 1969, Factors affecting voluntary alcohol consumption
in the albino rat. Ann. Zool. Fennici 6:227.

ERIKSSON, K., 1971a, Inheritance of behaviour towards alcohol in
normal and motivated choice situations in mice. Ann. Zool.

Fennici 8:400.

ERIKSSON, K., 1971b, Rat strains specially selected for their
    alcohol consumption. Ann. Med. Exp. Biol. Fenn. 49:67.

ERIKSSON, K., 1972, Behavioral and physiological differences among
    rat strains specially selectet for their alcohol consumption.
    Ann. N. Y. Acad. Sci. 197:32.

ERIKSSON, K. & MALMSTRÖM, K. K., 1967, Sex differences in consump-
    tion and elimination of alcohol in albino rats. Ann. Med.
    Exp. Biol. Fenn. 45:389.

ERIKSSON, K. & PIKKARAINEN, P. H., 1968, Differences between the
    sexes in voluntary alcohol consumption and liver ADH-activity
    in inbred strains of mice. Metab. Clin. Exp. 17:1037.

FALCONER, D. S., 1964, Introduction to quantitative genetics.
    Oliver & Boyd, Edinburgh, 365.

FENNA, D., SCHAEFER, O. & GILBERT, J. A. L., 1971, Ethanol metab-
    olism in various racial groups. Can. Med. Ass. J. 105:472.

FIALKOW, P. J., THULINE, H. C. & FENSTER, L. F., 1966, Lack of
    association between cirrhosis and the common types of color
    blindness. N. Engl. J. Med. 275:584.

FORSANDER, O. & ERIKSSON, K., 1974, Förekommer det etnologiska
    skillnader i alkoholens ämnesomsättningen. (in swedish).
    Alkoholpolitik 37:115.

FREUND, G., 1969, Alcohol withdrawal syndrome in mice. Arch.
    Neurol. (Chicago) 21:315.

FREUND, G., 1973, Alcohol, barbiturate and bromide withdrawal
    syndromes in mice. Ann. N. Y. Acad. Sci. 215:224.

FULLER, J. L., 1964, Measurement of alcohol preference in genetic
    experiments. J. Comp. Physiol. Psychol. 57:85.

GOLDSTEIN, D. B., 1972, Relationship of alcohol dose to intensity
    of withdrawal signs in mice. J. Pharmacol. Exp. Ther. 180:203.

GOLDSTEIN, D. B., 1973, Inherited differences in intensity of
    alcohol withdrawal reactions in mice. Nature (London) 245:154.

GOODWIN, D. W., SCHLUSINGER, F., HERMANSEN, L., GUZE, S. B., &
    WINOKUR, G., 1973, Alcohol problems in adoptees raised apart
    from alcoholic biological parents. Arch. Gen. Psychiat. 28:238.

GORELL, G. J. & THULINE, H. C., 1967, Inheritance of alcoholism.
    Lancet 1:274.

HIRSCH, J., 1967, Behavior-Genetic analysis. McGraw Hill, New
    York, 522.

JACOBY, M. G., 1967, Alcoholism and color-blindness. Lancet
    1:113.

JELLINEK, E. M., 1960, The disease concept of alcoholism. Hill-
    house Press, New Haven. 246.

JINKS, J. L. & FULKER, D. W., 1970, Comparison of the biometrical
    genetical, mava, and classical approaches to the analysis
    of human behaviour. Psychol. Bull. 73:311.

JONSSON, E. & NILSSON, T., 1968, Alkoholkonsumption hos monozygota
    och dizygota tvillingar. (in swedish). Nord. Hyg. Tidskr.
    49:21.

KAIJ, L., 1960, Alcoholism in twins. Studies on the etiology and
    sequels of abuse of alcohol. Diss., Univ. Lund, Almqvist
    & Wiksell, Stockholm 144.

KAKIHANA, R. & MCCLEARN, G. E., 1963, Development of alcohol pre-
    ference in BALB/c mice. Nature (London) 199:511.

KELLER, M. & ROSENBERG, S. S., 1971, Alcohol and health. First
    special report of the U. S. Congress on alcohol and health
    from the secretary of health, education and welfare.
    DHEW Publication No. 73-9031, reprinted 1972.

LESTER, D., 1966, Self-selection of alcohol by animals, human
    variation and the etiology of alcoholism. Quart J. Stud.
    Alc. 27:395.

LIEBER, C. S. & DECARLI, L. M., 1968, Ethanol oxidation by hepatic
    microsomes: Adaptive increase in ethanol feeding. Science
    162:917.

LOEHLIN, J. C., 1972, An analysis of alchol related questionnaire
    items from the national merit twin study. Ann. N. Y. Acad.
    Sci. 197:117.

MARDONES, J., 1960, Experimentally induced changes in the free
    selection of ethanol. Int. Rev. Neurobiol. 2:41.

MARDONES, J. 1972, Evidnece of genetic factors in the appetite
    for alcohol and alcoholism. Ann. N. Y. Acad. Sci. 197:138.

MATHER, K. & JINKS, J. L., 1971, Biometrical genetics, the
     study of continuous variation. 2ned ed. Chapman & Hall,
     London, 382.

MCCLEARN, G. E., 1973, The genetic aspects of alcoholism. In
     alcoholism, progress in research and treatment. Ed. by P. G.
     Bourne and R. Fox, Academic Press, New York and London,
     337-358.

MCCLEARN, G. E. & RODGERS, D. A., 1959, Differences in alcohol
     preference among inbred strains of mice. Quart J. Stud.
     Alc. 20:691.

MCCLEARN, G. E. & RODGERS, D. A., 1961, Genetics factors in
     alcohol preference of laboratory mice. J. Comp. Physiol.
     Psychol. 54:116.

MURRAY, R. F. & MOTULSKY, A. G., 1971, Developmental variation
     in the isoenzymes of human liver and gastric alcohol
     dehydrogenase. Science 171:71.

HYRHED, M., 1974, Alcohol consumption in relation to factors
     associated with ischemic heart disease. A co-twin control
     study. Acta Med. Scand. Suppl. 567:93.

NORDMO, S. H., 1959, Blood groups in skizopreania, alcoholism and
     mental deficiency. Amer. J. Psychiat. 116:460.

OGATA, S. & MIZOHATA, M., 1972, Studies on atypical human liver
     dehydrogenase in Japanese. Report of 30th International
     Congress on Alcoholism and Drug Dependence, Amsterdam.

PARTANEN, J., BRUUN, K. & MARKKANEN, T., 1966, Inheritance of
     drinking behavior. A study on intelligence, personality,
     and use of alcohol of adult twins. The Finnish Foundation
     for Alcohol Studies 14:159.

RODGERS, D. A., 1966, Factors underlying differences in alcohol
     preference among inbred strains of mice. Psychosom. Med. 28:
     498.

RODGERS, D. A. & MCCLEARN, G. E., 1962, Mouse strain differences
     in preference for various concentrations of alcohol. Quart.
     J. Stud. Alc. 23:26.

ROE, A., 1944, The adult adjustment of children of alcohlic par-
     ents raised in foster homes. Quart J. Stud. Alc. 5:378.

SASSOON, H. F., WISE, J. B. & WATSON, J. A., 1970, Alcoholism and
     color vision: are there familial links? Lancet 2:367.

SATINDER, K. P., 1972, Behavior-genetic-dependent self-selection of alcohol in rats. J. Comp. Physiol. Psychol. 80:422.

SEIXAS, F. A. & EGGLESTON, S., 1973, Alcoholism and the central nervous system. Ann. N. Y. Acad. Sci. 215:389.

SCHLESINGER, K., KAKIHANA, R. & BENNET, E. L., 1966, Effects of tetraethylthiuramdisulfate (Antabuse) on the metabolism and consumption of ethanol in mice. Psychosom. Med. 28:514.

SCHUCKIT, M. A., 1972, Family history and halfsibling research in alcoholism. Ann. N. Y. Acad. Sci. 197:121.

SHEPPARD, J. R., ALBERSHEIM, P. & MCCLEARN, G. E., 1968, Enzyme activities and ethanol preference in mice. Biochem. Genet. 2:205.

SINCLAIR, J. D., 1974a, Rats learning to work for alcohol. Nature (London) 249:590.

SINCLAIR, J. D., 1974b, Morphine suppresses alcohol drinking regardless of prior alcohol access duration. Pharmacol. Biochem. Behav. 2:409.

SINCLAIR, J. D. & SENTER, R. J., 1968, Development of an alcohol-deprivation effect in rats. Quart. J. Stud. Alc. 29:863.

SINCLAIR, J. D., ADKINS, J. & WALKER, S., 1973, Morphine induced suppression of alcohol drinking in rats. Nature (London) 246:425.

SMITH, J. W., 1972, Color vision in alcoholics. Ann. N. Y. Acad. Sci. 197:143.

SPEISER, P., 1958, Krankheiten und Blutgruppen. Krebsarzt 4:208.

SWINSON, R. P. & MADDEN, J. S., 1973, ABO-bloodgroups and ABH-substance secretion in alcoholics. Quart J. Stud. Alc. 34:64.

THOMAS, K., 1969, Selection and avoidance of alcohol by two strains of inbred mice and derived generations. Quart, J. Stud. Alc. 30:849.

THULINE, H. C., 1972, Considerations in regard to a proposed association of alcoholism and color-blindness. Ann. N. Y. Acad. Sci. 197:148.

DE TOROK, D., 1972, Chromosomal irregularities in alcoholics. Ann. N. Y. Acad. Sci. 197:96.

WALD, G., 1968, The molecular basis of visual excitation. Nature (London) 219:800.

WALLGREN, H. & BARRY, H., III., 1970, Actions of alcohol. Vol. 1, Elsevier, Amsterdam, 400.

VAN THIELE, D. H., GAVALER, J. & LESTER, R., 1974, Ethanol inhibition of vitamin A metabolism in the testes: Possible mechanism for sterility in alcoholics, Science 186:941.

VARELA, N., RIVERA, L., MARDONES, J. & CRUZ-COKE, R., 1969, Color vision defects in non-alcoholic relatives of alcoholic parents. Brit. J. Addict.

WARTBURG, J-P. & PAPENBERG, J., 1966, Alcohol dehydrogenase in ethanol metabolism. Psychosom. Med. 28:405.

WARTBURG, J-P., PAPENBERG, J. & AEBI, H., 1965, An atypical human alcohol dehydrogenase. Can. J. Biochem. 43:889.

WARTBURG, J-P. & SCHÜRCH, P. M., 1968, Atypical human liver dehydrogenase. Ann. N. Y. Acad. Sci. 151:936.

VESELL, E. S., 1972, Ethanol metabolism: Regulation by genetic factors in normal volunteers under a controlled environment and the effect of chronic ethanol administration. Ann. N. Y. Acad. Sci. 197:79.

VESELL, E. S., PAGE, J. G. & PASSANANTI, G. T., 1971, Genetic and environmental factors affecting ethanol metabolism in man. Clin. Pharmacol. Ther. 12:192.

WHITNEY, G., 1972, Relationship between alcohol preference and other behaviors in laboratory mice. International Symposium Biological Aspects of Alcohol Consumption. Helsinki 1971. Ed by O. Forsander & K. Eriksson. Finnish Foundation for Alcohol Studies 20:151.

WILLIAMS, R. J., 1947, The etiology of alcoholism; A working hypothesis involving the interplay of hereditary and environmental factors. Quart. J. Stud. Alc. 7:567.

WINOKUR, G., 1967, X-borne recessive genes in alcoholism. Lancet 2, 466.

WINOKUR, G. & CLAYTON, P. J., 1968, Family history studies IV. Comparison of male and female alcoholics. Quart J. Stud. Alc. 29:885.

WINOKUR, G., REICH, T., RIMMER, J. & PITTS, F. N., 1970, Alcohol-
    ism III. Diagnosis and familial psychiatric illness in 259
    alcoholic propands. Arch. Gen. Psychiat. 23:104.

WOLFF, P. H., 1972, Ethnic differences in alcohol sensitivity.
    Science 175:449.

WOLFF, P. H., 1973, Vasomotor sensitivity to alochol in diverse
    mongoloid populations. Amer. J. Hum. Genet. 25:193.

NEUROLEPTIC-INDUCED MOVEMENT DISORDERS: PHARMACOLOGY AND TREATMENT

William E. Fann, M.D.

Baylor College of Medicine
Houston, Texas

C. Raymond Lake, M.D., Ph.D.

National Institute of Mental Health
Bethesda, Maryland

John L. Sullivan III, M.D.

and

Robert D. Miller, Ph.D., M.D.

Duke University Medical Center
Durham, North Carolina

CONTENTS

INTRODUCTION

Since 1952, when Delay & Deniker introduced chlorpromazine (Thorazine), the prototype of the group of major tranquilizers known as neuroleptics, psychiatrists and neurologists have been aware that patients sometimes develop aderse neurological conditions as side effects of these drugs. It is our purpose in

this discussion to examine some current theories concerning the
pharmacology of neuroleptic-induced movement disorders - primarily
parkinsonism, and the dyskinesias - and to consider some of the
recent thinking regarding their treatment. We have conducted in
our laboratory a series of studies testing the clinical efficacy
of adrenergic and cholinergic compounds in relieving symptoms
of various drug-induced movement disorders. We will here report
on some of these investigations and subsequently consider them
in the wider context of work done throughout the field of drug-
related extrapyramidal disorders.

REPORTS

Drug-induced Parkinsonism

Drug-induced parkinsonism can imitate, in all ways, the idiopathic or post-encephalitic types of the disease (Fann & Lake,
1974). Cases of moderate severity will display mild rigidity,
tremor, and a slowing of movement (bradykinesia). The most severe
cases will involve stooped posture, a marked pill-rolling tremor,
a mask-like fixed facial expression, increased salivation with
drolling, cog-wheeling rigidity, and an involuntary tendency to
shorten speed in walking (marche petit pas).

In our study of the condition, forty-one hospitalized subjects,
21 males and 20 females, diagnosed by two clinicians as having drug-
induced parkinsonism, were initially given physical examinations,
clincal history, and laboratory screens, including EKG. No contra-
indication to a stimulant-type antiparkinson agent was discovered.
The ages ranged from 17 to 72 years, with an average of 43 years.
All had developed drug-induced extrapyramidal symptoms while being
treated with anti-psychotic medication for illnesses diagnosed as
follows: schizophrenia (N = 36), senile psychosis (N = 2), manic-
depressive psychosis (N = 1), postpartum psychosis (N = 1) and
chronic brain syndrome associated with syphillis (N = 1). Pregnant females and patients with parkinsonism were excluded from the
study. The patients were randomly assigned to two groups, (a→s)
and (s→a). Group (a→s) received trihexyphenidyl as coded
medication for two weeks; Group (s→a) received amantadine as
coded medication for two weeks. Severity of parkinsonism and side
effects were measured at baseline (just before coded medication),
and at examinations scheduled for the first, third, seventh, tenth,
and fourteenth day of medication. After 14 days, placebo was sub-
stituted for coded medication. Those patients in whom significant
parkinsonism occurred on placebo were given the alternate to their
first coded medication for a second two-week period, during which
they were scheduled for examination as before. Both periods of
coded medication were double blind. The placebo period was single

blind.

Practical exigencies precluded strict adherence to the planned examination schedule. Examinations following within the day
of the specified time were accepted in lieu of missing examinations.
Some examinations were missed, but sufficient data were obtained
for a meaningful analysis. The severity of parkinsonism was rated
on the Simpson-Angus rating scale of each examination.

Both the trihexyphenidyl and amantadine were effective treatments for drug-induced parkinsonism. Their efficacies according
to our preliminary data were equivalent.

Of patients who completed the second period of coded medication, 20 experienced recurrence of significant parkinsonism on
placebo. Of this group, which included 9 of the 20 in the (a→s)
group and 11 of the 22 in the (s→a) group, the data elicited
by baseline placebo and 14 day examinations on both coded medications were evaluated. Again, in this group, the data are consistent with trihexyphenidyl and amantadine being of equivalent efficacy in treatment of drug-induced parkinsonism.

Side effect incidence was approximately the same for both compounds. Slightly more anticholinergic activity (i.e., dry mouth)
was attributable to the trihexyphenidyl than to amantadine. Tardive dyskinesia, seen in three of the subjects who also experienced drug-induced parkinsonism (i.e., cogwheel rigidity), was
mildly aggravated by both compounds.

Tardive Dyskinesia

Tardive dyskinesia is a syndrome characterized by involuntary
choreoathetoid movements of the face, mouth, tongue, extremities
and trunk muscle groups. The onset is usually late in the course
of antipsychotic drug treatment (after approximately one year
high dose neuroleptic therapy), and persists in many cases months
to years after withdrawal of the drug (Crane, 1968). In some
cases, it is irreversible. This condition is severely disfiguring,
and can be disabling to the extent that it renders the person unable to feed or otherwise care for himself.

Because TD is similar in many of its features to the hyperdopaminergic heredodegenerative disease, Huntington's Chorea, it
has been speculated that TD is also due to a hyperdopaminergic
state (Klawans & Rubovitz, 1972). This rationale is based on
observance of the actions of neuroleptics on CNS neuronal mechanisms. Among the effects of neuroleptic agents in the CNS is
the antagonization of dopamine through competitive blockade of the

postsynaptic dopamine receptor site, resulting in an increase
in dopamine synthesis or a functional hypersensitivity of the
postsynaptic neuron through prolonged blockade of the neuron
receptor site (Klawans, 1973).

In a trial of physostigmine in tardive dyskinesia, seven
chronic state mental hospital patients (six female and one male)
were accepted for study after providing informed consent and
after physical examination, clinical history and laboratory screen,
including EKG, revealed no contraindications to the medication.
All had been diagnosed by two physicians as having tardive dyskinesia. All carried a diagnosis of schizophrenia, though organic brain disease could not be ruled out in three. The patients
ranged in age from 55 to 70 years. In the past, each had been
treated at various times with several phenothiazines, haloperidol
and antiparkinson agents, but none was receiving medication other
than phenothiazines at the time of the study. Because several
subjects had multiple past hospital admissions, including two at
hospitals from which complete records were not available, the
total hospitalization time could not be accurately tabulated.
Nevertheless, all of the subjects had been hospitalized for a
total of at least three years, and had been on long-term neuroleptic therapy. Each was administered physostigmine, 40 μg/kg
intravenously, in amount and method previously demonstrated to
provoke changes in the involuntary movements of Huntington's
disease (Klawans, 1973; Aquilonius & Sjostrom, 1971) and Parkinsonism (Duvoisin, 1967). The injections were given slowly over
a period of three to five minutes per individual. Peripheral
cholinergic action was blocked by concomitant administration of
methylscopolamine, a quarternary anticholinergic salt which does
not cross the blood-brain barrier. The latter was mixed in the
syringe with the physostigmine. The dose of this agent ranged
from 0.25 to 0.5 mg, according to the dose of physostigmine. In
this manner, the peripheral effects of physostigmine were reduced
without interfering with its enhancement of central acetylcholine
activity. All three subjects were maintained on their phenothiazine medication.

Each subject was videotaped immediately before being given
the physostigmine, 45 minutes and 24 hours after injection. The
videotaping procedures for all subjects were uniform in all respects. Each subject was allowed an adjustment period of approximately 10 minutes in the room, and was then directed through a
standard examination routine (Fann et al., 1974). The taped sequences, 10 minutes per subject, were re-run randomly and rated
on a blind basis by two faculty neurologists, who assessed symptoms on a global estimation of severity on the following five
parameters: hand-fingers, feet, head, mouth-lip, tongue. The
tapes were played again for recheck at the request of the raters

during their individual sessions. The estimation of severity of
the body part dyskinesia was made on a 100 point scale, with 0
reflecting absence of movement and 100 the most severe the neurol-
ogist had ever seen.

In a trial of methylphenidate, a group of 30 hospitalized
patients, diagnosed independently by other clinicians as having
tardive dyskinesia, were taken into the study. Electrocardiogram,
physical examination, blood studies and urinalysis were performed
before and after the treatment. Blood pressure and pulse readings
were recorded. Patients were housed on their regular treatment
wards, and were escorted once a week to the office of the rater,
where they were examined 10 minutes each and rated on Crane's
neurological scale. This method has proven highly reliable in
our laboratory. Nurses' Observation Scale for In-patient Evaluation (Nosie-30) forms were completed weekly by the ward staff.
Global ratings of the patients' overall functioning and ability
to carry out activities of daily living were made from reports
systematically collected from members of the ward staff and other
observers (e.g., vocational rehabilitation counselors, occupational
therapists). Videotapes were made of each subject before, during,
and after treatment. These were re-run in random sequence, and
rated blind. One-half of the subjects were randomly placed in
the placebo group and one-half received the active drug. All subjects began by receiving 20 mg of methylphenidate per day (or its
placebo equivalent), and the dosage increased for each patient
by equal weekly increments to a maximum of 80 mg/day. At the end
of six weeks, the two groups crossed over. All subjects continued
to receive the prescribed neuroleptics: 200-800 mg of chlorproma-
zine/day, or its equivalent. Phenothiazines were the only neuroleptics used.

In a trial of orally administered deanol, a cholinergic agent
(Pfeiffer et al., 1959), thirteen hospitalized, chronically mental-
ly ill patients, diagnosed by three psychiatrists as having TD,
were scored by these three physicians on four parameters: mouth-
lip, tongue, hand-finger, feet. The rating was done on a 100 point
scale with 0 reflecting no movement and 100 the worst the rater
had ever seen. Each patient was escorted to a room with the three
raters present and subjected to a standard rating procedure (Fann
et al., 1974). The subjects were rated prior to the drug treatment and after five days on deanol 500 mg per day in divided
doses. The raters did not communicate their assessments to one
another until the ratings were completed and the score sheets
submitted. Because the possibility of investigator bias exists
on an open trial, assessments of the three raters were subjected
to the Kendall Coefficient of Concordance for determination of
inter-rater reliability. No special laboratory work was conducted,
in view of deanol's long history of safe clinical use in treatment

of hyperkinesis. Blood pressure was monitored and recorded four
times daily.

In the physostigmine study (Tables 1, 2 and 3), some decreases
in the severity of the movements could be detected after 45 minutes.
In the five of seven subjects who showed abnormal tongue movements,
all five were judged by at least one rater to have improved; in
three there was complete inter-rater agreement. This decline in
comparison to control was significant by t-test (p < 0.025). Six
of seven subjects showed abnormal mouth-lip movements. Three of
the six were rated as improved. All seven of the subjects showed
involuntary hand-finger movements. Only two of these were rated
as displaying less hand-finger movement after 45 minutes lapse
time. The changes were non-significant for the group (t-test).
At 24 hours, tongue movement was decreased in five subjects with
highly significant (p < 0.005) inter-rater agreement. Mouth-lip
motion was decreased in five of the six (p < 0.0005). Six of the
seven showing abnormal hand-finger motion were given lower values
after 24 hours (p < 0.01). In the head and feet parameters, abnormal movements were not present in enough of the subjects and,
where present, were of insignificant magnitude to make a statistical comparison.

Side effects of the physostigmine included mild abdominal
cramps in three subjects, acute moderate diarrhea in two, and
nausea in two, all of which abated within two hours after the injection. No changes in alertness or psychopathology were noted in
any of the subjects. A several-week follow-up of each subject revealed no side effects or sequelae related to the physostigmine.

In the methylphenidate trials, 17 of the 30 subjects completed the 12 weeks of the study. Of the remaining 13 patients,
five displayed an increase in psychiatric symptoms becoming un-
ruly or hyperactive. These five were removed from the methylphenidate treatment. Eight others were removed for administrative
reasons (e.g., discharged at family requests or transferred to other
units). Seventeen who completed the study were compared on serial
ratings between methylphenidate and placebo.

The Nosie scales for those patients remaining on the study
showed no significant changes. No differences were found from
serial assessment of the videotape. The weekly blind ratings
showed no definite or consistent changes in the neurological symp-
tomatoloty for either group at any time. On the global weekly
neurological ratings by the nurse and ward staff, six patients
showed some increase in hyperkinesia, eight showed no change,
and three were judged to have improved while taking methylphenidate. These three became able to feed themselves, tie their shoe
strings, carry cafeteria trays and dress themselves. This im-

Table 1

Effects of physostigmine on tongue movement
in tardive dyskinesia

Patient	Rater	Pre-drug	45 min.	24 hr.
1	A	50	20	20
	B	20	10	5
3	A	60	40	40
	B	30	40	10
4	A	50	10	20
	B	10	5	5
5	A	50	40	20
	B	10	10	5
6	A	60	50	40
	B	25	20	10
			$P<0.025$	$P<0.005$

Values given by two raters to severity of body part movement
expressed in raw numbers at 45 min. and 24 h. after IV physostigmine. P in comparison to control (t-test); N.S. = nonsignificant
(t-test); 100 = most severe; 0 = no movement.

Table 2

Effects of physostigmine on mouth-lip movements
in tardive dyskinesia

Patient	Rater	Pre-drug	45 min.	24 hr.
1	A	90	60	60
	B	10	20	10
3	A	80	80	70
	B	30	50	10
4	A	40	10	20
	B	45	5	20
5	A	100	100	80
	B	25	30	5
6	A	80	60	40
	B	30	15	5
9	A	40	30	20
	B	20	15	10
			N.S.	$P<0.001$

Values given by two raters to severity of body part movement
expressed in raw numbers at 45 min. and 24 h. after IV physostigmine. P in comparison to control (t-test); N.S. = nonsignificant
(t-test); 100 = most severe, 0 = no movement.

provement was lost when methylphenidate was withdrawn.

Table 3

Effects of physostigmine on hand-finger movements
in tardive dyskinesia

Patient	Rater	Pre-drug	45 min.	24 h.
1	A	100	100	100
	B	60	75	50
2	A	30	30	3
	B	15	20	5
3	A	30	5	5
	B	5	5	5
4	A	5	5	5
	B	10	5	10
5	A	50	40	20
	B	10	10	5
6	A	30	10	2
	B	15	5	2
9	A	30	20	3
	B	20	10	8
			N.S.	$P<0.01$

Values given by two raters to severity of body part movement expressed in raw numbers at 45 min and 24 h after IV physostigmine. P. in comparison to control (t-test); N.S. = nonsignificant (t-test); 100 = most severe, 0 = no movement.

Side effects included a transient (five day) rise of 20 mm
Hg in the systolic blood pressure of one patient, transient-moder-
ate (trace-2+) protein urea in five women patients, and EKG
changes that had no corresponding clinical symptoms in three.

In the deanol study, ten subjects completed the five day
course of therapy. One subject was dropped from the study because
of an increase in blood pressure, which returned to normal upon
withdrawal of the drug. Two others dropped out, refusing to continue taking the medication. This appeared to be associated with

their chronic suspicion and hostility rather than with any dis-
comfort caused by the study medication. Table 4 summarizes the
decrease in dyskinetic movements in the ten subjects after com-
pletion of treatment with deanol. All ten achieved some or
total relief of their involuntary movements after five days on
deanol. Data was analyzed by Wilcoxin Matched-Pairs Signed Rank
test (Table 5). One subject (Patient 9) showed mildly increased
severity of a slight parkinsonian hand tremor.

DISCUSSION

There are several types of neurons within or relating to the
striatum which are thought to play a role in normal extra-pyramidal
system neurological function. These neurons are usually classified on the basis of their transmitter substance in the following
manner: (1) the dopaminergic, neurons that are dependent upon
dopamine as a transmitter substance; (2) cholinergic, neurons
that are dependent upon acetylcholine as their transmitter substance; (3) serotonergic neurons, those neurons which are dependent upon serotonin - sometimes called 5-hydroxytryptamine or 5-HT.
The dopaminergic and cholinergic neurons have been the ones most
extensively studied, although several investigators, including
Prange and his group, have shown definite effects on clinical
manifestations of these systems brought about by enhancing serotonin (Prange et al., 1973). In the normal function of striatal
neuronal systems theoretically there exists a balance between
the dopaminergic and acetylcholine-dependent systems (Klawans &
Rubovitz, 1972; Klawans, 1973). A relative diminution of activity of the dopamine system or a dominance of the acetylcholine
systems brings about the parkinson-like syndrome. Conversely,
hyperactivity of the dopamine systems or a relative diminution of
acetylcholine activity results in a choreo-athetoid type syndrome
of which tardive dyskinesia or even the heredo-degenerative condition, Huntington's Disease, would be examples (Fann & Lake, 1974).
More simply stated, a decreasing dopamine and increasing acetylcholine activity results in motor hypoactivity, whereas reversing
these states (i.e., decreasing acetylcholine and increasing dopamine activity) results in hyperactivity.

Neuroleptics are known to block dopamine activity within the
central nervous system. It is through this mechanism - the lowering of dopamine activity in the central nervous system at certain
striatal neuron receptor sites - that a parkinson-like state in
subjects treated with these agents is created. In this manner,
they bring about an imbalance between the dopamine and the acetylcholine systems, allowing a relative dominance of the acetylcholine
system. Because of this, the sound pharmacological treatment is
to prescribe an agent which would lower the acetylcholine activity,

Table 4

EFFECTS OF DEANER IN TARDIVE DYSKINESIA

Patient	Rater	Mouth/Lip Pre	Post	Tongue Pre	Post	Hand-Finger Pre	Post	Feet Pre	Post
1	A	50	10	40	10	20	10	10	0
	B	50	20	50	0	35	0	10	0
	C	70	15	70	5	30	10	5	0
2	A	30	10	10	10	0	10	0	0
	B	25	0	25	0	0	0	0	0
	C	30	15	10	0	20	5	5	0
3	A	0	0	5	0	15	0		
	B	0	20	0	0	25	20		
	C	10	0	10	0	10	0		
4	A	50	10	10	5	5	5	0	0
	B	50	25	10	0	0	0	0	0
	C	30	5	20	0	20	0	10	0
7	A	0	5	20	5	20	5		
	B	0	20	10	0	0	0		
	C	15	10	35	0	10	0		
9	A	0	0	20	0	0	5		
	B	0	0	25	0	0	15		
	C	20	0	30	0	0	f.t.*		
10	A	0	5	25	5	20	10	15	0
	B	0	0	25	20	25	0	25	0
	C	5	0	30	5	20	f.t.*	15	0
11	A	30	20	30	10	25	0	10	10
	B	70	25	70	25	50	0	25	25
	C	50	15	50	15	50	25	20	5
13	A	30	20	10	10	0	5	0	0
	B	50	25	50	15	0	5	0	0
	C	40	15	25	10	0	f.t.*	10	0
14	A					5	10	5	0
	B					10	0	25	0
	C					0	0	10	0

Values given by three raters to severity of body part movement
expressed in raw numbers, before drug and after five days on oral
deanol, 500 mg/day. 100=most severe hyperkinesia the rater has
ever seen; 0=no hyperkinetic movement.

*fast tremor

Table 5

EFFECTS OF DEANER IN TARDIVE DYSKINESIA: LEVEL OF SIGNIFICANCE

	Rater Agreement* Pre	Rater Agreement* Pre Minus Post	Improvements**
Hand-Finger	.05	.05	N.S.
Tongue	.001	.05	.01
Feet	.01	N.S.	.02
Mouth-lip	.02	.01	.05

* Kendall Coefficient of Concordance
** Wilcoxin Matched-Pairs Signed Rank Test

and thereby bring the two systems back into balance. Nearly all
of the anti-parkinson agents now marketed and used are strong anti-
cholingerics; that is, they block the activity of central nervous
system acetylcholine in striatal neuronal mechanisms (Duvoisin,
1967).

Trihexyphenidyl, or Artane, is a prominent and effective anticholinergic antiparkinson agent. Amantadine is an antiparkinson
agent of another sort. Generally prescribed as an anti-viral,
amantadine is known to enhance CNS dopamine (Herblin, 1972; Heimans et al., 1972; Heikkila et al., 1972). Our study, comparing
the effectiveness of trihexyphenidyl and amantadine in drug-induced
parkinsonism, was based on the assumption that a therapy which enhanced one system was preferable to one which retarded the other
in an attempt to restore balance to striatal dopamine and acetylcholine. Our finding that the two drugs were equally effective
in relieving the condition, with fewer side effects from amantadine,
tends to support this reasoning.

It is well-known that the neuroleptics possess strong anticholinergic properties; that is, they are able to block the activity of CNS acetylcholine as a transmitter substance. In view of
this, the manner in which they bring about a parkinsonoid state
in certain individuals is not known, but it is probable that there
are individual susceptibilities to the differential effects of
anticholinergic and antidopaminergic activity. It is possible
that since acute drug-induced neurological conditions may assume
a broad spectrum of manifestations, certain individuals are more
susceptible to the anticholinergic effects (thereby bringing on an

acute hyperkinetic disorder, as is sometimes seen) and in other
patients the sensitivity to dopamine blocking is predominant
(thereby bringing on a hypokinetic or parkinson-like state). Complicating this picture is the fact that the dopamine-dependent
neurons are thought to be both inhibitory and facilitory and
that blocking the one type might bring about a facilitation of
striatal neuronal activity, whereas blocking the other would
bring about hypoactivity of these mechanisms (Klawans, 1973).

Current theories of drug-induced dyskinesias posit a putative
imbalance between CNS acetylcholine and dopamine neuronal mechanisms with a consequent dominance of dopamine activity (Klawans,
1973). Chronic administration of neuroleptics blocks post-synaptic
DA receptor sites, and causes either a "functional" denervation-
type hypersensitivity of these neurons, or, through an undefined
feedback mechanism, stimulates excessive synthesis of DA by the
pre-synaptic neuron. In this manner, a hyperdopaminergic state
is developed which results in manifestations of tardive dyskinesia.
In Huntington's Chorea, an analogous hyperkinetic condition,
there is a presumed diminution of striatal dopaminergic neurons
with a normal amount of total DA, suggesting a hyperdopaminergic
condition appearing clinically as hyperkinesis (Klawans & Rubovitz,
1972). There may exist, however, a hypocholinergic state in TD
as a result of the anticholinergic effects of neuroleptics. Mc-
Geer and collaborators (1973) have reported that choline acetylase
activity in the caudate nucleus and putamen of post-mortem brain
tissue of Huntington's patients was markedly less than in normal
controls or in any other disease group tested (McGeer et al.,
1973).

The finding that methylphenidate increased the symptoms of
tardive dyskinesia is consistent with these theories (Fann et al.,
1973). TD, according to some theories, is a result of excessive
dopamine activity in the striatum. Thus, the neuroleptics block
postsynaptic dopamine receptor sites, stimulating an increase in
turnover and a subsequent increase in dopamine synthesis, with a
possible accompanying functional hypersensitivity of the postsynaptic neuronal receptor site through chronic blocking of the
receptor site. Either or both of these conditions (i.e., an excess amount of the transmitter agent or an excessively sensitive
receptor site) would result in the postulated hyperdopaminergic
state. Our data, however, suggest that a malfunction of acetylcholine-dependent systems may obtain in tardive dyskinesia. Subjects given physostigmine, whose action lasts approximately two
hours in man, exhibited a greater suppression of movement after
24 hours than at 45 minutes, a finding which suggests that the
systems are not only suppressed but that they may be "revitalized"
to function normally for at least a short time.

Our finding that a putative oral cholinergic agent, deanol,
also suppresses the movement of tardive dyskinesia would tend to
further corroborate this theory and suggest that our approach to
the treatment of tardive dyskinesia, through enhancement of striatal acetylcholine, is correst, particularly as opposed to suggestions that tardive dyskinesia be treated by increasing the dose
of the offending neuroleptic (Kazamatsuri et al., 1973; Peters,
et al., 1972; Singer, 1971). The neuroleptics, by blocking the
dopamine receptor sites, will decrease dopamine effect and thereby suppress tardive dyskinesia. Since these compounds are implicated in the genesis of tardive dyskinesia, however, we would
clearly be risking more damage to the insulted neuronal systems
rather than relieving the syndrome.

A more extensive trial of deanol in tardive dyskinesia is
currently underway in our laboratory. Subsequent investigations
of the cholinergic hypothesis of drug-induced dyskinesia will involve consideration of the tricyclic antidepressants, which are
known to the potent anticholinergics. Although the tricyclics
have not been widely implicated in the epidemiology of movement disorders, we have observed several cases in which they have
apparently aggravated latent or minimal phenothiazine-related
dyskinesias. If further inquiry substantiates these observations,
they will constitute additional support for the etiological paradigm we have here described.

REFERENCES

AQUILONIS, J. M. & SJOSTROM, R., 1971, Cholinergic and Dopaminergic
    Mechanisms in Huntington's Chorea. Life Sciences 10:405.

CRANE, G. E., 1968, Dyskinesia and Neuroleptics. Arch. Gen. Psy-
    chiat. 19:700.

DUVOISIN, R. C., 1967, Cholinergic-Anticholinergic Antagonism in
    Parkinsonism. Arch. Neurol. 17:124.

FANN, W. E., DAVIS, J. M., & WILSON, I. C., 1973, Methylphenidate
    in Tardive Dyskinesia. Amer. J. Psychiatry 130:922.

FANN, W. E., LAKE, C. R., 1974, Drug-induced Movement Disorders
    in the Elderly, in "Drug Issues in Geropsychiatry," ed.,
    Fann, W. E. & Maddox, G. L., Williams & Wilkins Co., Balti-
    more, 41-48.

FANN, W. E., LAKE, C. R., GERBER, C. J., MCKENZIE, G. M., 1974,
    Cholinergic Suppression of Tardive Dyskinesia. Psycho-
    pharmacologia 37:101.

HEIKKILA, R. E. & COHEN, G., 1972, Evaluation of amantadine as
    a releasing agent or uptake blocker for H^3-dopamine in rat
    brain slices. Eur. J. Pharmacol. 20:156.

HEIMANS, R. L., RAND, M. J. & FENNESSY, M. R., 1972, Effects of
    amantadine on uptake and release of dopamine by a particulate
    fraction of rat basal ganglia. J. Pharmacol. 24:875.

HERBLIN, W. F., 1972, Amantadine and catecholamine uptake. Bio-
    chem. Pharmacol. 21:1993.

KAZAMATSURI, H., CHIEN, C., & COLE, J. L., 1973, Long-term treat-
    ment of tardive dyskinesia with haloperidol and tetrabenazine.
    Am. J. Psychiatry 130:479.

KLAWANS, H. L., JR., 1973, The pharmacology of tardive dyskinesia.
    Am. J. Psychiatry 130:82.

KLAWANS, H. L., JR., & RUBOVITZ, R., 1972, Central cholinergic-
    anticholinergic antagonism in Huntington's Chorea. Neurol.
    22:107.

MCGEER, P. C., MCGEER, E. G., & FIBIER, H. C., 1973, Choline
    acetylase and glutamic acid decarboxylase in Huntington's
    Disease. Neurology 23:912.

PETERS, H. A., DALEY, R. F., SATO, S., 1972, Reserpine for tardive
    dyskinesia, N. E. J. M. 286:106.

PFEIFFER, C. C., GROTH, D. P. & BAIN, J. A., Choline vs. dimethyl-
    amino-ethanol (deanol) as possible precursors of cerebral
    acetylcholine, in: Masserman, J. H., Ed.: "Biological Psychi-
    atry," New York, Grune & Stratton, Inc., 1959, p. 259.

PRANGE, A. J., JR., WILSON, I. C., & MORRIS, C. E., 1973, Pre-
    liminary experience with tryptophan and lithium in treat-
    ment of tardive dyskinesia. Psychopharmacology Bulletin 9:
    36-37.

SINGER, K., 1971, Thiopropazate HCL in persistent dyskinesia.
    Brit. Med. J. 4:22.

PHARMACOGENETICS: CLINICAL AND EXPERIMENTAL STUDIES IN MAN

Gilbert S. Omenn, Ph.D. & A. G. Motulsky, M.D.

Department of Medicine, Division of Medical Genetics,
University of Washington, School of Medicine, Seattle,
Washington 98195

CONTENTS

INTRODUCTION

As the array of behavior-modifying drugs has grown, physicians employing these agents have become aware of the striking differences among individuals in therapeutic effectiveness and side-effects of the drugs (Omenn and Motulsky, 1973). These differences may be caused by variable rates of biotransformation, elimination of the pharmacologically active moeity, by different susceptibility of enzymes, or of specific cell receptors to drug action. Occasionally, different mechanisms may produce an apparently uniform psychiatric syndrome so that a given drug may not be effective in all patients. Drugs, of course, represent only one of several classes of exogenous agents which may have variable effects in different subjects; this larger subject is now termed "eco-genetics" (Brewer, 1971; Omenn and Motulsky, 1975).

In this chapter, several types of experimental approaches to the study of genetically-determined differences in the response of individuals to psychopharmacologic agents will be described. The use of pharmacologic responses in the investigation of particular psychiatric syndromes will also be discussed. Pharmacogenetics is potentially a heuristic approach to many aspects of behavioral sciences with its explicit focus on gene-environment interaction, in contrast with outmoded controversies about predominance of nature or nurture.

METHODS OF ANALYSIS IN PHARMACOGENETICS

Population Surveys

When a drug is tested in a general population sample or is used therapeutically in patients with any given diagnosis, considerable variability in effectiveness and in side effects is commonly noted. When drug potency, mode of administration, and pertinent dietary factors are carefully standardized, three sources of variation still must be expected. First, some individuals will need a larger or a smaller dose than the average in order to attain the same effect, or same plasma concentration of drugs; some individuals may fail to show the desired effect at any reasonable dose. Second, some patients may fail to respond because the diagnosis is incorrect, or because the diagnostic category comprises two or more distinct entities, only one of which is responsive to the drug therapy provided. Third, especially when response is measured by subjective behavioral symptoms, the attitudes and expectations of patients and volunteers may be highly variable; this source of variability, however, should be controllable with careful double-blind and crossover protocols for administration of the drug and appropriate placebos. The operation of genetic factors may be inferred when different frequencies of drug reaction or different rates of drug metabolism are found in various ethnic or racial groups in the population.

Family Studies

If a bimodal distribution of response, side effects or blood level is obtained in the population survey, families of individual probands from each of the modal subpopulations should be tested. A simple inherited pattern may emerge from such family studies as in the case of autosomal recessive inheritance for slow acetylation of isoniazid (below). Family studies have the major advantage that the same mechanism for unusual response to the drug or for a particular behavioral syndrome is more likely to be responsible in all affected members of one family than in a random group of individual patients. For example, investigations of the causes of mental retardation were hopelessly frustrating until subgroups of affected youngsters could be defined by associated clinical or laboratory findings and until family studies revealed specific inborn errors of metabolism in at least some cases. It is to be hoped that similar family and kindred studies provide clues to the expected heterogeneity of the common psychiatric syndromes. When the pattern of

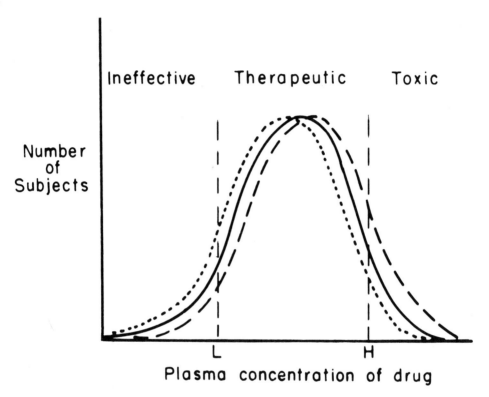

Fig. 1. Distribution curve of steady-state plasma concentration of
a drug, resulting from administration of a standard dose to a sample
of normal individuals. Twin studies indicate that most of this
variation is due to genetic factors. Family studies suggest that
polygenic inheritance is responsible, especially for commonly used
drugs. Persons above the threshold H will be at high risk for
toxic effects associated with high drug concentrations. Persons
with blood levels below threshold L will not have therapeutic benefit on usual dose. With polygenic inheritance, relatives of an
index case with low blood levels tend to have low levels (••••••••),
and relatives of someone with high blood levels tend to have higher
drug levels (▬ ▬ ▬) than the general population curve (▬▬▬▬).

variation is more nearly continuously distributed, searching for
distinctive subpopulations may be fruitful among individuals with
extreme values of blood level, urinary excretion rate or some other
measurable parameter. Studies of the families of such individuals
may reveal a bimodal distribution of that parameter, suggesting a
specific genetic mechanism occurring at too low a frequency in the
general population to produce a discernible "hump" in the distribution curve of the population. More commonly polygenic mechanisms
will be responsible. As illustrated in Figure 1, with polygenic
inheritance relatives of probands with extremely low or high drug
levels will have distribution curves shifted to low or to high
values, respectively.

Family studies may permit differentiation of environmental and
genetic sources of variation, as well. In the case of phenylbutazone (Whittaker and Evans, 1970), a series of normal subjects gave
a frequency distribution similar to Figure 1, but with a skew toward higher values. The regression of offspring values upon mid-
-parent values was significant. However, a positive correlation
was found also between husbands and wives, suggesting an environmental component to the variation in drug level. Since phenylbutazone is metabolized by enzymes in the liver microsomes which are
induced to a variable degree by food additives, foodstuffs, many
drugs, insecticides, and other agents, the authors pre-treated their
subjects with phenobarbitone. When all subjects were induced fully,
the skewed distribution was normalized, husband-wife correlation
became negligible, and the relative contribution of polygenic factors to the total variation was enhanced.

Twin Studies

Comparison of monozygotic (identical) and dizygotic (fraternal)
twins for rates of concordance of a trait or for intra-pair correlation in a quantifiable measurement, such as rate of elimination
of a drug, permits estimation of the extent to which variation is
due to inherited factors. The twin method does not provide evidence about the mode of inheritance. Nevertheless, clearcut evidence
for a remarkably high degree of genetic influence on rates of metabolism of such drugs as antipyrine, dicumarol, phenylbutazone,
ethanol and halothane have come from twin studies of Vesell and his
colleagues (Vesell and Page, 1968a, b, c; Vesell et al. 1971). The
contribution of environmental variables also can be assessed by
changing the environment, as in chronic versus acute administration
of the drug in retesting the same twin pairs, or by studying mono-

zygotic twin pairs reared apart and reared together. In studies of
monozygotic twins reared apart, which so far have been limited to
IQ and personality measures (Shields, 1962, 1973), the number of
twin pairs is so small that special care must be given to analysis
of the possible environmental variables in their placements. With
small numbers, rank-ordering, rather than overall descriptions, for
socio-economic and intellectual variables of the adoptive homes
might be correlated with behavioral and biochemical differences.

Biochemical Studies

The likelihood of defining specific genetic mechanisms increases as investigations reach closer to the primary gene product,
such as enzymes or proteins. Thus, a mutation in the gene for
plasma pseudocholinesterase or for red blood cell glucose-6-phos-
phate dehydrogenase is expressed directly by the altered properties
of these enzymes, but only indirectly by the adverse response to
certain drugs in the individual carrying such a mutation (see below).
Determination of qualitative patterns of metabolites may reveal the
enzymatic conversion (hydroxylation, glucuronidation, acetylation,
hydrolysis, etc.) responsible for inactivating or transforming the
drug. If rates of conversion are altered, the appropriate enzyme
activity mau be assayed in blood cells, fibroblasts, or liver biop-
sy, in decreasing order of feasibility. Electrophoretic and kinetic
properties of the enzyme may be demonstrably altered if a mutation
in the structural gene for the enzyme is the basis for the differential drug response. Differences may occur also in rate of absorption, renal clearance, and plasma protein binding. Finally,
differences in tissue responsiveness may be determined by genetic
alteration in receptor molecules. Although little has been learned
yet about specific drug receptor molecules, there is likely to be
variation among individuals at this site of drug action.

It is often dangerous to assume that other species metabolize drugs with the same pathway as does man. The patterns of
metabolites of amphetamines, for example, are quite different when
man is compared with dog, rabbit, and guinea pig (Davis et al.,
1971). In the case of the potent sedative glutethimide, the
clinical state after human overdosage correlates better with
concentration of a hydroxylated metabolite, which is twice as
potent as glutethimide itself in producing ataxia and death in mice
(Hansen et al., 1975). However, the hydroxylated derivative is not
detectable in plasma of dogs, rats or mice given intoxicating doses
of glutethimide, so there is no animal model that mimics the situa-

tion in man. Nevertheless, strain and species differences in the metabolism of specific drugs may provide useful models for the enzymatic steps involved and for correlation of metabolic degradation rates with therapeutic and adverse physiological or behavioral effects (Meier, 1963). Of course, the differences between animals and man represent a serious problem in interpreting practical tests of the effects and toxicity of new drugs.

GENE DETERMINED DIFFERENCES IN METABOLISM OF SPECIFIC DRUGS

Succinyl Choline (Suxamethonium)

Because of its rapid onset and short duration of action, this depolarizing muscle relaxant is used widely in premedication for anesthesia and for electroconvulsive therapy. However, suxamethonium will paralyze breathing for several hours in the one in 2500 Caucasians who has an abnormal form of the plasma enzyme pseudocholinesterase (PsChE). An otherwise perfectly normal individual is thus genetically susceptible to a drug-induced catastrophe because the enzyme required to inactivate the drug does not function properly. In the absence of the drug, there are no known abnormalities. Clear differentiation of homozygous normal, of heterozygous carriers, and of homozygotes for the abnormal or atypical gene is feasible with a variety of methods based upon the inhibition of pseudocholinesterase activity with enzyme inhibitors (Kalow, 1972). Several additional rather rare variant forms of pseudocholinesterase (PsChE) predisposing to suxamethonium sensitivity have been detected. Of particular interest is a very rare variant, PsChE-Cynthiana (Yoshida and Motulsky, 1969), which causes resistance to the action of suxamethonium; this enzyme variant is three times as active as the usual PsChE.

In clinical use of suxamethonium, inquiry regarding personal or family history of sensitivity may be helpful. Equipment for sustained artificial respiration should be available. Enzyme replacement therapy for this genetic defect can be accomplished by intravenous infusion of purified enzyme, or of normal plasma into patients with prolonged apnea. A simple screening test for PsChE sensitivity is available (Morrow and Motulsky, 1968). There is almost no need to test Negro or Oriental patients, since the frequency of the atypical PsChE gene is very low in these populations.

Phenelzine, Isoniazid and Dilantin: Acetylation in the Liver

The MAO (monoamine oxidase) inhibitor phenelzine, a drug used
to treat depression, together with the antituberculosis agent isoniazid, the antileprosy agent dapsone and the antihypertensive
agent hydralazine, are metabolically inactivated in the liver by
acetylation. The responsible enzyme is an N-acetyl-transferase.
The activity of this enzyme is determined by a single gene with
"slow acetylators" having a less active enzyme. The phenotype is
readily demonstrated by measurement of the serum concentration and
urinary excretion two or six hours after administration of isoniazid, or of a more easily assayed agent, sulfamethazine (Evans,
1969). Approximately 50% of Negroes and Caucasians, but only 15%
of Orientals, are slow acetylators.

Price-Evans et al. (1965) reported that adverse effects caused
by phenelzine were more common in slow acetylators than in rapid
acetylators, but observed no differences in the therapeutic effectiveness of the agent. By contrast, in a double-blind crossover
trial of phenelzine versus placebo, Johnston and Marsh (1973) described no excessive side effects, but found the drug to be more
effective than placebo only in slow acetylators. Although these
data with different patient groups give varying conclusions, it is
likely that the slow acetylators, with higher drug levels in the
plasma, would tend to have either a better therapeutic effect or
enhanced side effects.

Such conclusions are quite clearcut in the case of isoniazid.
Slow acetylators are much more likely to develop peripheral neuropathy and perhaps also such less common manifestations as acneform
eruptions (Cohen et al., 1974). When isoniazid is used to treat
tuberculosis with a daily dosage schedule, there is no difference
in therapeutic effectiveness between slow and rapid acetylators;
however, rapid acetylators do less well when the drug is given on
a two or three times per week schedule in ambulatory settings.
One of the most interesting aspects of isoniazid metabolism is interaction with diphenylhydantoin (Dilantin). Kutt (1971) found
that among tuberculous patients with seizure disorders who were
treated with dilantin and isoniazid, those who developed signs of
dilantin toxicity (nystagmus, ataxia snd drowsiness) were exclusively slow acetylators of INH. INH is one of several drugs (also
allopurinol, nortriptyline, and methylphenidate) which inhibit the
activity of the drug-metabolizing microsomal enzymes in the liver.

Dilantin itself is metabolized by hydroxylation followed by conjugation to form a glucuronide. A relationship has been found between Dilantin plasma levels and psychophysiological test parameters and self ratings of mood (Ideström et al., 1973). There is a wide range of drug levels among subjects, with blood levels of 3-18 micrograms/ml on a regular intake of 300mg/day. Induction or inhibition of microsomal hydroxylation by many drugs, food additives, and other compounds (Conney and Burns, 1972) contribute to this variation. In addition, there are some patients in several families who can metabolize only 2 mg/kg/day, whereas most subjects are capable of metabolizing up to 10 mg/kg dilantin per day (Kutt, 1971). This leads to continuous accumulation of unmetabolized drug in the body and toxic symptoms. The genetic mechanism for the defective hydroxylation has not been elucidated.

The polymorphic N-acetyl-transferase is not responsible for acetylation of all agents that are acetylated in the body. For example, p-amino-salicylic acid (PAS) is not acetylated by this system. There is uncertainty as to whether or not serotonin is acetylated by the polymorphic acetylating system (Schloot et al., 1969). With a purified enzyme preparation from human postmortem livers, White et al. (1969) failed to find a correlation between the acetylator phenotype determined with isoniazid and sulphamethazine and the ability to acetylate serotonin. Serotonin also is metabolized by the mitochondrial.

Nortriptyline

Nortriptyline has been studied extensively by Alexanderson and Sjoqvist (1971) and their colleagues. They have studied populations, twins, and famalies, and have examined absorption, plasma binding, volume of distribution, and elimination rate of this drug. Patients treated with the same dose of nortriptyline showed wide differences in the steady state plasma levels, ranging between 10 and 275 ng per ml (Sjoqvist et al., 1968). There was very little intra-individual variation when subjects were tested again two years after the first determination. Studies of plasma levels of nortriptyline in 19 monozygotic and 20 dizygotic twin pairs not previously exposed to the drug showed very much greater intra-pair differences for the dizygotic twins, consistent with a large genetic contribution to the observed variance in plasma level. Family studies (Asberg et al., 1971) of three probands with very high plasma nortriptyline levels showed no simple Mendelian pattern of transmission for slower metabolism of the drug; instead, analysis

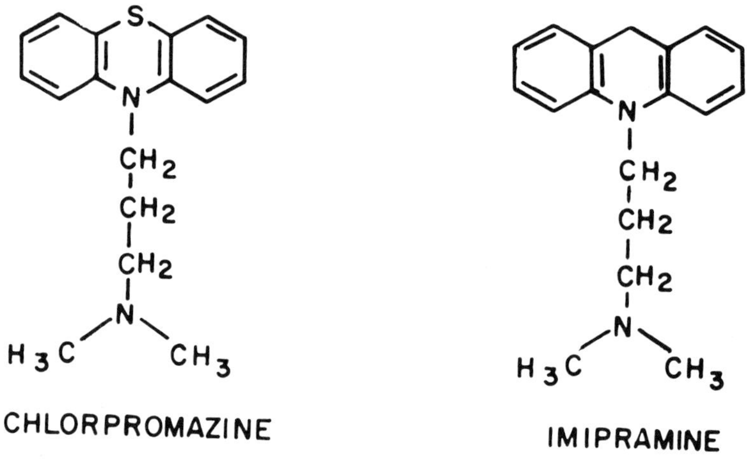

Fig. 2. Structural similarity of chlorpromazine and tricyclic anti-depressant imipramine. Note that chlorpromazine and other phenothiazines resemble tricyclic antidepressants in structure and may share some metabolic conversions.

of the data indicated polygenic control of the metabolism of this agent. The distribution of drug levels in relatives of "high" probands was shifted to higher values than in the general population sample, as illustrated schematically in Figure 1. This pattern of polygenic control of individual differences in drug level or action is probably much more common than the single-gene-mediated pattern exemplified by the atypical PsChE and slow acetylation.

The primary metabolic conversion appears to be hydroxlyation, but several different metabolic conversions may be involved in inactivation of nortriptyline. Thus, Alexanderson and Borga (1973) found variation in the pattern of metabolites between individuals. Levels of the main metabolite (10-hydroxy-nortriptyline) varied considerably in different subjects and should be studied for possible single gene control of this metabolic step. Other commonly used tricyclic antidepressants including amitriptyline (Braithwaite el. al., 1972), imipramine (Walter, 1971; Zeidenberg, 1971), and desmethylimipramine (Sjoqvist et al., 1968), also showed marked individual variations in plasma concentration on a given daily dose. In a crossover study (Alexanderson, 1972), there was a significant correlation between the steady state plasma levels of nortriptyline and desmethylimipramine in the same individuals.

Phenothiazines

There are substantial differences in serum levels of chlorpromazine in chronically treated patients, with a biological half-life ranging from 2 to 36 hours (Curry and Marshall, 1968; Perry et al., 1970). Chlorpromazine is degraded to a large number of metabolites. There is considerable inter-individual difference in the excretion rate of polar metabolites in schizophrenic patients, and there are different patterns of metabolites in individual patients, possibly correlated with therapeutic effectiveness (Green et al., 1965; Kaul et al., 1972b; March et al., 1972). Despite this pharmacologic and clinical evidence for inter-individual variability, there have been no genetic studies of phenothiazine metabolism. It may be noted (Figure 2) that chlorpromazine and other phenothiazines resemble tricyclic antidepressants in structure and may share some metabolic conversions. With regard to the important side-effects of Parkinsonism caused by phenothiazines, there is evidence that a hereditary predisposition is involved (Myrianthopoulos et al., 1962, 1967).

Ethanol

Vesell et al. (1971) demonstrated in a study of monozygotic
and dizygotic twins, that the rate of ethanol elimination from the
blood was largely determined by genetic factors. In an effort to
assess effects of chronic ingestion of alcohol, the same authors
tested healthy prisoners before and after three months of alcohol
intake and found little intra-individual variation. It is thought
that the major enzymatic step is the oxidation of ethanol to acetaldehyde by liver alcohol dehydrogenase. Mixed function oxidases
in liver microsomes and possibly other oxidazing enzymes such as
catalase may also contribute to ethanol oxidation. Alcohol dehydrogenase (ADH) has been studied extensively by electrophoretic
methods. Smith et al. (1973) demonstrated that there are three
ADH loci in the liver producing multiple bands on starch gel elec-
trophoresis. Previously, it was noted by Von Wartburg and Schürch
(1968) that 15-20% of European Caucasian subjects had an atypical
liver alochol dehydrogenase when compared with other subjects.
Their test involved assay of quantitative enzyme activity at pH
8.8 and 11.0; the atypical ADH pattern was associated with several-
-fold higher in vitro activity at pH 8.8. Edwards and Price Evans
(1967) were unsuccessful in an attempt to correlate the presence
of an atypical liver alcohol liver dehydrogenase pattern with the
rate of alcohol metabolism in vivo. Smith et al. (1973) have now
correlated the difference in quantitative activity associated with
the atypical ADH with electrophoretic variation at the ADH-2 locus.
In Japanese subjects, the frequency of the atypical ADH pattern is
very much higher, approaching 90% of subjects tested on liver spec-
imens at autopsy (Fukui and Wakasugi, 1972; Stamatoyannopoulos et
al., 1975).

There are also significant ethnic differences in the rate of
alcohol elimination. Fenna et al. (1971) investigated the observations in police reports that native Indians and Eskimos in
Edmonton, Alberta, required longer times to "sober up" after a
drinking bout than did Caucasians. Alcohol was administered intravenously to Eskimo, Indian, and Caucasian male subjects. The
rates of metabolism were 145 mg/kg/hour for 17 Caucasian subjects,
101 mg/kg/hour for 27 Indian subjects, and 110 mg/kg/hour for 21
Eskimo subjects. These differences were highly significant.
Neither diet nor previous alcohol ingestion could account for the
observed differences, which may very well reflect genetically determined variation in alcohol dehydrogenase or other oxidizing
enzymes. Since Eskimos and Indians probably share the high fre-

quency of the atypical ADH phenotype, as found in other Mongoloids, it is surprising that the rate of ethanol elimination is slower than that for Caucasians. Thus far, there have not been analyses of the ADH phenotypes of Eskimos and Indians, nor of the ethanol elimination rates for Japanese. Indians share the propensity of Japanese to flush immediately after ingestion of ethanol (see below).

Aryl hydrocarbons

The first metabolic conversion of some drugs _activates_ rather than inactivates their biological effects. For example, the enzyme aryl hydrocarbon hydroxylase (AHH) activates a variety of exogenous hydrocarbon compounds, including many drugs, insecticides, steroids, and chemical carcinogens (Heidelberger, 1973). Polycyclic hydrocarbons found in cigarette smoke and automobile exhaust are hydroxylated to highly reactive epoxides. The substrates induce an increase in AHH activity, but the extent of induction varies widely among individuals. Studies in human and animal liver and in human lymphocytes suggest that the extent of induction may be determined by a single autosomal gene, allowing classification of people as low, intermediate and high inducers (Kellerman et al., 1973a). As might be predicted, smokers who are high and intermediate inducers carry a greatly enhanced risk of developing carcinoma of the lung (Kellerman et al., 1973b). For other types of cancer, not thought to be induced by cigarette smoking or polycyclic hydrocarbons, no shift from general population frequencies for AHH inducibility was observed.

Some drugs with behavioral effects also may be activated by hydroxylation. For example, it is possible, though not tested, that the hydroxylation of glutethimide to a potent metabolite (see page 6 above) is carried out by this inducible liver enzyme system.

GENETICALLY DETERMINED DIFFERENCES IN TISSUE SENSITIVITY

Susceptibility of Red Blood Cells to Hemolysis by Oxidizing Agents.

Glucose-6-phosphate-dehydrogenase (G6PD) is the first enzyme of the energy-generating pentose-phosphate shunt pathway, essential to maintain the integrity of the red blood cell. Deficiency of G6PD occurs with significant frequency in many population groups originating in subtropical and tropical countries such as Africans, Southeast Asians, Indians and Mediterraneans. Many drugs, includ-

ing primaquine and 8-aminoquinoline antimalarials, sulfas, nitro-
furan derivatives, phenacetin, and probenecid, can precipitate
acute hemolytic anemia in these otherwise healthy but genetically
predisposed individuals (Motulsky, 1972). The drug does not interact directly with the abnormal enzyme; rather, the red cells are
more susceptible to drug injury. Many different mutations affecting G6PD cause enzyme deficiency. The Mediterranean type G6PD
deficiency is more severe than the Negro type, and a larger number
of drugs are a threat (Motulsky, 1972). Hemolytic anemia caused
by eating fava or broad beans (favism) occurs only in some G6PD-
-deficient persons. Apparently, a second genetic abnormality is
required to produce susceptibility to favism.

Recent population and family studies indicate that the second
abnormality involves defective glucuronidation (Cassimos et al,
1974). Interestingly enough, long before G6PD deficiency was known,
the Pythagoreans were said to have surrendered to their enemies
rather than flee through a field of fava beans. Also, in Greek
mythology, a particular sect allowed women but not men to eat the
fava beans (Graves, 1955), consistent with the X-linked recessive
inheritance of G6PD deficiency. G6PD in the brain is determined
by the same gene as G6PD in red and white blood cells (Cohen et
al., 1973).

Susceptibility to Cyanosis from Methemoglobinemia

Many of the same oxidizing drugs which can produce hemolysis
in G6PD-deficient individuals may produce methemoglobinemia in
individuals with mild methemoglobin reductase deficiency (Cohen
et al., 1968). Such persons are heterozygous carriers for the
autosomal recessive type of methemoglobinemia, a rare defect causing marked cyanosis early in life. Parents of such patients are
obligatory carriers and have normal or almost normal methemoglobin
levels under the usual living conditions. However, when challenged by methemoglobin-inducing drugs, such carriers have relatively
insufficient enzyme to reduce methemoglobin and methemoglobinemic
cyanosis results. Conceptually, this situation is a very important
type of drug reaction, since simple arithmetic indicates that even
for a rare autosomal recessive disease there are many carriers in
the population. For example, if a disease frequency is one per
10,000, 2% of the population would be carriers; with a disease frequency of one in 40,000, 1% of the population would be carriers.
There are a great many different inborn errors in metabolism and
other autosomal recessive diseases. Although each one is rather

rare, it is likely that many individuals in the normal population
are carriers for one or perhaps several of these abnormal genes
and may be susceptible or resistant to certain drugs or other environmental agents as a result.

Malignant Hyperthermia from Anesthesia

A single autosomal dominant gene makes otherwise healthy individuals susceptible to malignant hyperthermia from inhalational
anesthetics (halothane, methoxyglurane, ether) or muscle relaxants
(succinylcholine). The drugs trigger a rapid rise in temperature
(as high as 112°F), progressive muscular rigidity, tachycardia,
hyperventilation, myoglobinuria, metabolic and respiratory acidosis,
hyperkalemia, and--in two-thirds of reported cases--death from cardiac arrest (Britt and Kalow, 1970). Britt et al. (1973) and
Moulds and Denborough (1974) showed that halothane inhibits calcium
storage capacity of isolated sarcoplasmic reticulum and releases
calcium into the myoplasm, causing contracture in muscle biopsies
from survivors, to an extent far greater than in biopsies from normal persons. These muscle preparations are also more sensitive
than normal to rigor induced by succinylcholine, potassium chloride,
or caffeine. The underlying defect is not known, but a family has
been reported recently in which the mother and a sister of two
children who died with malignant hyperthemia were completely deficient in adenylate kinase (myokinase) activity in muscle (Schmitt et
al., 1974). This enzyme may be important in regulation of intra-
cellular ATP content, which is related to calcium uptake, myosin
ATPase, and oxidative phosphorylation. There is no specific therapy for malignant hyperthermia yet proved effective in man; however,
intravenous adminstration of procaine has been recommended, based
upon the knowledge that procaine can block the effects of caffeine
on calcium binding by sarcoplasmic reticulum and resulting induction of muscle rigor. Procaine was effective in preventing and
reversing this syndrome in a group of susceptible Landrace pigs in
South Africa (Harrison, 1971). For relatives of a proband with
malignant hyperthermia, an in vitro test with biopsied muscle for
increased sensitivity to halothane-induced contracture has been
recommended (Moulds and Denborough, 1974). Some susceptible persons have a significant elevation of serum CPK (creatine phospho-
kinase) levels, but this test is not specific. Despite the "path-
opharmacological" effects of caffeine in vitro, no case has been
reported in which ordinary use of caffeine has produced the clinical state of malignant hyperthermia.

Caffeine-Induced Wakefulness

Caffeine in the form of pills or coffee or tea will arouse some but not all individuals. Goldstein (1964) and Goldstein et al. (1965) reported large inter-individual differences in healthy volunteers in the degree of wakefulness after caffeine ingestion. Each subject received 300 mg of caffeine or lactose in random order and under double blind conditions. In eight of 20 subjects, there was no significant difference between caffeine and placebo in the delay of onset of sleep. In each of the remaining 12 subjects, caffeine produced significant wakefulness compared with placebo. There was no correlation between plasma levels of the agent at one, two or three hours after administration and the effects upon soundness of sleep. There was no striking difference among individuals who habitually drank more coffee than others. Presumably, these interindividual differences reflect differences in sensitivity of sites of action in the brain. It would be of interest to correlate these effects with parameters measurable during sleep EEG recordings and with age of subjects.

Susceptibility to the effects of ethanol

There is considerable evidence, though not analyzed genetically, for individual variation and susceptibility to the acute effects of alcohol on the central nervous system in man (Omenn and Motulsky, 1972; Omenn 1974). Although there are significant correlations between blood alcohol concentration and such psycho-physiological test parameters as flicker fusion frequency, tapping speed, reaction time, coordination, and standing steadiness, there are considerable inter-individual differences (Idestrom and Cadenius, 1968). In other tests, such as sensory motor coordination, correlation between blood alcohol concentration and the measured effect has been minimal (Munkelt et al., 1962). At the level of EEG observations, Ahrens (1971) described three patterns of response after acute alcohol ingestion: a) sensitive subjects with pronounced EEG changes even with blood alcohol concentration of less than 0.8 mg %, accounting for 25% of probands; b) responsive subjects who develop major alterations, especially increase of theta waves, but only at high blood alcohol levels; c) bioelectrically indifferent subjects who showed no major EEG changes even with higher blood alcohol concentrations. CNS sensitivity to the effects of alcohol has been extensively studied in mice. The time until sleeping after a single anesthetic dose of ethanol was found to be three times as long for BALB/cJ mice as for C57BL/J mice, for example, although the rates of alcohol elimination were nearly identical in the two strains (Kakihana et al., 1966; McClearn, 1972). The strains in which a higher brain resistance was found also showed a greater preference for alcohol in studies of drinking choice when mice were provided two bottles in water/alcohol cage situations.

Striking ethnic differences, presumably due to genetic factors, have been observed in the vasomotor response to acute alcohol ingestion. Adults of Oriental background typically respond to even small amounts of alcohol with a marked visible facial flushing reaction, increased peripheral pulse pressure and increased skin temperature. Wolff (1972) investigated this reaction in newborn Chinese infants. Nineteen of 20 newborns of Oriental background gave dramatic flushing reactions, while only one of 20 Caucasian babies did the same. In a later study (Wolff, 1973), the vasomotor responses of American Indians and of racially hybrid population groups in Hawaii were investigated. Vasomotor sensitivity was found also in these individuals. It is not known whether these differences reflect differences at the level of the autonomic nervous system or in the blood vessels themselves. It is possible that the highly active atypical alcohol dehydrogenase (ADH) demonstrated in a high proportion of livers from Japanese subjects (Fukui and Wakasugi, 1972; Stamatoyannopoulos et al., 1975) leads to rapid appearance of acetaldehyde in sufficient concentration to produce the vasomotor reactions.

Taste Sensitivity

The ability to taste a particular concentration of phenylthiocarbamide (PTC) is a common human genetic polymorphism. Non-tasters (30% of Caucasians; 2-10% of Negroes) are homozygous for a recessive gene, while tasters are heterozygous or homozygous for the dominant taster allele. More detailed studies of "threshold" for tasting a series of concentrations of PTC have shown, however, that multiple genes are involved in the overall variation in sensitivity to this agent (Stern, 1973). Differences in sensitivity of receptors in taste buds may take on more significance if such differences can be shown to be correlated with differences in sensitivity of receptors in the peripheral and central nervous system. Joyce et al. (1968) have claimed significant correlations between taste sensitivity and responses of the heart and salivary glands to hyoscine N-butylbromide. Knopp et al. (1966) reported that patients who are most sensitive to the extrapyramidal effects of

trifluoperazine (a phenothiazine) have lower taste thresholds to
quinine.

Reactions of the Autonomic Nervous System

Marked individual differences in the effects of atropine on
heart rate and of phenylephrine on pupillary dilatation are examples
of differing responsiveness of the autonomic nervous system (see
Smith and Rawlins, 1973, pp 2-3). Genetic analyses of these variations have not been performed. However, with such easily measured
peripheral signs of sympathetic and parasympathetic nervous system
response, it would be of interest to determine the genetic component in variation and to attempt to correlate such variation with
central nervous system behavioral effects. With current application of powerful biofeedback techniques, which are probably mediated through the autonomic nervous system, assessment of genetically
determined differences in the sensitivity of individuals to biofeedback training may be particularly interesting.

Highly sensitive and specific assays have now been developed
to assess biochemically the activity of the sympathetic nervous
system. Plasma norepinephrine levels and urinary excretion rates
of dopamine and norepinephrine metabolites have been determined.
Furthermore, measurement of the activity of dopamine beta-hydroxy-
lase (DBH) in plasma may be a good indicator of the activity of
the sympathetic nervous system. This enzyme catalyzes the last
step of norepinephrine synthesis, converting dopamine to norepinephrine in the adrenal medulla and the sympathetic nervous system
nerve terminals. The enzyme is released from merve terminals together with the catecholamines, on a stoichiometric basis, and is
then detectable in the blood plasma. There is wide inter-individual variability in the plasma levels of DBH, for example ranging
from 4 to 340 units in a sample of 34 individuals (Planz and Palm,
1973). Twin studies (Ross et al., 1973) and family studies
(Weinshilboum et al., 1975) demonstrate that genetic factors substantially affect plasma DBH levels and that very low levels of
plasma DBH activity may be determined by a single autosomal recessive gene. It is not known whether these genetically determined
differences reflect differences in specific activity per molecule
of the enzyme or differences in rate of release of norepinephrine
plus DBH as a sign of sympathetic nervous system activity.

Monoamines in Platelets and Brain

The peripheral blood platelet is coming to be recognized as a potential "window" on the central nervous system. The platelet contains monoamine oxidase (MAO) with properties similar to those of brain mitochondrial MAO (Omenn and Cheung, unpublished). Furthermore, platelets take up the neurotransmitter substances serotonin (5-hydroxytryptamine) and dopamine; the K_m for uptake and the K_i's for inhibition by drugs such as phenothiazines, tricyclic antidepressants, amphetamines and reserpine are in the same range as the K_m and K_i's for the reuptake of these neurotransmitters in serotoninergic and dopaminergic nerve terminals (synaptosomes) from brain (Pletscher, 1968; Sneddon, 1973; Tuomisto, 1974).

Twin studies indicate a major genetic component to the variance in quantitative activity of platelet MAO. In both depressed and schizophrenic patient groups, decreased platelet MAO has been reported (Murphy and Weiss, 1972; Wyate et al., 1973). The significance of these observations is not yet apparent. Genetic analyses of platelet uptake of neurotransmitters and its inhibition by drugs are in progress (Omenn). Decreased amount of uptake in such genetic disorders as Huntington's disease (Aminoff et al., 1974), Duchenne's muscular dystrophy (Murphy et al., 1973), and Down's syndrome (Boullin and O'Brien, 1973) has recently been reported. These investigations suggest that the blood platelet may prove useful for indirect studies of reactions in the inaccessible brain, especially for family investigations.

We have studied brain monoamine oxidase activity for evidence of variation in susceptibility of the MAO to inhibition (Omenn and Cheung, unpublished). MAO is well-suited for pharmacogenetic analysis because an array of substrates and different types of inhibitors can be employed to explore the properties of the enzyme. Kynuramine was used as substrate in a fluorimetric assay (Kraml, 1965); pargyline was used as an irreversible or non-competitive inhibitor and D-amphetamine as a reversible or competitive inhibitor. Brain samples were obtained from frontal cortex and basal ganglia at autopsy in 46 adult cases, including 26 suicides (depressed) and 20 "controls". Mean values for the inhibition constants were 1.8×10^{-7}M for pargyline and 1.4×10^{-4}M for amphetamine. Standard deviations were relatively small, and no individuals gave inhibition constants markedly deviant from the mean values. Thus, in this study of total MAO without subfractionation to isozymes, we could find no evidence for sufficient variation in the inhibition

constant of MAO in brain to account for the strikingly different
effectiveness of MAO inhibitors among patients treated for depression. No cases were available for which treatment response to MAO
inhibitors among patients treated for depression. No cases were
available for which treatment response to MAO inhibitor was known.

PHARMACOGENETICS IN THE MAJOR BEHAVIORAL DISORDERS

Affective Disorders

Twin and family studies indicate that depression and especially manic-depressive illness is conditioned by genetic factors
(Winokur et al., 1969; Gershon et al., 1971). Recent linkage
studies with the X-chromosome gene markers for color blindness and
blood group Xg^a suggest that in some families with manic-depressive
illness a single X-linked dominant gene may be largely responsible
for the affective disorder (Mendlewicz and Fleiss, 1974). A comprehensive pathophysiologic hypothesis involving biogenic amine metabolism has been formulated on the basis of multiple, but indirect,
pharmacologic effects in patients with depression and mania. In
brief, depression appears to be associated with decreased action or
turnover of norepinephrine (and serotonin), while manic states are
associated with increased biogenic amine turnover (Schildkraut,
1969). Drugs which deplete norepinephrine from nerve terminals (reserpine) or interfere with its biosynthesis (alpha-methyl-tyrosine,
alpha-methyl dopa) precipitate depression in some patients. Drugs
which enhance biosynthesis of norepinephrine (NE) (L-dopa) can induce hypomanic states, and agents which prolong the action of norepinephrine by inhibiting intraneuronal monoamine oxidase (MAO inhibitors) or the neuronal reuptake of norepinephrine released into
the synapse (tricyclics) are effective antidepressants. Finally,
electroconvulsive shock acts to increase tyrosine hydroxylase activity and norepinephrine turnover (Musacchio et al., 1969). Shock
therapy, like treatment with reserpine, MAO inhibitors, or tricyclic antidepressants, alters serotonin as well as catecholamine
metabolism (Cooper et al., 1968). Lapin and Oxenkrug (1969) have
proposed that the mood-elevating component of anti-depressant drugs
and of shock therapy is related to increase of brain serotonin,
while enhancement of central adrenergic mechanisms accounts for
psycho-energizing and motorstimulating effects. This hypothesis is
consistent with the report (Bunney et al., 1972) that six of seven
depressed manic-depressive patients with psychosis became hypomanic on large doses of L-dopa (dopamine and norepinephrine increased),
while only one of the six showed elevation of the depressed mood

serotonin unchanged or decreased).

    Two sets of clinical observations suggest significant pharma-
cogenetic approaches. Pare et al. (1962) reported that two groups
of depressed patients could be differentiated by their response to
either MAO inhibitors or tricyclic compounds. In their hands and
without placebo comparisons, patients who responded to one class
of antidepressant tended not to respond to the other. When the
patients suffered subsequent episodes of depression, perhaps precipitated by quite different life stresses, their pharmacologic
responsiveness was the same as before in 27 of 28 cases. Even more
impressively, relatives of the proband patients who also had affective disorders and were treated with antidepressants shared the
same pattern of responsiveness and unresponsiveness to these classes
of drugs (Pare and Mack, 1971). Angst (1964) used only imipramine
and found 34 relatives concordant with the proband for a positive
antidepressant response, four concordant for lack of response, and
only five of the 41 first-degree relatives discordant. There is
some skepticism about the distinctiveness of response to treatment
in these studies. Pairs concordant for positive response might reflect, at least in part, the frequent favorable outcome with placebo administration in depressed patients (King, 1970). Rarely
were relatives and probands both tested with both classes of drugs.
As noted above, there are significant genetic differences in the
rates of metabolism of phenelzine and of tricyclic compounds, which
might account for the differential therapeutic effectiveness.
However, the unproved conclusion of Pare and his colleagues that
the underlying mechanisms of the depression are different and that
the treatment responsiveness is a means of clinical delineation
cannot be dismissed. The hypothesis that patients who do not respond are less susceptible to the action of the drug at its site
of action than those who do respond can be tested: individuals
having monoamine oxidase with a higher K_i would not be inhibited
by usual doses of MAO inhibitors; similarly, individuals who because of genetic variation had a reuptake mechanism with a higher
K_i for tricyclic compounds might be unresponsive to the drugs for
that reason.

    The second clinical observation of pharmacogenetic interest
is the risk that about 10 percent of patients treated for high
blood pressure with the Rauwolfia alkaloid reserpine will develop
depression (Harris, 1957; Muller et al., 1955). These patients
tend to have a personal history of affective disorder more often
than do the 90 percent of reserpine-treated patients who do not

develop depression (Muller et al., 1955). Reserpine, in animals, is known to deplete neuronal stores of norepinephrine and serotonin and to induce an increase in activity of tyrosine hydroxylase, the rate-limiting step for biosynthesis of norepinephrine. It is conceivable that individuals differ in their capacity to step up norepinephrine biosynthesis or that individuals with low-normal stores of norepinephrine might be more severely depleted at similar doses of reserpine. Whatever the mechanism, reserpine most likely unmasks a predisposition to depression.

So general a phenotype as "depression" or even the better-delineated subcategory encompassing manic-depressive illness is likely to be mediated by multiple genetically-determined mechanisms, even if alterations in biogenic amine metabolism serve as a common pathogenetic pathway. Differential responses to therapy and differential susceptibility to precipitation of attacks with drugs such as reserpine, alpha-methyl-dopa or ACTH may provide insights and investigational "handles" into the heterogeneous causes of affective disorders.

The platelets and red blood cells in the peripheral blood may offer opportunities to assay certain properties of the nervous system. We noted above (page 22) that MAO activity and inhibition can be determined in platelets and that serotonin and dopamine uptake can be assessed for affinity and inhibitability in platelets. More work is needed to characterize the platelet and synaptosomal systems and determine whether or not the same genes specify the properties of the MAO and the properties of the uptake process in these two different tissues. One of the most elegant means of demonstrating identical properties is to find a genetic variant in one or more individuals and show that a simply-inherited trait is expressed identically in both platelets and nervous system. Effectiveness of MAO inhibitors (which many psychiatrists are bringing back into clinical use, especially for hostile older patients with depression) may be correlated with the baseline level of platelet MAO activity, with the inhibition constant of the MAO for inhibition by the drug chosen, and with later platelet MAO levels after in vivo administration of the drug. Analogous studies can now be carried out for tricyclic antidepressants affecting the serotonin uptake process in platelets.

Besides mitochondrial MAO and the reuptake process in the presynaptic membrane, the enzyme catechol-O-methyl transferase (COMT), which is located in the synapse, serves to inactivate norepinephrine and dopamine. COMT activity can be measured in the red blood cell, though it is not yet established whether its properties can be distinguished from those of COMT in the brain. Cohn et al. (1970) and Dunner et al. (1971) claimed that red blood cell COMT activity is decreased in certain groups of women with affective disorder. Very interestingly, the distribution of COMT activity among the control group of women without affective disorders (Cohn et al., 1970) suggested a subgroup with lower COMT activity, possibly representing a predisposed subgroup in the "normal" population. Weinshilboum et al. (1974) also observed a bimodal distribution of COMT activity in red blood cells in a survey of normal adolescents and found a highly significant correlation for siblings (r = 0.485). The properties of the enzyme from subjects with lower or higher activity have not yet been investigated.

Some caution must be exercised in the interpretation of results with enzyme or receptor studies in peripheral tissues. For example, a report of DOPA decarboxylase activity in red blood cells (Tate et al., 1971) had to be retracted a year later when the activity was shown to be due to non-enzymatic catalysis (Tate et al., 1972).

Alcoholism: A Psycho-Pharmco-Genetic Disorder

Studies of families with affective disorder show that women are much more likely than men to have affective disorders. However, there is a large excess of chronic alcoholism among the male relatives (Pitts and Winokur, 1966; Winokur et al., 1969). Thus, it is possible that alcoholism is related to manic-depressive and depressive illness in the spectrum of affective disorders. Laymen, of course, have the quite appropriate intuition that at least some people who are depressed turn to alcohol. As we have noted previously, genetic factors may be important with regard to alcoholism in the acute intoxicating effects, in the metabolism of ethanol, in the likelihood of addictability, in the premorbid personality, and in the susceptibility of tissues to medical and neuropsychiatric complications of alcoholism (Omenn and Motulsky, 1972; Omenn, 1974).

The crucial issue in alcoholism and other addiction syndromes is the nature of central nervous system addictability--physical and psychological dependence, with withdrawal symptoms. It is possible by selective breeding to develop strains of rats and mice which are addiction-prone or addiction-resistant to morphine or alcohol (Nichols, 1972). Further work is needed to test whether a final common pathway of addictability exists which manifests as dependence and tolerance in individual cells of the nervous system. It is conceivable that different agents trigger addictive behavior differently, but that the response at the cellular level is similar. An analogy can be cited in the action of polypeptide hormones, which interact with hormone-specific receptors in the membrane of target cells, then trigger an intra-cellular response mediated in each case by cyclic AMP (Sutherland, 1970).

Alcoholism affects some ten million people in the United States and is clearly a disorder in which the diagnosis cannot be made without the environmental exposure of a genetically predisposed individual to the agent, ethanol. Recent adoption studies have shown that the excess of familial incidence of alcoholism lies in the biological relatives rather than adoptive or foster parents (Goodwin et al., 1973), a surprising finding to those who have assumed that only the social environment molds the difficulties of alcohol persons. Just as reserpine precipitates depression in only 10 percent of hypertensive patients treated with this srug, chronic abuse of alcohol and poor diet leads to cirrhosis of the liver in only 10-15 percent of patients and leads to chronic pancreatitis, cerebellar degeneration and Wernicke-Korsakoff psychosis in even smaller proportions. Virtually nothing is known yet about the factors in liver, pancreas and brain regions which determine susceptibility to these complications, except for the Wernicke's component of nystagmus, opthtalmoplegia and ataxia, which is due to depletion of thiamine. An old observation of Chvostek (1922) that men who developed alcoholic cirrhosis tended to have less body hair prior to the onset of cirrhosis was confirmed by Muller (1952) and might implicate male hormones as one factor affecting liver susceptibility.

Among children born to mothers who were chronic alcoholics a striking new malformation syndrome has been recognized (Jones et al., 1973, 1974). These children have retarded intrauterine and postnatal physical and mental development, microcephaly, decreased width to the palpebral fissure causing the eyes to appear rounded, and variable limb and cardiac malformations. The degree of linear growth deficiency was more severe than the deficit of weight at birth, which is quite uncommon. The mechanism of toxicity and the genetic and environmental factors that affect the risk are not yet resolved.

Schizophrenia

In comparison with the delineation of unipolar and bipolar
categories of affective disorders and the formulation of the biogenic amine hypothesis, clinical and biochemical investigations of
schizophrenic patients have made less progress. Nevertheless,
carefully organized adoption studies have demonstrated that genetic
factors are highly significant in the predisposition to schizophrenia (Heston, 1966; Kety et al., 1971). Longitudinal followup of
individual patients and family studies thus far fail to support
clinical subtypes as a basis for sorting the presumed heterogeneity
of schizophrenias (Rosenthal, 1970). Furthermore, despite claims
to the contrary, there is little evidence that certain phenothiazines are relatively better than other phenothiazines for different forms of schizophrenic illness (Hollister, 1970). Nevertheless,
the relative effectiveness of various anti-psychotic agents may yet
prove a useful variable in attempts to delineate biologically, meaningful classifications of schizophrenia.

It seems reasonable to wonder whether individuals who have a
schizophrenia-like reaction to amphetamine (Ellinwood, 1969) or a
persistent 'bad-trip' from LSD are genetically predisposed to such
psychotic reactions and would have been at relatively high risk
for development of "spontaneous" schizophrenia. Even without such
drugs, some one percent of adults in the age group of 15-40 years
develop chronic schizophrenia. Amphetamine-induced psychosis provides special opportunities for pharmacological deductions about
possible neurotransmitter mediation of at least some types of
schizophrenia. The active groups of potent anti-psychotic phenothiazines, when viewed in a three-dimensional molecular model,
appear to resemble the molecular conformation of dopamine (Horn
and Snyder, 1971). Amphetamines also act on biogenic amines, primarily through inhibition of the neuronal reuptake mechanism. In
vitro studies of isolated synaptosomes from dopamine-rich and from
norepinephrine-rich regions of rat brain have shown that D-amphetamine and L-amphetamine are equipotent in their action on dopamine
reuptake (dopamine lacks an optically active beta-carbon), whereas
D-amphetamine is ten times more potent than its L-stereoisomer on
norepinephrine reuptake (both amphetamine and norepinephrine have
an asymmetric, optically active beta-carbon). A locomotor activity
measure thought to be mediated by norepinephrine in rats is enhanced in vivo at a ratio of 10:1 by D and L amphetamine, whereas a
stereotyped gnawing behavior thought to be mediated by dopamine is
elicited at a 1:1 ratio (Snyder et al., 1970). Finally, D and L

amphetamine appear to be equipotent in inducing amphetamine psychosis, many features of which resemble schizophrenic syndromes
(Angrist et al., 1971). It should be noted that Ferris et al.
(1972) have challenged the experimental basis for correlation of
D- and L-amphetamine relative potency with norepinephrine or DA.

The importance of considering heterogeneity of underlying
mechanism and of using family studies to delineate different types
of schizophrenia may be illustrated by reference to the study by
Slater er al. (1963) of the so-called "epileptic psychosis".
Their 69 patients had all the cardinal features of schizophrenia,
although affective responsiveness was preserved relatively well
and late deterioration of personality seemed not to occur. The
mean age of onset for the psychosis was 30 years, following a history of epilepsy lasting, on the average, for 14 years. Eighty
percent had evidence of temporal lobe dysfunction, and all had incomplete control of the seizures at the time they became psychotic.
The most convincing element of these histories was the low incidence of schizophrenia in the first-degree relatives of these patients, suggesting that their familial predisposition was to a
special type of seizure disorder rather than to the usual types of
schizophrenia.

Minimal Brain Dysfunction/Hyperactivity Syndrome

The category of childhood behavioral disorders called "hyperactivity syndrome" or "minimal brain dysfunction" (MBD) almost
certainly comprises many different underlying mechanisms. In
analogy with the dozens of specific causes of "mental retardation"
now identified, we may anticipate that hyperactive behavior may
reflect various genetic abnormalities, intrauterine or postnatal
viral infections, birth injuries, environmental toxins ranging
from food additives to subclinical lead poisoning, and sociopsych-
ological influences (Omenn, 1973, 1975). Proof that any one of
these factors accounts for the behavior problem in a given child
or family is not yet available. However, good evidence of a significant role for genetic factors in the predisposition to hyperactive behavior has appeared (Morrison and Stewart, 1971; Cantwell,
1972). Compared with relatives of non-hyperactive children, the
parents of 109 hyperactive children in the two studies had a significantly increased incidence of alcoholism, hysterical behavior,
and sociopathic behavior; these relatives also more frequently
gave a history suggesting hyperactivity in their own childhood.
Morrison and Steward (1973) separated the familial excess inciden-

ce into inherited and environmental factors by use of the adoption
technique pioneered in studies of schizophrenia. Unlike the biological parents of hyperactive kids, foster parents of hyperactive
children who had been adopted early in life had no increase in
alcoholism, hysteria or sociopathy.

The most promising "handle" for investigating MBD may be the
central nervous system stimulating drugs used therapeutically in
some of these children. The serious ethical constraints on experimentation with drugs in children can be fully respected, since it
is very much in the child's interest to determine whether the drug
being prescribed is actually helping him significantly. In the
process of evaluating proper dosage and comparing the chosen agent
with placebo and alternative agents, the physician should be tail-
oring more rational therapy to the needs of the particular patient.
Without such individualized attention, the child may be taking a
drug of limited or no benefit, when another agent or greater non-
-drug therapy would be more effective. Since these stimulant
drugs, amphetamines and methylphenidate, are administered usually
for months or years up to puberty, any toxic effects—including
effects on growth and development—must be viewed with concern,
all the more so if definite benefit cannot be demonstrated. Even
when the child does improve, there is uncertainty whether the drug
effect persists (Sroufe and Stewart, 1973). Indeed, deterioration
of performance reported when children are temporarily withdrawn
from medication may be evidence of behavioral dependence, rather
than of positive drug effects.

In several reports between 1937 and 1950, Bradley documented
the effectiveness of Benzedrine (D,L-amphetamine) and Dexedrine
(D-amphetamine) in the treatment of hyperactivity syndromes and
other behavioral syndromes in children. Bradley's conclusion
(1950) that Dexedrine was twice as potent as Benzedrine suggested
that the L-isomer had negligible activity. However, he noted that
the D,L-mixture was better than Dexedrine alone in some children,
raising the possibility of individual differences in response,
such that L-amphetamine had an independent action or acted syner-
gistically with D-amphetamine in some patients. The excitatory
effects of sedative doses of phenobarbital in hyperactive children
also has been known for a long time (Lindsley and Henry, 1942).
It is not known whether the extent of excitation by phenobarbital
correlates with the degree of hyperactivity or with the likelihood
of positive response to stimulant drugs. As noted in the discussion of schizophrenia, the analysis of the relative potency of D-

and L-amphetamine may be applied to MBD as well. Arnold et al.
(1973) reported a double-blind cross-over comparison of the two
isomers in 11 hyperactive children. D-amphetamine was only slightly more effective than L-amphetamine. When the data were reanalyz-
ed in light of Fish's subclassification (1971) of children with
MBD, L-amphetamine seemed equally as effective in calming aggressive children, but much less effective than the D-amphetamine in
reducing anxiety or hyperactivity. Admittedly these conclusions
are based upon very few cases thus far.

Weber and Sulzbacker (1975) found that among hyperactive
children the best responders to amphetamine or methylphenidate gave
lower amplitudes in auditory-evoked potentials before drug administration and larger differences induced by drug than did the children who were poor responders according to behavioral measures. In
another neurophysiological study, Satterfield et al. (1973) contrasted the six best responders and five worst responders among 31
hyperkinetic boys given methylphenidate. The good responders had
higher mean amplitudes and greater range of amplitude in the rest-
ing EEG, more movement artefacts (presumably indicating hyperactivity), lower mean skin conductance, and larger auditory-evoked
cortical responses. Knopp et al. (1972) measured the extent of
pupillary contraction electronically before and after a 5 mg test
dose of amphetamine in 22 children. The greater the deviation of
the child's light-reactive pupillary contraction from the normal
mean before medication and the closer it approached the mean after
medication, the better the correlation with a good behavioral response to D-amphetamine. None of these measures can be utilized
reliably in an individual patient to assess the likelihood of a
good clinical response, since all the differences represent group
comparisons. Nevertheless, these neurophysiological measures provide an intermediate level of observation, together with clinical
assessment and analysis of drug metabolism, to evaluate the relative effectiveness of stimulant drugs versus placebo, of D- versus
L-amphetamine, of amphetamines versus methylphenidate, of various
dosages of any effective drug, and of responses due to familial
predisposition rather than an altered response secondary to the behavior disorder (Omenn, 1973).

Seizure Disorders

The normal pattern of electrical activity in the brain, as reflected in the electroencephalogram (EEG) is determined almost entirely by genetic factors in a polygenic system (Vogel, 1970). In

TABLE I

Variants of the Normal Human EEG[a]

Rhythm	Genetic basis	Population frequency	
Normal alpha (8–13 cps)	Polygenic		
Low voltage alpha	Auto Dom	7.0%	
Quick alpha (16–19 cps)	Auto Dom	0.5%	
Occipital slow (4–5 cps)	??	0.1%	?Psychopathy
Monotonous tall alpha	Auto Dom	4.0%	?Assortative Mating
Beta waves	Multifactorial	5–10.0%	Sex, age
			?Assortative Mating
Frontal beta groups (25–30 cps)	Auto Dom	0.4%	
Fronto-precentral beta (20–25 cps)	Auto Dom	1.4%	

[a]After Vogel, 1970.

addition, however, several single-gene mediated "variants" of the normal EEG have been described, affecting altogether about 15 percent of the general population (Table 1). The clinical significance of these variants is unknown, and no studies have yet been performed with groups of individuals having different baseline EEG patterns to see whether they have different responses to various psychopharmacologic agents. One study of phenobarbital effects did find induction of beta waves in 13 of 18 similarly treated subjects (Essig and Fraser, 1958). All thirteen became tolerant by clinical criteria, but six of the 13 failed to show reversal to normal EEG activity (EEG tolerance). Withdrawal of phenobarbital caused EEG abnormalities in only five of the 18 subjects; none had preexisting or permanent EEG changes. It is likely that similar differences among individuals occur with alcohol and meprobamate withdrawal.

Population, twin, and family studies indicate polygenic predisposition to seizure disorders in man (Pratt, 1967). For the 3 cps spike-and-wave "centrencephalic" pattern of childhood petit mal seizures, the underlying EEG abnormality is inherited as an autosomal dominant trait expressed primarily between ages five and 16 years (Metrakos and Metrakos, 1969). A variety of anti-convulsive agents has been employed in clinical seizure disorders, without biochemical elucidation of the mechanisms of therapeutic effectiveness. There is some specificity in the types of seizure disorders that can be recognized from the selective effectiveness of particular drugs (Pincus and Tucker, 1974). In brief, phenobarbital is the most commonly used agent, usually effective in all types of seizure disorders. Diphenylhydantoin (Dilantin), which controls grand mal, focal and psychomotor seizures in children and adults, is ineffective in petit mal and myoclonic seizures. Primidone (Mysoline) is most useful in psychomotor seizures. Ethosuccimide (Zarontin) is the drug of choice in petit mal, but of essentially no value in other seizure disorders. Acetazolamide (Diamox), which may be effective in many types of seizures, is especially effective in minor motor and petit mal seizures. Finally, ACTH is highly useful in infantile spasms and juvenile minor motor seizures, but can actually trigger seizures in other types.

SIMPLY-INHERITED BEHAVIORAL DISORDERS WITH SPECIAL VULNERABILITY TO DRUGS

The Hepatic Porphyrias

These genetically-heterogeneous metabolic disorders of hepatic heme biosynthesis are transmitted vertically through families as autosomal dominant traits. The clinical syndromes occur in episodes of colicky abdominal pain with constipation (due to autonomic neuropathy), peripheral neuropathy, and variable central nervous system involvement, including flaccid paralysis, agitated and paranoid depression, and schizophrenic behavior (Marver and Schmid, 1972). Porphyria may have been the cause of the intermittent "madness" of King George III of England (MacAlpine and Hunter, 1969). In the Swedish type, or intermittent acute porphyria, biochemical diagnosis during the acute attack is highly reliable. However, increased urinary excretion of porphyrin precursors may not be present before puberty or between attacks. In the South African type, called porphyria variegata, there is continuous fecal hyperexcretion of protoporphyrins and coproporphyrins, with symptoms and signs similar to the Swedish type and with photosensitive dermatitis in addition. Several common drugs induce higher activity of the delta-aminolevulinic acid (ALA) synthetase, the rate-limiting enzyme in liver, and thus precipitate attacks in these predisposed individuals. The drugs include barbiturates, certain sulfonamides, the antifungal agent griseofulvin, and possibly general anesthetics, ethanol, and chloroquine (Marver and Schmid, 1972). Often the underlying disease has not been suspected before the drug-precipitated attack, so the diagnosis may be missed.

Familial Dysautonomia (Riley-Day Syndrome)

This autosomal recessive inherited disorder causes protean manifestations of neurogenic origin. Infants have difficulty swallowing and lack of overflow tears, followed by slow achievement of developmental milestones and recurrent pneumonia. Periodic crises of vomiting, abdominal pain, fever, flushing, sweating, and emotional lability dominate childhood. Sensitivity to pain is diminished, taste discrimination is defective (fungiform papillae are absent), and mortality risks of surgery are increased (Brunt and McKusick, 1970). Infusion of norepinephrine into dysautonomic patients produces a very exaggerated hypertensive response without bradycardia. Conversely, the parasympathomimetic drug methacholine gave an excessive hypotensive response without increase in heart rate, plus abdominal cramps, sweating, and overflow tears (Dancis, 1968). These youngsters lack the radiating pains and flare response to intradermal histamine, unless pretreated with methacholine. Also they compensate poorly in conditions of decreased oxygen saturation. The relationship between autonomic nervous system imbalance and emotional lability is not at all elucidated.

Lesch-Nyhan Syndrome

This X-linked recessive condition of young boys is characterized clinically by choreoathetosis, spasticity, mental retardation,
and a bizarre, compulsive behavior disorder with selfmutilation of
lips, fingers, and eyes (Lesch and Nyhan, 1964). Biochemically,
there is hyperuricemia and excessive production of uric acid, due
to complete deficiency of an enzyme in purine metabolism, hypoxan-
thineguanine phosphoribosyl transferase (HGPRT). Tophaceous gout
and uric acid nephropathy leading to uremia may result. The HGPRT
activity is normally highest in the brain, particularly in the
basal ganglia, providing a correlation with the choreoathetosis.
However, the basis for the behavioral disorder is altogether unknown. Certain drugs which are normally transformed by the same
phosphoribosyl transferase are handled differently in HGPRT-defic-
ient individuals. The anti-neoplastic agent 6-mercaptopurine
(6-MP) must be converted to its ribonucleotide by HGPRT to be
active in vivo. The immunosuppressive agent azathioprine (Imuran)
is first converted to 6-MP and then activated similarly. Allopurinol is a valuable drug in the treatment of hyperuricemia and gout,
since it blocks the conversion of hypoxanthine and xanthine to uric
acid, which is less soluble than xanthines and forms renal stones.
Allopurinol normally decreases purine synthesis, so that total
xanthine excretion is less than that of uric acid. In HGPRT deficiency, allopurinol ribonucleotide is not formed, so purine synthesis is not inhibited. As a result, these patients are liable to
formation of xanthine stones (Kelley and Wyngaarden, 1972).

Huntington's Disease

This autosomal dominant neurologic and psychiatric disorder
is one of the major problems in genetic counseling in medicine.
The age of onset of involuntary movements is usually in the 30's
or 40's, but may be delayed even longer. Thus, individuals at
risk (50 percent if a parent is affected) have a dual misery of
not knowing whether they will be transmitting the disease to their
children and of worrying that any "normal" twitches or behavioral
problems may be the early signs of the disease. Over a period of
10 to 20 years, the affected person undergoes progressive deterioration of personality and of mental function, usually requiring
institutionalization because of psychotic behavior or dementia or
both. The pathophysiology is unknown, and no specific diagnostic
test has yet been devised. However, a pharmacological challenge
has been proposed: since L-dopa administration to patients with

Parkinsonism may induce involuntary choreiform movements, it was speculated that carriers of the gene for Huntington's chorea might manifest such movements at a lower dose of L-dopa than do normal people or Parkinsonism patients (Klawans et al., 1972). The proportion of false-positives and false-negatives is simply not known, and it is conceivable that the symptoms induced in the preclinical stage might not be reversible. Unlike laboratory tests with body fluids or cultured cells, this type of test allows the subject to judge for himself whether or not he will likely develop the dread disease; individuals at risk differ greatly in their desire to know whether they will be affected later.

SUMMARY

Psychopharmacogenetics consists of investigations of the differences among individuals in the therapeutic and adverse affects of behavior-modifying drugs. Clinically significant examples of well-delineated genetically-determined differences in metabolism of drugs and in tissue sensitivity to drug action are now known. Although single-gene mechanisms are prominent among these examples, it should be emphasized that polygenic inheritance appears to be the more common manner in which genes influence the absorption, metabolism, and tissue action of many other drugs.

Pharmacologic agents also provide valuable probes for the analysis of complex behavioral phenotypes, such as the affective disorders, alcoholism and other addiction syndromes, minimal brain dysfunction, schizophrenia, and seizure disorders. Pharmacogenetics contains good models for the interaction of genetic and environmental factors, interactions which underlie the panoply of normal and abnormal behavior in man.

REFERENCES

AHRENS, R. 1971. On the forensic-psychiatric significance of alcohol loading tests under EEG control. Electroenceph. Clin. Neurophysiol. 30:269.

ALEXANDERSON, B. 1972. Pharmacokinetics of desmethylimipramine and nortriptyline in man after single and multiple oral doses - a cross-over study. Europ. J. Clin. Pharmacol. 5:1.

ALEXANDERSON, B., & BÖRGA, O. 1973. Urinary excretion of nortriptyline and five of its metabolites in man after single and multiple oral doses. Europ. J. Clin. Pharmacol. 5:174.

ALEXANDERSON, B., & SJÖQVIST, F. 1971. Individual differences in the pharmacokinetics of monomethylated tricyclic antidepressants: role of the genetic and environmental factors and clinical importance. Ann. N.Y. Acad. Sci. 179:739.

AMINOFF, M. J., TRENCHARD, A., TURNER, P., WOOD, W. G., & HILLS, M. 1974. Plasma uptake of dopamine and 5-hydroxytryptamine and plasma catecholamine levels in patients with Huntington's chorea. Lancet 2:1115.

ANGRIST, B. M., SHOPSIN, B., & GERSHON, S. 1971. The comparative psychotomimetic effects of stererosomers of amphetamine. Nature 234:152.

ANGST, J. 1964. Anti-depressiver Effekt and genetische Faktoren. Arzneim. Forsch. 14:496-500.

ARNOLD, L. E., WENDER, P. H., McCLOSKEY, K., & SNYDER, S. H. 1972. Levoamphetamine and dextroamphetamine comparative efficacy in the hyperkinetic syndrome. Assessment by target symptoms. Arch. Gen. Psychiat. 27:816.

ASBERG, M., PRICE EVANS, D. A., & SJÖQVIST, F. 1971. Genetic control of nortriptyline plasma levels in man: a study of the relatives of propositi with high plasma concentration. J. Med. Genet. 8:129.

BOULLIN, D. J., & O'BRIEN, R. A. 1973. The metabolism of 5-hydroxytryptamine by blood platelets from children with mongolism. Biochem. Pharmacol. 22:1647.

BRADLEY, C.   1937.   The behavior of children receiving benzedrine.
    Amer. J. Psychiat. 94:577-585.

BRADLEY, C.   1950.   Benzedrine and Dexedrine in the treatment of
    children's behavior disorders.   Pediatrics 5:24.

BRAITHWAITE, R. A., GOULDING, R., THEANO, G., BAILEY, J., & COPPEN,
    A.   1972.   Plasma concentration of amitriptyline and clinical
    response.   Lancet 1:1297.

BREWER, G. J.   1971.   Annotation: Human ecology, an expanding role
    for the human geneticist.   Amer. J. Hum. Genet. 23:92.

BRITT, B. A., & KALOW, W.   1970.   Malignant hyperthermia.   A stat-
    istical review.   Aetiology unknown.   Canad. Anaesth. Soc. J.
    17:293.

BRITT, B. A., KALOW, W., GORDON, A., HUMPHREY, J. G., & REWCASTLE,
    M. B.   1973.   Malignant hyperthermia: an investigation of
    five patients.   Canad. Anaesth. Soc. J. 20:431.

BRUNT, P. W., & McKUSICK, V. A.   1970.   Familial dysautonomia: a
    report of genetic and clinical studies, with a review of the
    literature.   Medicine 49:343.

BUNNEY, W. E. JR., GOODWIN, F. K., MURPHY, D. L., HOUSE, K. M. &
    GORDON, E. K.   1972.   The "switch process" in manic-depressive
    illness.   Arch. Gen. Psychiat. 27:304.

CANTWELL, D. P.   1972.   Psychiatric illness in families of hyper-
    active children.   Arch. Gen. Psychiat. 27:414.

CASSIMOS, C., MALAKA-ZAFIRIU, K., & TSIURES, J.   1974.   Urinary
    D-glucaric acid excretion in normal and G-6-PD-deficient
    children with favism.   J. Pediatr. 84:871.

CHVOSTEK, F.   1922.   Klinische Vorträge.   Zur pathogenese der
    Leberzirrhose.   Wiener. Klin. Wochenscrift. 35:381.

COHEN, F. R., SACHS, J. R., WICKER, D. J., & CONRAD, M. E.   1968.
    Methemoglobinemia provoked by malarial chemoprophylaxis in
    Viet Nam.   New Eng. J. Med. 279:1127.

COHEN, L. K., GEORGE, W., & SMITH, R. 1974. Isoniazid-induced acne and pellagra - occurrence in slow inactivators of isoniazid. Arch. Dermatol. 109:377.

COHEN, P. T. W., OMENN, G. S., MOTULSKY, A. G., CHEN, S-H., & GIBLETT, E. R. 1973. Restricted variation in the glycolytic enzymes of human brain and erythrocytes. Nature (New Biol.) 241:229.

COHN, C. K., DUNNER, D. L., & AXELROD, J. 1970. Reduced catechol--O-methyl transferase activity in red blood cells of women with primary affective disorder. Science 170:1323.

CONNEY, A. H., & BURNS, J. J. 1972. Metabolic interactions among environmental chemicals and drugs. Science 178:576.

COOPER, A. J., MOIR, A. T. B., & GULDBERG, H. C. 1968. Effect of electroconvulsive shock on cerebral metabolism of dopamine and 5-hydroxytryptamine. J. Pharm. Pharmacol. 20:729.

CURRY, S. H., & MARSHALL, J. H. L. 1968. Plasma levels of chlorpromazine and some of its relatively nonpolar metabolites in psychiatric patients. Life Sci. 7:9.

DANCIS, J. 1968. Altered drug response in familial dysautonomia. Ann. N.Y. Acad. Sci. 151:876.

DAVIS, J. M., KOPIN, I. J., LEMBERGER, L., & AXELROD, J. Effects of urinary pH on amphetamine metabolism. Ann. N.Y. Acad. Sci. 179:493.

DUNNER, D. L., COHN, C. K., GERSHON, E. S., & GOODWIN, F. K. 1971. Differential catechol-0-methyl transferase activity in unipolar and bipolar affective illness. Arch. Gen. Psychiat. 25:348.

EDWARDS, J. A., & PRICE-EVANS, D. A. 1967. Ethanol metabolism in subjects possessing typical and atypical liver alcohol dehydrogenase. Clin. Pharmacol. Ther. 8:824.

ELLINWOOD, E. H. JR. 1969. Amphetamine psychosis: a multi-dimensional process. Semin. Psychiat. 1:208.

ESSIG, C. F., & FRASER, H. F. 1958. Electroencephalographic changes in man during use and withdrawal of barbiturates in moderate doses. Electroencephalogr. Clin. Neurol. 10:649.

EVANS, D. A. P. 1969. An improved and simplified method of detecting the acetylator phenotype. J. Med. Genet. 6:405.

FENNA, D., MIX, L., SCHAEFER, O., & GILBERT, J. A. L. 1971. Ethanol metabolism in various racial groups. Canad. Med. Assoc. J. 105:472.

FERRIS, R. M., TANG, F. L. M., & MAXWELL, R. A. 1972. Comparison of the capacities of isomers of amphetamine, deoxypipradrol and methylphenidate to inhibit the uptake of tritiated catecholamines into rat cerebral cortex slices, synaptosomal preparations of rat cerebral cortex, hypothalamus and striatum and into adrenergic nerves of rabbit aorta. J. Pharmacol. Exp. Ther. 181:407.

FISH, B. 1971. The "one child, one drug" myth of stimulants in hyperkinesis. Arch. Gen. Psychiat. 25:193-203.

FUKUI, M., & WAKASUGI, C. 1972. Liver alcohol dehydrogenase in a Japanese population. Jap. J. Legal Med. 26:46.

GERSHON, E. S., DUNNER, D. L., & GOODWIN, F. K. 1971. Toward a biology of affective disorders. Genetic considerations. Arch. Gen. Psychiat. 25:1.

GOLDSTEIN, A. 1964. Wakefulness caused by caffeine. Naunyn--Schmiedebergs Arch. Pharmacol. 248:269.

GOLDSTEIN, A., WARREN, R., & KAIZER, S. 1965. Psychotropic effects of caffeine in man. I. Individual differences in sensitivity to caffeine-induced wakefulness. J. Pharmacol. Exp. Ther. 149:156.

GOODWIN, D. W., SCHULSINGER, F., HERMANSES, L., GUZE, S. B. & WINOKUR, G. 1973. Alcohol problems in adoptees raised apart from alcoholic biological parents. Arch. Gen. Psychiat. 28: 238.

GRAVES, R. 1955. The Greek Myths. Baltimore, Penguin, Vol. I, p. 348.

GREEN, D. E., FOREST, I. S., FORREST, F. M., & SERRA, M. T. 1965. Inter-patient variation in chlorpromazine metabolism. Exp. Med. Surg. 23:278.

HANSEN, A. R., KENNEDY, K. A., AMBRE, J. J., & FISCHER, L. J. 1975. Glutethimide poisoning: a metabolite contributes to morbidity and mortality. New Eng. J. Med. 292:250.

HARRIS, T. H. 1957. Depression induced by Rauwolfia compounds. Amer. J. Psychiat. 113:950.

HARRISON, G. G. 1971. Anaesthetic-induced malignant hyperpyrexia: a suggested method of treatment. Brit. Med. J. 3:454.

HEIDELBERGER, C. 1973. Current trends in chemical carcinogenesis. Fed. Proc. 32:2154.

HESTON, L. L. 1966. Psychiatric disorders in foster home reared children of schizophrenic mothers. Brit. J. Psychiat. 112:819.

HOLLISTER, L. E. 1970. Choice of antipsychotic drugs. Amer. J. Psychiat. 127:186.

HORN, A. S., & SNYDER, S. H. 1971. Chlorpromazine and dopamine: conformational similarities that correlate with the anti--schizophrenic activity of phenothiazine drugs. Proc. Nat. Acad. Sci. U.S. 68:2325.

IDESTRÖM C-M., & CADENIUS, B. 1968. Time relations of the effects of alcohol compared to placebo. Psychopharmacologia (Berl.) 13:189.

IDESTRÖM, C-M., SCHALLING, D., CARLQVIST, V., & SJÖQVIST, F. 1972. Acute effects of diphenylhydantoin in relation to plasma levels. Psychol. Med. 2:111.

JOHNSTONE, E., & MARCH, W. 1973. Acetylator status and response to phenelzine in depressed patients. Lancet 1:567.

JONES, K. L., SMITH, D. W., STREISSGUTH, A. P., & MYRIANTHOPOULOS, N. C. 1974. Outcome in offspring of chronic alcoholic women. Lancet 1:1076.

JOYCE, C. R. B., PAN, L., & VARONES, D. D. 1968. Taste sensitivity may be used to predict pharmacological effects. Life Sci. 7:533.

KAKIHANA, R., BROWN, D. R., McCLEARN, G. E., & TABESHAW, J. R. 1966. Brain sensitivity to alcohol in inbred mouse strains. Science 154:1574.

KING, L. J. 1970. Chemotherapy of mental depression. Ann Rev. Med. 21:367.

KALOW, W. 1972. Pharmacogenetics of drugs used in anesthesia, in Human Genetics, Proceedings Fourth International Congress of Human Genetics, Paris, September.1971, Excerpta Medica, Amsterdam, pp. 415.

KAUL, P. N., TICKU, K. K., & CLARK, M. L. 1972. Chlorpromazine metabolism. V. Disposition of free and conjugated metabolites in blood fractions of schizophrenic patients. J. Pharm. Sci. 61:1753.

KELLERMAN, G., LUYTEN-KELLERMAN, M., & SHAW, C. R. 1973a. Genetic variation of aryl hydrocarbon hydroxylase in human lymphocytes. Amer. J. Hum. Genet. 25:327.

KELLERMAN, G., SHAW, G. R., & LUYTEN-KELLERMAN, M. 1973b. Aryl hydrocarbon hydroxylase inducibility and bronchogenic carcinoma. New Eng. J. Med. 289:934.

KELLEY, W. N., & WYNGAARDEN, J. B. The Lesch-Nylan syndrome, in The Metabolic Basis of Inherited Disease, 3rd edition, J. B. Stanbury, J. B. Wyngaarden & D. S. Fredrickson, (Eds.), New York, McGraw-Hill, pp. 969.

KETY, S. S., ROSENTHAL, D., WENDER, P. H., & SCHULSINGER, F. 1971. Mental illness in the biological and adoptive families of adopted schizophrenics. Amer. J. Psychiat. 128:302.

KLAWANS, H. L. JR., PAULSON, G. W., RINGEL, S. A., & BARBEAU, A. Use of L-dopa in the detection presymptomatic Huntington's chorea. New Eng. J. Med. 286:1332.

KNOPP, W., ARNOLD, L. E. ANDRAS, R. L., & SMELTZER, D. J. 1972. Electronic pupillography predicting amphetamine response in hyperkinetic children. Abstract, APA meetings.

KNOPP, W., FISCHER, R., BECK, J., & TEITELBAUM, A. 1966. Clinical implications of the relation between taste sensitivity and the appearance of extrapyramidal side effects. Dis. Nerv. Syst. 27:729.

KRAML, M. 1965. A rapid microfluorimetric determination of mono-amine oxidase. Biochem. Pharmacol. 14:1684.

KUTT, H. 1971. Biochemical and genetic factors regulating Dilantin metabolism in man. Ann. N.Y. Acad. Sci. 179:705.

LAPIN, I. P., & OXENKRUG, G. F. 1969. Intensification of the central serotoninergic processes as a possible determinant of the thymoleptic effect. Lancet 1:132.

LESCH, M., & NYHAN, W. L. 1964. A familial disorder of uric acid metabolism and central nervous system function. Amer. J. Med. 36:561.

LINDSLEY, D. B., & HENRY, C. E. 1942. The effect of drugs on behavior and the electroencephalogram of children with behavior disorders. Psychosom. Med. 4:140.

MACALPINE, I., & HUNTER, R. 1969. Porphyria and King George III. Sci. Amer. 221:38.

MARCH, J. E., DONATO, D., TURANO, P., & TURNER, W. J. 1972. Interpatient variation and significance of plasma levels of chlorpromazine in psychotic patients. J. Med. 3:146.

MARVER, H. S., & SCHMID, R. 1972. The porphyrias, in The Metabolic Basis of Inherited Disease, 3rd ed, J. B. Stanbury, J. B. Wyngaarden, D. S. Fredrickson (Eds.), New York, McGraw--Hill, pp. 1087.

MCCLEARN, G. E. 1972. Genetics as a tool in alcohol research. Ann. N.Y. Acad. Sci. 197:26.

MEIER, H. 1963. Experimental pharmacogenetics, in Physiopathology of Heredity and Pharmacologic Responses, New York-London, Academic Press.

MENDLEWICZ, J., & FLEISS, J. L. 1974. Linkage studies with X chromosome markers in bipolar (manic-depressive) and unipolar (depressive) illnesses. Biol. Psychiat. 9:261.

METRAKOS, J. D., & METRAKOS, K. 1969. Genetic studies in clinical epilepsy, in Basic Mechanisms of the Epilepsies, H. H. Jasper, A. A. Ward, Jr., & A. Pope (Eds.), Boston, Little Brown, pp. 700.

MORRISON, J. R., & STEWART, M. A. 1971. A family study of hyperactive child syndrome. Biol. Psychiat. 3:189.

MORRISON, J. R., & STEWART, M. A. 1973. The psychiatric status of the legal families of adopted hyperactive children. Arch. Gen. Psych. 28:888.

MORROW, A. C., & MOTULSKY, A. G. 1968. Rapid screening method for the common atypical pseudocholinesterase variant. J. Lab. Clin. Med. 71:350.

MOTULSKY, A. G. 1972. History and current status of pharmacogenetics. Proceedings Fourth International Congress of Human Genetics, Paris 6-11, Excerpta Medica, pp. 381.

MOTULSKY, A. G. 1964. Pharmacogenetics. Prog. Med. Genet. 3:49.

MOULDS, R. F. W., & DENBOROUGH, M. A. 1974. Biochemical basis of malignant hyperthermia. Identification of susceptibility to malignant hyperthermia. Brit. Med. J. 2:241.

MÜLLER, G. 1952. Der erbkonstitutionelle Hypogenitalismus des Mannes als Dispositionsfaktor der Lebercirrhose. Med. Klin. 47:71.

MULLER, J. C., PRYER, W. W., GIBBONS, J. E., & ORGAIN, E. S. 1955. Depression and anxiety occurring during Rauwolfia therapy. J. Amer. Med. Assoc. 159:836.

MUNKELT, P., LIENERT, G. A., FRAHM, M., & SOEHRING, K. 1962. Geschlechtsspezifische Wirkungsunterschiede der Kombination von Alkohol und Meprobamat auf psychisch stabile und labile Versuchspersonen. Arzneim-Forsch 12:1059.

MURPHY, D. L., MENDELL, J. R., & ENGEL, W. K. 1973. Serotonin and platelet function in Duchenne muscular dystrophy. Arch. Neurol. 28:239.

MURPHY, D. L., & WEISS, R.   1972.   Monoamine oxidase: reduced
    activity in blood platelets from bipolar depressed patients.
    Amer. J. Psychiat. 128:35.

MUSACCHIO, J. M., JULOU, L., KETY, S. S., & GLOWINSKI, J.   1969.
    Increase in rat brain tyrosine hydroxylase activity produced
    by electroconvulsive shock.   Proc. Nat. Acad. Sci. USA
    63:1117.

MYRIANTHOPOULOS, N. C., KURLAND, A. A., & KURLAND, L. T.   1962.
    Hereditary predisposition in drug-induced Parkinsonism.
    Arch. Neurol. 6:5.

MYRIANTHOPOULOS, N. C., WALDROP, F. N., & VINCENT, B. L.   1967.
    A repeat study of hereditary predisposition in drug-induced
    Parkinsonism.   Excerpta Medical International Congress Series
    175:486.

NICHOLS, J. R.   1972.   The children of addicts: what do they
    inherit? Ann. N.Y. Acad. Sci. 197:60.

OMENN, G. S.   1973.   Genetic issues in the syndrome of minimal
    brain dysfunction. Sem. Psych. 5:5.

OMENN, G. S.   in press.   Alcoholism: a pharmacogenetic disorder.
    Modern Problems in Pharmacopsychiatry.

OMENN, G. S.   1975.   Pharmacogenetic aspects of treating behavioral
    disorders in children with drugs, in Studies on Psychiatric
    and Psychological Problems of Childhood, D. V. S. Sankar (Ed.),
    New York, PJD Publications Ltd.

OMENN, G. S., & MOTULSKY, A. G.   1972.   A biochemical and genetic
    approach to alcoholism. Ann. N.Y. Acad. Sci. 197:16.

OMENN, G. S., & MOTULSKY, A. G.   1973.   Pharmacogenetics. Year
    Book of Drug Therapy, Chicago, Year Book Medical Publishers,
    pp. 5.

OMENN, G. S., & MOTULSKY, A. G.   1975.   Eco-Genetics: genetic
    variation in the susceptibility to environmental agents, in
    Genetic Issues in Public Health, B. Cohen, (Ed.), Johns
    Hopkins.

PARE, C. M. B., & MACK, J. W. 1971. Differentiation of two genetically specific types of depression by the response to antidepressant drugs. J. Med. Genet. 8:306.

PARE, C. M. B., REES, L., & SAINBURY, M. J. 1962. Differentiation of two genetically specific types of depression by the response to anti-depressants. Lancet 2:1340.

PERRY, H. M. JR., TAN, E. M., CARMODY, S., & SAKAMOTO, A. 1970. Relationship of acetyltransferase activity to antinuclear antibodies and toxic symptoms in hypertensive patients treated with hydralazine. J. Lab. Clin. Med. 76:114.

PINCUS, J. H., & TUCKER, G. 1974. Behavioral Neurology, New York, Oxford University Press.

PITTS, F. N. JR., & WINOKUR, G. 1966. Affective disorders. VII. Alcoholism and affective disorder. J. Psych. Res. 4:37.

PLANZ, G., & PALM. D. 1973. Acute enhancement of dopamine-β-hydroxylase activity in human plasma after maximum work load. Europ. J. Clin. Pharmacol. 5:255.

PLETSCHER, A. 1968. Metabolism, transfer and storage of 5-hydroxytryptamine in blood platelets. Brit. J. Pharmacol. 32:1.

PRATT, R. T. C. 1967. The Genetics of Neurological Disorders, Oxford, Oxford University Press.

PRICE-EVANS, D. A., DAVIDSON, K., & PRATT, R. T. C. 1965. The influence of acetylator phenotype on the effect of treating depression with phenelzine. Clin. Pharmacol. Ther. 6:430.

ROSENTHAL, D. 1970. Genetic Theory and Abnormal Behavior, New York, McGraw-Hill.

ROSS, S. B., WETTERBERG, L., & MYRHED, M. 1973. Genetic control of plasma dopamine-β-hydroxylase. Life Sci. 12:529.

SATTERFIELD, J. H., CANTWELL, D. P., LESTER, L. I., & PODOSIN, R. L. 1972. Physiological studies of the hyperkinetic children. Amer. J. Psych. 128:1418.

SCHILDKRAUT, J. J. 1969. Neuropsychopharmacology and the affective disorders. New Eng. J. Med. 281:197.

SCHLOOT, W., TIGGES, F-J., BLAESNER, H., & GOEDDE, H. W. 1969.
N-acetyltransferase and serotonin metabolism in man and other
species. Hoppe-Seylers Z. Physiol. Chem. 350:1353.

SCHMITT, J. J., SCHMITT, K., & RITTER, H. 1974. Hereditary malignant hyperpyrexia associated with muscle adenylate kinase
deficiency. Humangenetik 24:253.

SHIELDS, J. 1973. Heredity and psychological abnormality, in
Handbook of Abnormal Psychology, H. J. Eysenck (ed.), London,
Pitman Medical, pp. 540.

SHIELDS, J. 1962. Monozygotic Twins Brought Up Apart and Brought
Up Together. Oxford, Oxford University Press.

SJÖQVIST, F., HAMMAR, W., IDESTRÖM, C-M., LIND, M., TUCK, D., &
ASBERG, M. 1968. Plasma level of monomethylated tricyclic
antidepressants and side-effects. Excerpta Medica International Congress Series 145:246.

SLATER, E., BEARD, A. W., & GLITHERO, E. 1963. The schizophrenia-
-like psychoses of epilepsy. Brit. J. Psychiat. 109:95.

SMITH, M., HOPKINSON, D. A., & HARRIS, H. 1973. Studies on the
properties of the human alcohol dehydrogenase isozymes determined by the different loci ADH_1, ADH_2 and ADH_3. Ann. Hum.
Genet. 37:49.

SMITH, S. E., & RAWLINS, M. D. 1973. Variability in Human Drug
Response, London, Butterworth.

SNEDDON, J. M. 1973. Blood platelets as a model for monoamine-
-containing neurones. Prog. Neurobiol. 1:151.

SNYDER, S. H., TAYLOR, K. M., COYLE, J. T., & MEYERHOFF, J. L.
1970. The role of brain dopamine in behavioral regulation and
the actions of psychotropic drugs. Amer. J. Psychiat. 127:117.

SROUFE, L. A., & STEWART, M. A. 1973. Treating problem children
with stimulant drugs. New Eng. J. Med. 289:407.

STAMATOYANNOPOULOS, G., CHEN, S-H., & FUKUI, M. Submitted for
    publication. Genetic factors in alochol sensitivity: evid-
    ence from studies in Japanese.

STERN, C. 1973. Principles of Human Genetics, 3rd ed, San
    Francisco, W. H. Freeman and Company, pp. 161.

SUTHERLAND, E. W. 1970. On the biological role of cyclic AMP.
    J. Amer. Med. Assoc. 214:1281.

TATE, S. S., ORLANDO, J., & MEISTER, A. 1972. Decarboxylation of
    3,4-dihydroxyphenylalanine (DOPA) by erythrocytes: a reaction
    promoted by methemoglobin and other ferriheme proteins. Proc.
    Nat. Acad. Sci. USA 69:2505.

TATE, S. S., SWEET, R., MCDOWELL, F. H., & MEISTER, A. 1971.
    Decrease of the 3,4-dihydroxyphenylalanine (DOPA) decarboxylase
    activities in human erythrocytes and mouse tissues after ad-
    ministration of DOPA. Proc. Nat. Acad. Sci. USA 68:2121.

TUOMISTO, J. 1974. A new modification for studying 5-HT uptake
    by blood platelets: a reevaluation of tricyclic antidepress-
    ants as uptake inhibitors. J. Pharm. Pharmacol. 26:92.

VESELL, E. S., & PAGE, J. G. 1968a. Genetic control of drug
    levels in man: phenylbutazone. Science 159:1479.

VESELL, E. S., & PAGE, J. G. 1968b. Genetic control of drug
    levels in man: antipyrine. Science 161:72.

VESELL, E. S., & PAGE, J. G. 1968c. Genetic control of dicumarol
    levels in man. J. Clin. Invest. 47:2657.

VESELL, E. S., PAGE, J. G., & PASSANANTI, G. T. 1971. Genetic
    and environmental factors affecting ethanol metabolism in man.
    Clin. Pharmacol. Ther. 12:192.

VON WARTBURG, J. P., & SCHURCH, P. M. 1968. Atypical human liver
    alcohol dehydrogenase. Ann. N.Y. Acad. Sci. 151:936.

VOGEL, F. 1970. The genetic basis of the normal human electroen-
    cephalogram (EEG). Humangenetik 10:91.

WALTER, C. J. 1971. Clinical significance of plasma imipramine levels. Proc. Roy. Soc. Med. 64:282.

WEBER, B. A., & SULZBACHER, S. I. In press. Use of CNS stimulant medication in averaged electroencephalic audiometry with children with minimal brain dysfunction. J. Learning. Disabilities.

WEINSHILBOUM, R. M., RAYMOND, F. A., ELVEBACK, L. R., & WEIDMAN, W. H. 1974. Correlation of erythrocyre catechol-0-methyltransferase activity between siblings. Nature 252:490.

WEINSHILBOUM, R. M., SCHROTT, H. G., RAYMOND, F. A., WEIDMAN, W. H., & ELVEBACK, L. R. Submitted for publication. Inheritance of very low serum dopamine-βhydroxylase activity.

WHITE, T. A., JENNE, J. W., & PRICE-EVANS, D. A. 1969. Acetylation of serotonin in vitro by a human N-acetyltransferase. Biochem. J. 113:721.

WHITTAKER, J. A., & EVANS, D. A. P. 1970. Genetic control of phenylbutazone metabolism in man. Brit. Med. J. 4:323.

WINOKUR, G., CLAYTON, P. J., & REICH, T. 1969. Manic-Depressive Illness, St. Louis, Mosby.

WOLFF, P. H. 1972. Ethnic differences in alcohol sensitivity. Science 175:449.

WOLFF, P. H. 1973. Vasomotor sensitivity to alcohol in diverse mongoloid populations. Amer. J. Hum. Genet. 25:193.

WYATT, R. J., MURPHY, D. L., BELMAKER, R., COHEN, S., DONNELLY, C. H., & POLLIN, W. 1973. Reduced monoamine oxidase activity in platelets: a possible genetic marker for vulnerability to schizophrenia. Science 179:916.

YOSHIDA, A., & MOTULSKY, A. G. 1969. A psuedocholinesterase variant (E Cynthiana) associated with elevated plasma enzyme activity. Amer. J. Hum. Genet. 21:486.

ZEIDENBERG, P., PEREL, J. M., KANZLER, M., WHARTON, R. N. & MALITZ, S. 1971. Clinical and metabolic studies with imipramine in man. Amer. J. Psychiat. 127:1321.

THE ROLE OF GENOTYPE IN BEHAVIORAL RESPONSES TO ANESTHETICS

Merrill F. Elias, Ph.D.

and

Clyde A. Pentz, A.B.[1]

Department of Psychology and
All-University Gerontology Center
Syracuse University
Syracuse, New York   13210

[1]Clyde A. Pentz is a graduate student in the Department of Psychology
and the All-University Gerontology Center. He is supported by a
grant from the National Institute of Child and Human Development
(HD-08220) to MFE.

CONTENTS

THE ROLE OF GENOTYPE IN BEHAVIORAL
RESPONSES TO ANESTHETICS

Research on the behavioral effects of anesthetics falls into
two general categories: (1) studies which deal with the effects
of anesthetics on memory, and (2) studies which are concerned
with the more general question of the long term influence of anesthetics on a variety of behaviors. Memory studies typically
involve descriptions of the anterograde or retrograde amnestic effects of anesthesia. These studies employ the pharmacological
properties of various anesthetics as a tool for studying the input, consolidation and retrieval characteristics of learning
and memory. Studies concerned with the more general effects of
anesthesia on performance have been concerned with a wide range
of behaviors, including those involving memory processes. Moreover, they deal with the long and short term behavioral effects
of acute or chronic exposure to anesthetic vapors.

For some period of time, investigators have been concerned
with long and short term behavioral effects of anesthesia and
pre-anesthetic medication on surgical patients (Cherkin & Harroun,
1971; Choy & Parkhouse, 1969; Gruber & Reed, 1968). These clinically oriented studies have been important from a descriptive standpoint, but generally speaking they have not contributed substantially to understanding of memory input, consolidation, and retrieval processes. In part, this is related to the confounding
of anesthetic effects with effects of premedication, surgical
stress and pre-existing disease processes. Studies which have
controlled for one or more of these factors have generally failed
to utilize experimental paradigms that permit separation of input,
consolidation, and retrieval processes. Experiments on chronic
effects of exposure to anesthetic vapors are few in number, and
memory consolidation studies with animals have been plagued with
methodological problems including (1) failures to establish drug-
dose relationships prior to experimentation; (2) failure to control anesthetic administration procedures in many instances where
volatile anesthetics have been used; (3) use of only one inbred
strain of mice or rats or failure to specify the strain or
stock of animals utilized; (4) failure to control for stressful
effects of anesthetics which may influence behavior via mechanisms
other than those involved in memory (e.g. negative reinforcement
of specific responses); (5) a high degree of interstudy variation
in dose level, duration, and type of anesthetic delivered, as
well as interstudy variations in learning tasks and the intervals
between input of information and administration of the anesthetic.
Interstudy variations of this nature make it very difficult to

specify methodological differences among studies which might account
for divergent results.

Despite these methodological difficulties, it is quite clear
from a great number of studies (Porter, 1972) that anesthetics administered after input, e.g. a learning trial or trials, can cause
retrograde amnesic effects, although sometimes low doses of some
anesthetics result in memory facilitation (e.g. Wimer, 1968). The
major problem created by methodological differences among studies
is that it is difficult to establish precisely the time course of
effective anesthetic treatment. The latter consideration is of
considerable importance with regard to the testing of theories
regarding memory consolidation.

Methodological problems inherent in memory consolidation research with anesthetics, particularly inhalation anesthetics, may
have contributed to a decrease in the number of studies which
have been published in the last few years. Despite the diminish-
ing number of anesthetic studies designed to test memory consolidation theories, there has been a modest revival of interest in
the effects of anesthetics on behavior in general. This renewed
concern has been related to recent observations of physiological
and behavioral changes in surgical personnel subjected to anesthetic vapors (Bruce et al., 1974; Gruce et al., 1968; Cohen, et
al., 1971).

The applied basis of this renewed interest places a premium
on methodological sophistication, because results of basic experiments may have important implications for policies with regard
to anesthetic administration, e.g., agents, duration, safeguards.
While human studies will undoubtedly address these questions, increased tightening of controls with regard to the use of human subjects in potentially harmful medical and psychopharmacological experiments will, of necessity, elevate the animal model in importance. Thus, it seems important to correct methodological problems
which have been associated with past research; and, it seems imperative that animal models be utilized in a more productive manner.

One unique virtue of the animal model is that it permits the
manipulation and control of genotype in a manner which is not possible with humans. In some instances, it may be possible to establish a relationship between specific genes on particular chromosomes and behavioral responses to the various anesthetics. Use
of animal models in this manner may constitute a particularly productive approach to the understanding of how anesthetics influence
behavior, because gene-behavioral "linkages" permit exploration
of physiological mechanisms which intervene between genes and behavior. Here, we use the term linkage to refer to the relationship

between a specific gene and behavior rather than the relationship
between two genes on a given chromosome.

It is the thesis of this chapter that optimal utilization of
genetic materials and methods is central to the psychopharmacogenetic approach, that is, study of anesthetic effects on behavior
with genetically available animal models. No attempt has been made
to review the literature for all anesthetics, nor does this chapter
deal with studies of memory consolidation or the physiological
bases of memory. Excellent reviews of these topics are available
elsewhere (Deutsch, 1962; Jarvik, 1964, 1968; Porter, 1972), and
a general discussion of the methodological aspects of memory research with drugs may be found in McGaugh and Petrinovich, 1965.
For the most part, the chapter deals with inhalation anesthetics
with an emphasis on the non-hydrogen bonding anesthetics as they
are defined by Porter (1972). However, other anesthetic agents
and non-anesthetic agents are discussed in the context of a central
focus on inhalation anesthetics.

                            MEMORY CONSOLIDATION

The rationale underlying the use of anesthetics in the study
of memory is essentially the same as that underlying the use of
electroconvulsive shock (ECS), hypothermia, metabolic inhibitors,
and other amnesia producing agents. These treatments are employed
to disrupt a hypothetical perserveration-consolidation process
which permits sensory input to be stored for later recall.

Muller and Pilzecker (1900) were the first investigators to
suggest a perseveration process which could be adversely affected
by interference. Burnham (1903) added the concept of consolidation
to the idea of perserveration, and related them both to retrograde amnesia resulting from head trauma. The basic idea is that
some sort of memory trace must be maintained for a sufficiently
long period of time so as to permit it to become consolidated or
"fixed" into permanent memory. During the period of perserveration
and consolidation this hypothetical trace is vulnerable to disruption. Basic support for this model comes from the finding that
amnesia resulting from application of amnestic agents is retrograde in nature, i.e., magnitude of memory impairment increases
as the interval between information input and anesthetic treatment
decreases.

                            The Memory Trace

The precise nature of the memory trace which is presumed to
be susceptible to disruption has never been specific. Miller and
Springer (1973) point out that early models featuring disruption

of a perserveration-consolidation process as a source of retrograde amnesia suggested that stimulus input is uniquely encoded
in short-term memory in the form of electrochemically active,
neural reverberatory circuits that are terminated either by decay
or interference processes (Hebb, 1949). The continued action of
these circuits over time was believed to give rise to a more permanent long-term memory of an "energetically, passive, chemical-
structural format (Miller & Springer, 1973, p. 70)."

More recent, but basically similar, theories regarding the
electrophysiological nature of memory consolidation can be found
in the contemporary literature (Galambos, 1967). One hypothesis
is that short term memory represents electrophysiological conduction of impulses through an assembly of neurons and that a gradual
entry of DNA-dependent chains of biochemical events fixes the
activity in a permanent manner (Galambos, 1967, p. 642). Amnestic
agents would thus interupt or interfere with the electrophysiological and neurochemical characteristics of the memory trace prior to
the time that they were fixed in permanent form. In this event,
new chains of neuronal activity necessary for permanent storage
are either not formed or are formed in a weakened state. The nature of the biochemical events which constitute a memory trace is
yet unknown, but there seems little question that biochemical e-
vents such as a change in the quantity of messenger RNA and protein synthesis are involved in memory storage (Agranoff et al.,
1965; Hyden, 1967).

Models for memory consolidation include a variety of two and
three stage theories. The three stage theories (McGaugh, 1966)
suggest not only short- and long-term memory storage processes, but
an intermediate state as well. It has been proposed that amnestic
agents disrupt the shorter term processes before long-term memory
storage takes place (McGaugh, 1966; Barondes & Cohen, 1968).

There seems to be general agreement that it is the short term
memory storage processes that are affected by posttrial anesthetization, although alternative explanations for behavioral effects
such as conditioned fear (Chorover & Schiller, 1966) and negative
reinforcement (Elias & Simmerman, 1971a) have been suggested. Furthermore, the wide range of posttrial treatment intervals over
which anesthetics have been effective (Porter, 1972) is inconsistent with the hypothesis that only short-term memory processes are
vulnerable to anesthetic treatments. In general, however, a number of studies controlling factors implicit in the fear or negative
reinforcement explanations of impaired memory have provided evidence which is consistent with consolidation theory (see Glickman,
1958; McGaugh & Petrinovich, 1965), and an impressive amount of
data support a retrograde amnesic interpretation of impaired learning and performance as a function of posttrial administration of

anesthetic agents.

Memory Consolidation Paradigms

There are some common features of the design paradigms employed to test short-term memory consolidation models. Information input is controlled in some manner, and the amnestic agent is administered at various intervals <u>after</u> input has occurred. Some times, the amnestic agent is administered after a single learning trial. Alternatively, a number of trials are given with long intertrial intervals. In the latter case, the amnestic agent is administered between trials and care is taken so as not to confound posttreatment effects for one trial with pretreatment effects on the next. This precaution is particularly important for anesthetics with long or unknown clearance times. In some studies, amnestics are presented before a learning trial. This "pretrial paradigm" does not permit separation of anesthetic effects on sensory input from those which are related to memory. It does constitute a useful control condition (Elias & Simmerman, 1971b) when results are to be interpreted in terms of posttrial anesthetic effects.

If memory consolidation is completely blocked by a strong amnestic agent, retention or recall in a single trial paradigm should be zero. For the multiple trial paradigm, performance from trial-to-trial should show no improvement. On the other hand, a weak amnestic agent may fail to block consolidation, but may slow its rate so that retention scores are lower in a single trial paradigm or learning progresses more slowly in a multiple trial paradigm. Of course, performance trends or recall scores for treated groups are compared with those for untreated controls, and a number of posttrial treatment intervals are utilized, if the major objective of the study is to test a short-term memory consolidation model.

The memory consolidation paradigm has been used with a variety of performance tasks, although some are not suitable for memory consolidation studies because they do not permit separation of stimulus input and motor output factors from memory storage <u>per se</u>. Human research studies have employed tasks ranging from informal recitation of events occurring prior to anesthetization to more formal laboratory tasks such as serial and rote learning. Tasks used for animal studies include maze, bar press, discrimination, and avoidance learning. Passive avoidance learning appears to be particularly susceptible to posttrial anesthetic treatments (Porter, 1972). In the passive avoidance task, evidence for retrograde amnesic effects is provided by failure to refrain from jumping into a punishing stimulus such as shock. Thus, it

has played an important role in the arguments <u>against</u> explanations
of retrograde amnesic effects of anesthetics in terms of negative
reinforcement and punishment. However, demonstration that punishing effects of amnestic agents do not always account for performance impairment does not indicate that aversive properties of anesthetics do not contribute to retrograde amnesia, nor does it
eliminate reinforcement explanations of performance impairment in
many studies in which the nature of the task does not permit separation of anesthetic effects on <u>non</u>-memory aspects of performance
from direct anesthetic effects on memory <u>per se.</u>

ANIMAL STUDIES

Retrograde Amnesia

Single strain studies within species far outweigh studies
which employ strain comparisons in order to evaluate the influence
of genotype on behavioral response to anesthetics. More studies
have been done with the rat and mouse than any other species with
the exception of man. In some cases the strain of mouse or rat
used has not been specified, although in the majority of the
studies reported this information is given.

Studies with inbred strains permit genetic control because subjects within the strain may be considered to be genetically identical units. On the other hand, single strain studies provide no
information with regard to the interaction of genotype and the
treatments under investigations, and they do not permit generalizations to the species as a whole. These limitations are not
serious when certain treatment effects are uniformly observed for
all strains of a species and for a variety of species. However,
one can never be sure that this is the case unless a wide sampling
of inbred strains has been undertaken for the phenotype in question.
Even when this has been accomplished, characteristics of inbred
strains as opposed to outbred strains may limit the extent to
which data may be characteristics of a species. Henderson (1969)
has discussed the problems involved in research with inbred strains
of <u>Mus musculus</u> from the standpoint of generalizability of findings
for the species, and he has presented an argument for utilization
of hybrids formed by the complete intercrossing of several inbred
strains.

Despite the advantages of multiple strain studies or utilization of carefully specified outbred stocks, a minority of experimenters have elected to employ either of these strategies in memory
consolidation studies with animals. It may be possible to derive
some notion as to the extent to which findings may be expected to
generalize across strains and species by examining studies which

Table 1

Effects of Ether Anesthesia on Performance

Table Explanation

Animal: NS = strain is not stated.

Age: NS = not stated in report.

Task: Pass. Avd. = passive avoidance; Act. Avd. = active avoidance; T = trial.

Dosage: %I.A. = percent anesthetic vapor in inspired air; SAT = saturated; RT = room temperature as

reported by the author; NS = not specified.

TTI: Trial-Treatment Interval.

Results: Facilitation in learning as retention relative to controls; Decrement in learning as retention

relative to controls.

Author	Animal	Age (days)	Task	Duration (sec)	Dosage %I.A.	TTI (min)	Results
Ransmeier et al (1954)	Hamsters Strain NS	NS	Maze learning 24 hr retest	"anesthesia"[1]	NS/RT	1 & 2	No Difference
Abt et al (1961)	Mice Swiss Webster	28	Pass. Avd. 1 T 24 hr retest	40	NS/RT	0,2,4,6,8, 16,20,24	Decrement -Decreased latencies up to 8 min TTI
Essman et al (1961)	Mice Swiss Webster	21	Pass. Avd. 1 T	36	SAT/RT	0,60	Decrement -Decreased latencies for 0 TTI
Pearlman et al (1961)	Rats Sprague Dawley	90-120	Operant bar press 1 T Pass. Avd. 24 hr retest	35	SAT/RT	0.16,5,10	Decrement - Higher response rate the shorter the TTI
Gutekunst et al (1963)	Chick New Hampshire Red	1	Imprinting 24 hr retest	"anesthesia"[1]	NS/RT	0,15,30	Decrement - Chicks did not follow cube as well

Reference	Species/Strain		Task		Condition		Effect
(1963)	Rats (albino) Strain NS	90	Pass. Avd. 24 hr retest	300	NS/RT	0	No Difference
Herz et al (1966)	Mice Swiss Webster	420	Pass. Avd. 24 hr retest	40 & 70	SAT/30.5°C	0	Decrement -Decreased latencies for 70 sec group
Pearlman (1966)	Rats Sprague Dawley	110	Pass. Avd. 1 T 24 hr retest	60	SAT/RT	1,5,10, 15	Decrement -Decreased latencies of avoidance with 15 min TTI being longer than 1 min TTI
Alpern et al (1967)	Mice Swiss Webster	60	Pass. Avd. 1 T 24 hr retest	60	SAT/RT	0,60	No Difference
Black et al (1967)	Rats Hooded	NS	Discrimination Avoidance 24 hr retest	100 "deep anesthesia"[1]	SAT/RT	5	Facilitation - Increased latencies of avoidance
Suboski et al (1968)	Rats Long Evans	NS	Discrimination Avoidance 24 hr retest	100	SAT/37.7°C	1.66,53	Facilitation - Increased latencies of avoidance
Wimer (1968)	Mice C57BL/6J[2]	42	Act. Avd.	35	SAT/RT	0	Facilitation - When reserpine administered before learning trial, mice had shorter latencies
Herz (1969)	Mice Swiss Webster	60	Appetitive & aversive learning 24 hr retest	NS	SAT/30-35°C	0.01, 0.25, 0.5,1.0	Decrement -Increased latencies when water is a reinforcer. Decreased latencies when shock is a reinforcer
Dye (1969)	Rats Holtzman	1,330-360, 660-720	Discrimination 24 hr retest	180 "surgical anesthesia"[1]	NS/RT	3,15,30	Decrement - Running time is longer for the shorter TTI

[1] Subjective criteria

[2] Pretreated with reserpine

Table 2

Effects of Carbon Dioxide on Performance

Table Explanation

Animal: NS = strain not stated

Age: NS = not stated in report

Task: Pass. Avd. = passive avoidance; Act. Avd. = active avoidance; T = trial; D = day.

Dosage: %I.A. = percent inspired air; NS = not specified; atm. = atmospheres.

TTI = Trial-Treatment Interval

Results: Facilitation in learning as retention relative to controls; Decrement in learning as
retention relative to controls.

Author	Animal	Age (days)	Task	Duration (sec)	Dosage %I.A.	TTI (min)	Results
Quinton (1966)	Rats Spraque Dawley	90-110	Operant bar press (shock suppressed) 24 hr retest	120,240,900	30% & 50% 9.4 1/min	0	Decrement - the greater the concentration the greater the number of bar presses
Leukel et al (1964)	Rats (albino) Strain NS	90-180	Act. Avd. 1 T/D for 31 D	10 & 40	2.5 1/min NS	0.16,5,30,60	Decrement - greater number of trials necessary for learning

Reference	Species		Test		Gas source	Concentration	Result
Paolino et al (1966)	Rats Hotzman	90-120	Pass. Avd. 1 T 24 hr retest	10,15,25	gas from dry ice NS	0.03,1,2,3, 4,13,27	Decrement - decreased latencies for 15 & 25 sec duration
	Mice CF 1	63-70	Pass. Avd. 1 T 24 hr retest	10	gas from dry ice NS	3,5	Decrement - decreased latencies for 3 min TTI only
Taber et al (1966)	Mice CF 1	NS	Pass. Avd. 1 T 24 hr retest	10	gas from dry ice NS	0,5,15,30, 60, 120	Decrement - decreased latencies if CO_2 given up to 30 min TTI
Freckleton et al (1968)	Cockroach	NS	Pass. Avd. 22 hr retest	15	gas from compressed tank - NS	0.25	Decrement - decreased latencies of avoidance
Nachman et al (1969)	Rats Sprague Dawley	70	Pass. Avd. 1 T 24 hr retest	25	gas from dry ice NS	0.07	Decrement - decreased latencies of avoidance
Galluscio (1971)	Rats (albino) Strain NS	NS	Pass. Avd. 1 T 24 hr retest	40	gas from dry ice NS	0	No Difference
Porter (1974)	Chicks white leg horn	2	Pass. Avd. 1 T 3, 24 hr retest	60-300	0.45 atm- 0.90 atm	0	No Difference

have employed different strains and species. It is obvious that
cross-experiment strain comparisons are limited by interstudy
variations in procedure, and that species comparisons are severely
compromised by the fact that input and output mechanisms (modes
of sensing and responding) vary widely for species at different
points on the phylogenetic scale of development.

Tables 1, 2 and 3 provide a short summary of the results of
studies of ether, flurothyl, and CO_2, with single strains or stocks
of mice.

Each of the tables contains the following information:

1) author;
2) strain and species;
3) anesthetic dosage parameters and the criterion for
   anesthetization;
4) interval between trials;
5) trial-treatment interval (TTI);
6) the nature of the task and key task parameters;
7) general description of results.

In some studies, the strain or stock of mice utilized was
not given. In those studies in which it was specified, it was
assumed that mice identified as inbred were not randomly bred
in the experimenters' laboratory prior to experimentation.
Strictly speaking, CO_2 is not an inhalation anesthetic. It has
been included because it has been widely used to study memory
consolidation and it is a volatile gas which produces amnesia.

Rapid inspection of these tables reinforces the notion that
cross-species and between-strain comparisons are compromised by
interstudy variations in age, type of task, duration of anesthetization, dosage level and other factors. It is exceedingly difficult to resolve the discrepancies between these studies for
which impaired learning, no differences, or facilitation in learning have resulted from posttrial anesthetic treatment. Porter
(1972) performed a comparative statistical analysis of different
studies which suggests that posttrial anesthetization results in
impaired learning (presumably reflecting retrograde amnesia)
if the trial-treatment interval is sufficiently short, the dose level is sufficiently large and the treatment duration is extended.
However, there are exceptions to these findings. Black et al.
(1967) and Suboski et al. (1968) found that learning was facilitated rather than impaired by rather extended durations of anesthetic treatment in ether-saturated and ether-potentiated atmospheres (Suboski et al., 1968). It is tempting to resolve these
discrepancies between Black et al.'s findings and Suboski et al.'s
findings and other studies with ether in terms of variations in
critical task parameters. However, both of these investigators

used a strain of rats which was highly appropriate for discrimination studies, but different than that used in other studies.

The possibility that genotype was an important factor in
Black et al's and Suboski et al's findings if reinforced by strain
comparison studies. Table 4 summarizes strain comparisons for
ether and halothane. It is quite clear from brief examination of
this table, that genotype interacts with critical treatment parameters to influence performance in the direction of improvement or
decrement relative to nontreated controls. These studies dealing
with strain difference will be discussed in more detail in a later
section of this chapter.

Time Course of Retrograde Amnesia

Porter's (1972) comparative statistical analysis of the anes-
thetic-memory consolidation literature indicated that the trial-
-treatment interval factor was second only to dosage level as a
parameter influencing posttrial anesthetic treatment effects. In
fact, efficacy of anesthetic-induced facilitation and impairment
is increased with decreasing trial-treatment intervals. The exact
nature of the time gradient for effective posttrial treatment is a
critical issue from the standpoint of various memory consolidation
theories. Establishment of a point where trial-treatment interval
is so long that treatments are only partially effective, or completely ineffective, in producing retrograde amnesic symptoms (or facilitation) is critical to resolution of the time course of short
term memory consolidation. This assumes that only short and intermediate memory storage stages are vulnerable to disruption by amnestic agents, an assumption which may be tested by identifying
trial-treatment intervals.

Table 5 summarizes the studies which have employed comparisons
of trial-treatment intervals with regard to anesthetic effectiveness. Generally, shorter intervals are more effective, but it is
impossible to establish a specific time gradient because of variation in critical experimental parameters including genotype. Moreover, age varies considerably from study to study and is not specified in several studies. Anesthetic dosage levels are inadequat-
ely described in at least two studies and very loosely described
in many. Rarely do two studies contain exactly the same trial-
-treatment intervals. Similar problems are encountered when one
attempts to compare studies with the nonvolatile anesthetics, although dosage levels are more adequately and precisely described.

Table 3

Effects of Flurothyl on Performance

Table Explanation

Animal: NS = strain not stated

Age: NS = not stated in report

Task: Pass. Avd. = passive avoidance; T = trials

Duration: NS = duration not stated

TTI = Trial-Treatment Interval

Results: Facilitation in learning as retention relative to controls; Decrement in learning as retention
relative to controls

Author	Animal	Age (days)	Task	Duration (sec)	Dosage %I.A.	TTI (min)	Results
Alpern et al (1967)	Mice Swiss Webster	60	Pass. Avd. 1 T 24 hr retest	1	20 microliters in 250 ml flask[2]	0,60,120 240,1440	Decrement - decreased latencies of avoidance up to 240 min TTI

et al (1967)	CF 1		Pass. Avd. 1 T 24 hr retest	NS	20 microliters in 250 ml flask[2]	5,60,360 720	Decrement - decreased latencies of avoidance in 5 & 60 min group
Cherkin (1969)	Chicks white leg- horn	NS	Pass. Avd. 1 T 20-24 hr retest	1-16	range 0.43%v/v- 3.0% v/v[2]	4-2880	Decrement - the greater the dosage the shorter the latencies. The shorter the TTI the shorter the latencies
Riege et al (1973)	Goldfish	180-210	Pass. Avd. 1 T 1,4,16,64 hr retest	16	range 14 mg/l- 1200 mg/l[1]	3	Facilitation - longer latencies of avoidance
Porter (1974)	Chick white leghorn	2	Pass. Avd. 1 T 3,5,24 hr retest	9	0.017 atm[2]	0	Decrement - decreased latencies of avoidance

[1]Fish swan in solution of flurothyl

[2]Inhalation of flurothyl

Table 4

Strain Differences in Response to Inhalation Anesthetics

Table Explanation

Anesthetic: SAT = saturated chamber; RT = room temperature; I.A. = inspired air

Duration: NS = not specified

Criterion of anesthesia: LRR = loss of righting reflexes; HB = heavy breathing

Task: Act. Avd. = active avoidance; Pass. Avd. = passive avoidance; T = trial; D = day;

   Discrim. = spatial discrimination

Results: Facilitation in learning as retention relative to controls; Decrement in learning as retention

   relative to controls.

Author	Strains	Anesthetic	Duration (sec)	Criteria of Anesthesia	TTI (min)	Task	Results
Wimer et al (1968)	C57BL/6J DBA/2J	Ether SAT/RT	35	LRR & HB	0, 120, 240	Act. & Pass. Avd. 1 T/D	DBA/2J - Facilitation Act. & Pass. Avd. C57BL/6J - No Difference
Wimer (1973)	SJL/J BDP/J	Ether SAT/RT	40	LRR & HBB	0	Act. & Pass. Avd. 1 T/D	SJL/J - Facilitation Pass. Avd. BDP/J - Facilitation Act. Avd.
Wimer et al (1974)	C57BL/6J DBA/2J	Ether SAT/RT	9	No LRR & No HB	0	Act. Avd. 1 T/D	DBA/2J - Facilitation C57BL/6J - No Difference

Simmerman et al (unpublished)	C57BL/6J DBA/2J	Ether SAT/RT	35	LRR & HB	0	Spatial Discrim. Water Maze 5 T/D	DBA/2J - Facilitation C57BL/6J - No Difference
Elias et al (unpublished)	C57BL/6J DBA/2J	Ether SAT/29.5°C	15	LRR & HB	0	Spatial Discrim. Water Maze 1 T/6 hr	DBA/2J - Decrement C57BL/6J - No Difference
Elias et al (1971)	C57BL/6 DBA/2J	Ether SAT/RT	35	LRR & HB	0	Spatial Discrim. Water Maze 2 T/D	DBA/2J - No Difference C57BL/6J - No Difference
Elias et al (unpublished)	C57BL/6J DBA/2J	Ether SAT/RT	35	LRR & HB	0	Spatial Discrim. Water Maze 2 T/D	DBA/2J - No Difference C57BL/6J - No Difference
Simmerman et al (unpublished)	C57BL/6J DBA/2J	Halothane (6 to 7% I.A.)	10	LRR & HB	0	Spatial Discrim. Water Maze	DBA/2J - No Difference C57BL/6J - No Difference
Elias et al (unpublished)	RI Strains[1] {Bailey, 1971}	Halothane (6%)	15	LRR	0	Spatial Discrim. Water Maze 1T/D	CXBD and BALB/cBy - Decrement All others - No Difference
Heinze (1974)	B,I,J, Hybrid BI,BJ,JI	Ether SAT/RT	NS	LRR + 15 sec	15	Pass. Avd. 1T/D	Decrement - all mice showed shorter latencies with a difference between the different types of mice

[1]RI Strains - Recombinant Inbred Strains

This is related to the fact that dosage parameters are more easily measured and specified for anesthetics which are injected in aqueous solutions or suspensions.

The Locus and Mechanisms of Anesthetic Effects

The fact that a wide variety of anesthetics produce retrograde amnesia is disappointing in terms of identification of the mechanisms by which anesthetics influence memory and provides little hope for identification of physiological substrates of the memory trace using comparisons among anesthetic agents as a research strategy. The anesthetic agents listed in Tables 1 to 5 have similar and dissimilar effects on the peripheral and central nervous system, and they influence a wide range of both diffuse and specific physiological changes. These changes are influenced by dose and duration of anesthetic treatment as well as temperature, partial pressure and other critical parameters of effective dosage level. Thus, the mechanisms by which they impair memory are most likely different under some conditions and similar under others. In short, it is difficult to dissociate the effects of anesthetization from the diffuse effects of various anesthetic agents.

In very general terms, the nonhydrogen bonding anesthetics appear to impair memory consolidation via a general depression of CNS activity. However, Porter (1972) calls attention to the fact that Winters and Wallach's (1970) electrophysiological data indicate that non-hydrogen bonding anesthetics do not act solely through general depression of CNS functions. Winters and Wallach (1970) recorded EEG from both cortical and subcortical sites, as well as recording multiple unit activity in the midbrain reticular formation. Results indicated either CNS excitation (increased multiple unit activity) or depression (decreased multiple unit activity) can occur simultaneously with observed behavioral depression.

Table 6 summarizes various CNS and peripheral nervous system effects of the most widely employed non-hydrogen bonding anesthetics and CO_2. It is clear from inspection of this table that most agents show an initial excitement stage followed by either increasing depression (halothane, ether) or further excitation (CO_2).

Of the agents listed, ether and CO_2 have been among the most widely employed in animal studies of memory consolidation. Ether is felt to interfere with the process of memory consolidation via a reduction in amplitude and frequency of electrical activity

(Pearlman, Sharpless & Jarvik, 1961). However, depressant effects
and interference with memory consolidation are dependent on dosage
level. At a surgical level of anesthetization, the amplitude and
frequency of EEG is reduced, but with light ether anesthesia sensory stimulation results in a generalized increase in afferent discharges to the cerebral cortex which occur after spontaneous cortical activity has been depressed.

While the disparity between findings of performance facilitation with light doses of ether (Table 4), and retrograde amnesia
with heavy doses of ether (Table 1) seems to make perfect sense
when the influence of dose level on CNS stimulation and depression
are taken into consideration, it cannot be concluded that CNS
excitation is the mechanism underlying memory facilitation. If
this were true, all drugs with predominantly excitatory effects
might be expected to facilitate memory consolidation. This is
clearly not the case. For example, increased level of CO_2 are
associated with increased nervous system excitation, yet CO_2 did
not produce learning facilitation in any of the studies summarized
in Table 2. In fact, the general finding was behavioral impairment or no effect. Furthermore, it is clear from inspection of
Table 4 that not all inbred strains exhibit the facilitation phenomenon in response to low doses of diethyl ether. Thus, the
important factors relative to facilitation (or inhibition), and
the time gradient of posttrial treatment effectiveness appear to
be the multiple mechanisms of anesthetics.

Explanations of decrements or facilitation in terms of excitation or depression of nervous system activity are oversimplifica-
tions. For diethyl ether alone, there are a number of CNS and PNS
effects which may explain its facilitative retrograde effects on memory. Wimer (1968) points out that diethyl ether (1) is a lipid solvent
and may influence neuron permeability, and thus learning via alterations in neuron permeability and membrane structure; (2) produces
an increase in brain glucose which may be related to either decreased brain metabolism or changes in glucose transport factors
(Mayman, Gatfield & Breckenridge, 1964); (3) alters the activity of

two probable brain transmitter substances increasing release of
norepinephrine (Voght, 1954) and altering activity of acethylcho-
line (Crossland & Merrick, 1954; Elliott, Swank & Henderson, 1950;
Hosein & Ara, 1962).

In discussing the neural basis of ether anesthesia, French,
Verzeans and Margoun (1953) and Davis, Dillon, Collins and Randt
(1958) point out that at anesthetic depth ether results in (1) reduction or block of impulses conducted corticopetally through the
multisynaptic medial brain stem system; (2) depression of cortical
excitation by afferent volleys over lateral brain stem pathways;
(3) elimination of the normal influences of the central cephalic
brain-stem activating system on the diencephalic and cortical structures; (4) depression of two-neuron and multineuron reflexes; (5)
depression of the spontaneous rhythmic activity of both the inter-
nuncial neurons and the motor neurons.

The diffuse nature of anesthetic effects, and the problems
involved in separating effects of different anesthetics on memory
from effects of anesthesia seem to indicate that little in the way
of information about the underlying physiological basis of memory
consolidation can be gained from comparing anesthetics. Attempts
have been made to learn something of the locus of anesthetic effects on memory by comparing non-anesthetic treatments and anesthetic agents which affect memory. "Locus of effect" has been investigated by comparing results of spreading cortical depression and
diethyl ether. Spreading cortical depression (SD) (Marshall, 1959)
refers to a slowly moving depression of cortical activity in response to electrical stimulation or other forms of stimulation.
Under appropriate conditions in the cerebral cortex, it proceeds
in all directions from the point of origin.

An important feature of spreading depression is a marked reduction in spontaneous and evoked activity of the involved area.
There is evidence that the effects of SD are due to interference
with cortical function as effects of the treatment do not appear
to spread to subcortical or limbic areas (Bureš, 1959; Weiss &

Fifková, 1961). Pearlman (1966) found that the effects of diethyl
ether and cortical spreading depressing were identical for a passive avoidance task presented to male albino rats of the Sprague
Dawley strain (110 days of age). These findings are interpreted
as suggesting a neocortical locus of action of anesthetic drugs in
the disruption of consolidation. However, other experiments have
reported less deficit in retention with spreading depression (Bureš
& Burešová, 1963) then with ether. Moreover, whether or not similar or dissimilar effects for ether and spreading cortical depression are obtained is highly dependent on the task employed (e.g.
Black, Suboski & Freedman, 1967). In short, cortical spreading depression effects do not seem to be a great deal more specific than
those of inhalation anesthetics. Pearlman points out that evidence for a diminution in activity of hypothalamic and nonspecific
thalamic nuclei and altered frequency of discharge in many units
of the reticular formation precludes evaluation of the possible
role of reverberatory cortico-diencephalic or cortico-reticular
circuits in consolidation.

     In view of the emphasis on chains of neuronal circuits, and
alterations in the physiochemical activities and structure of synapses as possible physiological substrates of learning and memory,
the selective action of anesthetics on synapses and axons is of
particular interest to the psychopharmacogeneticist. Anesthetic
agents, in suitable concentrations, depress various functions of
the CNS and leave, relatively unimpaired, the capacity for activity in the peripheral nerve fibers, sensory nerve endings and various effector organs (Larrabee & Posternak, 1952). Larrabee and
Posternak (1952) point out that this selective action on the CNS
is usually explained by assuming that synaptic mechanisms "are
more readily modified by anesthetics than is conduction or excitation in the peripheral nerves or end-organs" (p. 91). These investigators examined the degree of selectivity of a variety of anesthetics on axonic conduction versus synaptic transmission. These
and other studies of anesthetic selectivity at the axonic and synaptic level cannot be reviewed in this paper, but they are highly
relevant to investigators who may wish to test and build models
for memory consolidation based on the selective actions of anesthetics at the neuronal level.

     In terms of structural changes at the neuronal level, a re-
cent experiment by Ungar and Keats (1973) is of particular interest. They used as the basis of their experimental paradigm, the
fact that chick embryo cells dissociated with trypisin reaggre-
gate within a 24 hour period. Addition of six volatile anesthetics (chloroform, halothane, methoxyflurane, trichlorethylene,
ether and nitrous oxide) and five nonvolatile anesthetics (pentobarbital, thipental, ketamine, chloralose and urethane) to the
embryonic brain cell suspensions inhibited reaggregation in a dose-
-related manner. This inhibitory action was reversed by removal of

We (Elias & Simmerman, unpublished)[2] attempted to evaluate
the potential "punishing" of ether and halothane side effects for
a water maze escape discrimination escape task. Loss of righting
reflexes was used as the criterion for "light" anesthetization in
both instances and an attempt was made to closely equate, for each
anesthetic, the length of anesthetic exposure necessary to produce
loss of righting reflexes. Ether (a much more aversive inhalation
anesthetic than was halothane) was more effective in reducing incentive to escape than halothane and a blast of air (aversive control) was even more effective than ether. Halothane did not appear
to influence incentive to escape (swimming time to choice point)
when compared with handled controls. However, this was true only
for inbred strain DBA/2J. For inbred strain C57BL/6J, diethyl
ether was more effective than the blast of air. Neither anesthetic
agent affected error scores significantly. Our decision not to pub-
lish this data was related to our inability to explain the strain
X anesthetic agent interaction and even more important, our realization that there was simply no completely effective way in which
to equate all relevant variables with regard to dose level and anesthetic side effects simultaneously. Induction and recovery times
were dissimilar for both strains and for the two anesthetics regardless of the attempt to equate induction times. A recent study
(discussed later in the chapter) in which we (Elias, Elias &
Eleftheriou, unpublished)[3] compared strains with regard to respiration, heart rate, and blood pressure indicates that use of less
subjective indices of anesthetic depth does not represent a solution.

Dose Dependence

Cherkin and Harroun (1971) have noted that "The effect of an
anesthetic upon a wide variety of biological functions depends so
markedly upon its concentration that its effect on memory should
also be dose-dependent" (p. 471). The validity of this hypothesis
has been confirmed by the literature. We have already discussed
the fact that learning facilitation following posttrial administration of non-hydrogen bonding anesthetics has been reported for some
strains of mice and rats. It has also been observed with phenobar-
bitol for rats (Steinberg & Tomkiewicz, 1968). However, subanesthetic concentrations in man appear to depress memory formation
(Parkhouse, 1960; Rosen, 1959; Robson, Burns & Welt, 1960;
Parkhouse, Henrie, Duncan & Rome, 1960).

---

[2]Elias, M. F. and Simmerman, S. J. Effects of halothane, ether and
air-blast on incentive to perform in a water maze for inbred strains
DBA/2J and C57BL/6J (Unpublished, partially reported in Elias &
Simmerman, 1971).

[3]Elias, P. K., Elias, M. F. and Eleftheriou, B. E. A genetic investigation of systolic blood pressure in the RI strains; an unpublished study performed at the Jackson Laboratory (in preparation).

There are several reasons for this apparent inconsistency.
(1) For animals, memory facilitation has been observed with ether,
but many studies of subanesthetic concentrations in man have been
done with nitrous oxide; (2) the retrograde amnesia paradigm has
been used with animals, but it has not been as widely employed with
humans. Thus, the nature of the designs used in human studies
makes it difficult to separate the variables of information input,
short-term storage, and recall. It is possible that light anesthetic doses depress or have a disorganizing effect on information input, but facilitate consolidation. The former effect may be more
pronounced than the latter. These hypotheses await resolution by
experiments using human research design paradigms that permit separation of input and memory factors as well as careful control of
premedication factors.

The mechanisms of action of anesthetic on sensory input mechanisms are difficult to separate from effects on memory consolidation and recall in studies which do not employ strict retroactive
amnesia paradigms. Nevertheless, these studies have important clinical implication. Light anesthetic doses are utilized for a number
of surgical procedures, e.g., heart surgery. In these instances,
it is highly desirable to eliminate unpleasant memories of traumatic experiences.

It is clear that general anesthesia does not result in a complete block of neural function. Cherkin and Harroun (1971) indicate that information processing for different sensory modalities
is affected selectively. For example, the auditory system of the
cat and the visual system of the mouse remain functional at planes
of anesthesia which depress the reticular formation to a level of
unconsciousness (Mori, Winters & Spooner, 1968; Domino, 1967).
During ether or barbiturate anesthesia in animals, painful stimuli
evoke electrical responses in the cerebral cortex, although they
are not observed in the reticular system (Arduini & Arduini, 1954).
In addition, data from studies by Berger (1970) and Lico, Hoffman
and Covian (1968) indicate that elementary forms of learning may
occur under anesthesia. Lico et al. (1968) demonstrated classical
conditioning at a "neurovegetative" level. Berger demonstrated
that simple associative learning might possibly occur under urethane anesthesia.

Comparison of the studies involving different dose levels of the anesthetics. Addition of these anesthetics to the cells after aggregation resulted in a break up of aggregates. Inhibition of aggregation was not produced by local anesthetics and several central nervous system stimulants and depressants; neither was it produced by acetylcholine, serotonin, histamine or their antagonists. In fact, these neurotransmitters resulted in an accelerated aggregation. The aggregation process was actually accelerated by epinephrine, norepinephrine, dopamine and, to a lesser extent, γ-aminobutyric acid (GABA).

These findings led Ungar and Keats (1973) to speculate that

"The remarkable specificity of the effect for general anesthetics of such diverse chemical composition, both volatile and nonvolatile, suggests some more direct relationship with anesthesia. One could speculate that anesthetics--which not only prevented aggregation but broke up preformed aggregates--can perhaps loosen synaptic connections either anatomically or, at least, functionally. Such an effect could adequately explain anesthesia by a loss of synaptic transmission. That the several central neurotransmitters studied exerted an opposite effect and accelerated aggregation might even support if one could find a gradient of sensitivity to anesthetic agents between cells taken from the higher and lower centers of the brain." (p. 369).

If such a gradient were to be obtained it would be consistent with the Hughlings Jackson Law (1884) which states that behaviors reflecting higher cortical functioning are depressed first, and then followed by lower order behaviors associated with subcortical structures. Not only are these data interesting in view of memory consolidation models which suggest physiological and chemical alterations in the synapse as a basis for retrograde amnesia (or facilitated learning), but they have implications for possible permanent structural and functional changes as a result of prolonged exposure to volatile anesthetics, particularly during very critical periods of development. Space does not permit further review of related studies, but the literature on cell reaggregation is of importance in view of the possible role of proteins in memory and learning. For example, studies indicate that specific proteins on cellular surfaces produce aggregation and that reaggregation of trypsin-disassociated cells does not take place in the presence of protein synthesis inhibitors (Moscona & Moscona, 1963; Nakanishi, Katao & Twasaki, 1963). These data are of interest in view of the growing amount of evidence that protein synthesis is in some way involved in long term memory consolidation (McGaugh, 1966), e.g. memory consolidation in mice and goldfish seems to be impaired by intercranial injections of the protein synthesis inhibitor, puromycin.

The literature dealing with functional responses and structural changes in the neurons may eventually lead to the description of memory consolidation processes in something other than purely hypothetical terms. However, characterization of the "physiology" of memory consolidation will not be possible unless functional and structural responses to anesthesia can be related to the time gradient of anesthetic effectiveness either in terms of facilitation or inhibition of memory consolidation. This is an extremely difficult task because not only are functional and structural responses to anesthesia influenced by genotype, but genotype interacts with environmental and developmental factors in such a complex fashion that it is difficult to design adequate descriptive studies let alone to establish relationships between behavioral change and physiological changes in response to anesthesia and to relate correlated physiological and behavioral phenomenon to specific genes.

The minimum qualifications for undertaking a research program designed to characterize the physiology of memory consolidation seems to be an understanding of the critical environmental-treatment and developmental factors which interact both with genotype and anesthetic parameters. Relatively few treatment or environmental factors do not interact with genotype, and thus one may generate a long list of potentially relevant parameters. It is possible to discuss a number of the most important environmental-treatment factors and developmental factors which play a major role in anesthetic effects on behavior.

Critical Environmental and Developmental Variables

Porter's (1972) comparative-statistical analysis of retrograde amnesia studies identified the following variables as particularly critical in terms of their influence on memory facilitation or amnesia resulting from administration of non-hydrogen bonding anesthetics: (1) anesthetic agent; (2) drug dose; (3) trial-treatment interval; (4) type of training task; (5) species; (6) type of task; (7) age; (8) sex; (9) interval between training and retention, and (10) other, e.g., a variety of environmental factors and circadian rhythms.

Amnestic Agent

Porter listed only two studies that compared different non-hydrogen bonding anesthetics in a single experiment. Mazzia and Randt (1966) compared effects of nitrous oxide, ether, halothane, and cyclopropane on man. Schmid (1964) compared effects of nitrous oxide, ether, carbon dioxide and chloroform on bees. Neither study showed differences in performance between treatment and control groups or differences among anesthetics. However, neither investigation employed a design that permitted an unconfounded evaluation of retrograde amnesia.

Anesthetic agents have been compared with other amnestic
agents within a single study. Paolino, Quartermain and Miller
(1966) found that the effective trial-treatment interval was
much shorter for ECS induced amnesia than for CO_2 induced amnesia.
Data by Galluscio (1971), among others, indicate that ECS is a
much more effective amnesic agent than CO_2, even under circumstances where both treatments produce seizures. In a study by
Pearlman, et al.(1961), pentobarbital was more effective than ether
in impairing retention and the treatment-trial effectiveness interval was longer. However, this finding may have been related to a
longer sleeping time with pentobarbital, or differences in anesthetic depth that could not be detected by examination of superficial reflexes. In this same study, a single pentylenetetrazol
convulsion resulted in marked impairment of retention up to eight
hours, and the effective trial-treatment interval was four days.
In contrast, the maximum trial-treatment effectiveness interval
for the anesthetics (ether and pentobarbital) was 15 min.

Porter (1972) performed statistical analyses designed to permit interstudy comparisons of anesthetic effectiveness and reported the following ordering in terms of "amnestic potency": carbon
dioxide, other (halothane, mixed anesthetics, and miscellaneous)
ether and nitrous oxide. He cautions the reader that the average
doses of nitrous oxide were generally low and that this factor
could account for their low level of amnestic potency. Clearly,
anesthetic effects on behavior are so highly dependent on dosage
that it is difficult to compare anesthetic effectiveness for studies using different dosages of different anesthetics. Many of
the studies reviewed by Porter (1972) are summarized in Tables 1
to 4. It is quite clear that they differed in many respects other
than anesthetic agent.

Comparison of anesthetic agents within a single study is not
a simple matter either. Dosage of different anesthetics are not
always specified in the same way and if they are specified in the
same way (percent concentration in inspired air) it is difficult
to equate percent concentrations of two anesthetics in terms of
effective concentrations. One solution is to use the animal's
vital signs, EEG, EKG, blood pressure, respiration, loss of righting reflexes, as criteria for effectiveness. This is a difficult
task because various anesthetics have unique effects on different
CNS and autonomic responses (Table 6) and time-to-induction as
measured by means of loss of righting reflexes does not guarantee
equal duration of effects for two different anesthetics. Moreover,
it is impossible to eliminate side effects such as those associated with administration of an anesthetic like diethyl ether, e.g.,
respiratory irritation, bronchial spasms. Many clinicians (e.g.,
M.B. Chenoweth in Bunker & Vandam, 1965) have commented on the un-
reliability of vital signs as a precise index of anesthetic depth.

the various anesthetics (Tables 1-3), Herz, Peeke and Wyers, 1966;
compared with Herz, 1962; Quinton, 1966; Alpern and Kimble, 1967
indicate that higher doses of amnestic agents are more likely to
produce amnesia. Increased duration of anesthetization is also
positively correlated with increased amnestic effect, as reflected
in the amount of information recalled (Herz, 1962; Herz et al., 1966;
Paolino et al., 1966; Quinton, 1966), although Porter's (1972) comparative analysis of the literature indicates that duration is less
strongly correlated with increasing amnesia than is dosage and
trial-treatment interval. It is difficult to separate the factors
of dosage and duration because effective dosage depends, in part,
upon duration and other factors such as the temperature of the volatile anesthetics (Cherkin, 1968b; Elias, Blenkarn, Simmerman &
Marsh, 1971). If consolidation continues for a finite period of
time after sensory input, anesthetics with prolonged durations
should be more effective consolidation blocking-agents than those
of short duration. Based on an observed correlation of 0.7 between
duration and behavioral effect in his statistical comparison among
studies, Porter (1972) has suggested that the drugs which saturate
the tissue slowly (e.g. ether) should provide clearer evidence of
duration-dependent behavioral effects than those which saturate
more slowly (nitrous oxide). However, the time course of memory
consolidation is difficult to establish by comparing different dosage levels of a single anesthetic because memory consolidation may
involve qualitatively different steps which are differentially affected by different anesthetic agents (Paolino et al., 1966).
Again, we see that the difficulty resides in the separation of
effects of anesthesia from the effects of anesthetics.

Time Gradient of Effectiveness

Inspection of Table 5 provides an indication of the trial-
-treatment interval of effectiveness for several anesthetic agents.
We have already noted that the increased probability of successful
inhibition or facilitation of behavioral response relative to controls is associated with decreased trial-treatment intervals. Regardless of dose level, effective treatments are most always observed with less than a 30 second interval. This finding is consistent with the hypothesis that memory consolidation is most vulnerable to disruption during a period which involves conduction of
neuronal impulses and biochemical alterations which are presumably
associated with perseveration of the hypothetical short-term memory
trace. However, depending on the dosage level, duration of anesthetization and other factors, amnesic effects have been observed

Table 5

Time Course of Anesthetic Effectiveness: Effective Treatment - Trial Intervals

Table Explanation

Strain: NS = strain not stated

Age: NS = not stated in report

Task: Pass. Avd. = passive avoidance; Act. Avd. = active avoidance; Disc. Avd. = discrimination avoidance.

Dosage: %I.A. = percent inspired air; NS = not stated; SAT = saturated; RT = room temperature

Effect: results as compared to controls

Time course: the effect of various Trial-Treatment intervals on behavior and performance.

0,5)10>15|20   Total effect at 0 and 5; partial effect at 10 which is greater than

15; no effect at 20.

Author	Anesthetic	Strain	Age (days)	Task	Dosage (time & %I.A.)	Effect	Time Course
Ransmeier et al (1954)	Ether	Hamsters	NS	Maze learning	"anesthesia"[1] NS/RT	No difference	1,2

Reference	Agent	Species/Strain		Task	Condition	Effect	Results
Abt et al (1961)	Ether	Mice - Swiss Webster	28	1T Disc. Avd.	40 sec NS/RT	Decrement	0,2,8}>16> 20|24
Pearlman et al (1961)	Ether	Rats - Sprague Dawley	90-120	Pass. Avd. of bar press	35 sec SAT/RT	Decrement	0.16> 5|10
Gutekunst et al(1963)	Ether	Chick - New Hampshire red	1	Imprinting	"anesthesia"[1] NS/RT	Decrement	0>15>30
Pearlman (1966)	Ether	Rats - Sprague Dawley	110	Pass. Avd.	60 sec SAT/RT	Decrement	1>5>10>15
Essman et al (1961)	Ether	Mice - Swiss Webster	21	Pass. Avd.	36 sec SAT/RT	Decrement	0}|60
Alpern et al (1967)	Potentiated ether	Mice - Swiss Webster	60	Pass. Avd.	60 sec SAT/RT	Decrement	0}>60>120>240 >1440
Wimer et al (1968)	Ether	Mice - C57BL/6J DBA/2J	30	Pass. Avd.	35 sec SAT/RT	Facilitation for DBA/2J; No effect for C57BL/6J	0|60,120
Suboski et al (1968)	Ether	Rats - Long Evans	NS	Maze learning	100 sec SAT/37.7°C	Facilitation	1.66>53

Study	Anesthetic	Species		Task	Conditions	Criterion	Results[1]
Herz (1969)	Ether	Mice – Swiss Webster	60	Appetitive adversive learning	NS SAT/30–35°C	Decrement	0.01>0.25 >0.5>1.0
Dye (1969)	Ether	Rats Holtzman	1,330–360,660–720	Disc. learning	180 sec NS/RT	Decrement	3>15>30
Taber (1966)	CO_2	Mice CF 1	NS	Pass. Avd.	Gas from dry ice	Decrement	0>5>15>30|60, 120
Leukel et al (1964)	CO_2	Rats NS	90–180	Act. Avd.	2.5 1/min for 10 & 40 sec	Decrement	0.16|5,30,60
Paulino et al (1966)	CO_2	Rats Holtzman	90–120	Pass. Avd.	25 sec; 15 sec; 10 sec	Decrement	0.03>1>2>3 4|5,30; 0.3>1>2|3, 4,5,30; 0.03,1,2, 4,5,30
Bohdanecky et al (1967)	Flurothyl	Mice CF 1	60–70	Pass. Avd.	20 microliter in 250 ml flask	Decrement	0>5>50> 360>700
Alpern et al (1967)	Flurothyl	Mice – Swiss Webster	60	Pass. Avd.	20 microliter in 250 flask for 60 sec	Decrement	0>60>120> 240|1440
Cherkin (1969)	Flurothyl	Chicks – white leg horn	2	Pass. Avd.	range 0.43% v/v 3.0%v/v for 1–16 min	Decrement	4>...>1440|2880

[1] **Subjective criteria**

up to a four hour posttrial-treatment interval. As noted previously, it is difficult to resolve the differences from study to study
in effective posttrial-treatment interval because different drugs
are used, different testing procedures are used, and different
strains and stocks of animals are employed.

Cherkin (1966a) has described a "probit analysis" method for
reducing the conflict regarding the values for effective posttrial
treatment. He suggests (1) the use of a consolidation half-time
(CT_{50}) which is defined as the interval at which the experimental
subjects emit one-half of the control responses, and (2) the use of
probit transformation for precise determination of CT_{50} and its
confidence limits.

Learning Task

In view of the fact that components of behavior, input, memory
consolidation, and retrieval, motor response, visual discrimination,
are differentially affected by anesthetics and in view of the fact
that higher cortical centers seem to be more readily affected by
given anesthetic doses than lower brain stem structures, it would
be quite unusual to find that task parameters do not play a major
role in results of anesthetic experiments.

Porter's (1972) interstudy analysis included an ordering of
tasks in terms of increasing amnesic susceptibility: human learning tasks, animal approach learning, multiple-trial avoidance
learning, 1-trial passive avoidance learning. He notes that while
partial correlations and step-wise regression confirmed this ordering of tasks, lowered incidence of amnesic effects on human learning tasks may be due to the wide spread use of low doses of nitrous
oxide for human subjects. We would add to this observation that
doses of anesthetics (e.g., halothane and other) for animal experiments generally exceed, by a considerable amount, the normal safe
levels used in human surgical procedures and controlled clinical
studies.

One-trial passive avoidance learning is not only the most susceptible type of learning (Porter, 1972), it offers some methodological advantages when used in the retroactive amnesia design paradigm. Amnesia is inferred from a failure to avoid punishment and
hence not easily explained in terms of the potentially negative reinforcing properties of posttrial anesthetization. Most important,
one exposure to the anesthetic is less likely to produce a situa-

Table 6

Some common effects of inhalation anesthetics used

in behavioral studies[1]

___

Ether

Circulation: Increased heart rate due to catecholamine release

             Decreased heart force with increasing dose

             Decreased peripheral resistance

             Normal blood pressure but decreases as anesthesia deepens

             Dilation of cerebral blood vessels

Respiration: Increased depth and rate

             Decreased amplitude as anesthesia becomes deeper

Central and peripheral nervous system: Increased sympathetic nervous system activity

             Decreased parasympathetic nervous system activity

             Cortex, brain stem activating system, reflex arcs in the spinal cord
             are all depressed

             EEG cortical activity is depressed in later stages of anesthesia

             Release of norepinephrine and epinephrine

Halothane

Circulation: Decrease blood pressure with increasing concentrations

             Peripheral vasodilation

             Decreased peripheral resistance

             Increased cerebral blood flow via direct vasodilation

Respiration: Decrease in rate and depth with increasing concentration

Central and peripheral nervous system: Depressed cortical centers and as the
             anesthesia deepens lower cerebral centers are affected

             Little emergence of excitement

             Decreases efferent sympathetic nervous activity

             Muscle relaxation more complete as deeper planes of anesthesia
             are reached

___

[1]The information for this table was taken from the following sources:

- A.M.A. Fundamentals of Anesthetics (1954);
- Gray and Nunn (1971);
- Woodbury, Rollins, Gardner, Hirschi, Hoyan, Rallison, Tanner and Brodie (1958);
- Goodman and Gilman (1970).

Table 6 (Cont'd)

N_2O

Circulation: No change in heart rate, rhythm, and output until the deeper planes
                of surgical anesthesia

                No change in blood pressure and peripheral resistance if no hypoxia

Respiration: Deeper and more rapid in early stages

                Less rapid and shallow in later stages

Central and peripheral nervous system: Minimal EEG changes

                No depression of reflexes

                Rapidly depressed cortical functions with all sense modalities
                affected

                Depression of thalamic centers but hypothalamic centers are not
                depressed

                No relaxation of muscles

CO_2[2]

Circulation: Increase in heart rate, cardiac output and pulse pressure

                Dilation of cerebral circulation

                Increase blood flow to brain and skin capillaries

                Increase in systolic blood pressure

Respiration: Increase rate and depth but above 10% concentration there is no increase

Central and peripheral nervous system: Excitation of sympathetic nerve endings

                Low concentrations depress the excitability of the cerebral cortex

                Excitation of the reticular activating systems and arousal of
                cerebral cortex

                Enhanced activity of neurons in the hypothalamus

                Progressive depression up to 150 mm Hg, excitation during which
                convulsions may occur when above 150 mm Hg and a progressive
                depression of cerebral activity when above 40% CO_2.

[2]Strictly speaking, not an inhalation anesthetic.

tion whereby (1) aversive properties of anesthesia are associated repeatedly with the behavioral response; (2) the cumulative effects of hypoxia or hypercarbia from poor anesthetic technique result in brain damage. However, it is obvious that the experimenter's battery of behavior tests cannot be limited to a single task if he is to sort out the various parameters which are affected by learning.

The ordering of tasks with regard to susceptibility to anesthesia suggests that fear-mediated responses may be highly vulnerable to disruption by anesthetic agents (Porter, 1972). On the other hand, animal approach learning tasks involving imprinting (Gutekunst & Youniss, 1963; Bloch, 1970) and drinking (Herz, 1969) are not impervious to retrograde amnesia effects.

Species

Differences between man and infrahuman subjects in behavior susceptibility to anesthetics is difficult to determine because the average doses used for animals would be unacceptable for safe use with humans. Comparisons among infrahuman subjects (Tables 1 to 4) are compromised by the fact that different species of animals use different modes of responding. Thus, swimming through flurothyl (Table 3) may be expected to have a different effect on behavior than flurothyl anesthetization in a closed chamber following a discrete learning trial. In the former case, it is difficult to separate sensory-input and motor-output effects from effects on memory consolidation per se.

In terms of findings of behavior decrements relative to controls, Porter's (1972) review of the literature on non-hydrogen bonding anesthetics revealed effects in a variety of species such as rats and mice, monkeys (Jarvik, 1964), chicks (Cherkin & Lee-Teng, 1965), and cockroaches (Freckleton & Wahlstein, 1968). Species differences exist in toxicity for various anesthetics such as chloroform and flurothyl (Cherkin, 1969). Anesthetics which are appropriate for use in human surgery for various procedures are not necessarily appropriate for animals lower on the phylogenetic scale such as mice[4].

---

[4] Combinations of drugs appropriate for surgery with man are often not the anesthetics of choice for rodents.

Buchsbaum and Buchsbaum (1962) point out that age differences in response to ether paralleled findings in previous studies with regard to age differences in rate of breathing, heart rate, and diffusing capacity of the lung. More rapid breathing, more rapid heart rate, and higher diffusing capacity of the lungs appear to produce faster intoxication in young mice than in older mice for which these processes are slower. The U-shaped curve for recovery times, and the absence of an induction-recovery correlation for the younger and older groups was explained in terms of variable physiological and behavioral responses in the extreme age groups as opposed to the middle aged group. The authors suggest that the response of mice to ether anesthesia can be used as a measure of physiological aging. We suggest that response to anesthesia may possibly reflect factors which themselves provide a reasonable index of functional aging. It is possible that responses observed by Buchsbaum and Buchsbaum (1962) were related to hypoxia-producing and aversive properties of ether which influenced the behavior of younger and older mice in such a way that physiological mechanisms were affected in a closed-loop feedback relationship. Thus, the correlations between physiological response and ether are confounded by correlations between behavioral response and ether. This confounding may be particularly serious when saturated dosages of ether are used as they may be highly aversive, and influence behavior via mechanisms which are partially unrelated to intoxication and detoxification mechanisms.

Dye (1969) tested male albino rats of the Holtzman albino strain, and found no age × treatment (ether) interaction for retention of a maze habit, although retention was poorer for the middle aged (11 to 12 months) than for the young (1 month) and old groups (22-23 months), all groups performed more poorly as the trial--treatment interval decreased. In contrast to Buchsbaum and Buchsbaum's (1962) findings with DBA/2J mice, the three age groups showed no differences in induction and recovery times. Thus, only meager evidence suggests a U-shaped relationship between recovery from anesthesia and age. Moreover, it seems that explanations in terms of hormonal differences with advancing age (Elias & Elias, 1975), aversive stimulation, and hypoxia or hypercarbia (Elias, Blenkarn, Simmerman & Marsh, 1971) are as reasonable as those which relate findings to lung permeability, breathing rate, and heart output. Failure to obtain treatment-age interactions for complex behavioral responses such as maze learning (Dye, 1969) may be related to the fact that the oldest group of rats tested was 23 months of age. Treatment × age interactions for anesthetics may

Age

With the exception of a study dealing with chronic exposure to halothane (discussed in a later section), there have been surprisingly few developmental studies at the lower end of the life-span. Studies at the aged end of the life-span have been few in number relative to single age group studies with young adult animals. This is surprising in view of the fact that short-term memory processes (registration and retrieval) may become less efficient with increasing age (Craik, 1968). From a clinical standpoint the combined stresses of anesthesia and surgery as they affect behavior in elderly persons is of considerable importance.

Direct tests of perseveration-consolidation theory with aged groups have been few in number. In a study by Thompson (1957), retention of a discrimination habit following posttrial ECS, young albino "Harlin rats" (30-42 days) were significantly inferior to adults (195-310 days) with a 15 sec. treatment-trial but not with a 30 sec. treatment-trial interval. Streicher and Garbus (1955) found sex and age differences in the recovery time of Sprague Dawley rats from hexobarbital. The sexually mature females remained under the effects of anesthesia four times as long as males of the same age. This difference was not observed for young or old mice. Differences are explained in terms of sex hormone levels.

Buchsbaum and Buchsbaum (1962) report a study by Sajner (1957) in which "ether consumption" of "juvenile and adult mice" was compared. Results indicated that the younger the animal the relatively greater is the resistance to ether per unit weight. However, Buchsbaum and Buchsbaum (1962) point out that expressing the results in terms of weight is not reasonable because the effective dosage is unknown and is determined by such factors as lung permeability, breathing rate and heart output. These investigators compared mice of inbred strain DBA/2 ranging in age from 2 weeks to 35 months. Animals were exposed to temperature-potentiated and saturated ether atmospheres in a closed chamber (29 to 33ºC). Induction times increased with increasing age. Females, 1 month and older, were generally more resistant than males. Recovery times were longer for younger (0.5 to 1.0 months) and older, (8 months to 20+ months) than for the middle aged mice (2 to 8 months). Older and younger mice were more variable than middle aged mice and showed lower anesthesia induction/recovery time ratios. In addition, induction time and recovery time were not correlated for very old and very young mice.

become apparent for older rats, for shorter lived strains, or for
rodents that are physiologically impaired, diseased, or subjected
to the joint stresses of surgery and anesthesia.

Sex

Aside from Buchsbaum and Buchsbaum's (1962) work, few studies
have dealt with sex differences in retrograde amnesic effects despite the fact that sex is a critical variable in drug sensitivity
and response (Goodman & Gilman, 1970). Porter (1972) commented
that the few data available for his review did not indicate sex
differences in memory sensitivity to the non-hydrogen bonding anesthetics. However, it would be surprising if the sex factor were to
be found unimportant in view of the literature on: (a) hormones,
aging and behavior (Elias & Elias, 1975); (b) ECS and the estrous cycle (Klemm, 1969); and (c) neuroendocrine based sex differences in cognition (Nash, 1970; Hutt, 1972; Freedman, Richart &
Van de Wiele, 1974); (d) differences in information processing strategies for males and females (Elias & Kinsbourne, 1974). The
importance of sex as a variable in memory and anesthetic research
clearly does not imply inferiority of either sex with regard to
memory processes, rather that the processing of information may be
somewhat different due to environmental and sex-linked biochemical
differences which may interact with differences in response to
drugs.

Circadian Rhythm

Circadian rhythm has long been recognized as a critical factor
in response to drugs (Nelson & Halberg, 1973; Munson, Mallrucci &
Smith, 1973; Matthews, Marte & Hallberg, 1964). A lethal dosage
at one period of the day-night cycle may result in no mortality at
another. Similarly, conculsion resulting from ether and other
drugs are influenced by circadian rhythms (Moore-Ede, 1973). The
reader may wish to consult a paper by Moore-Ede for a summary of
studies dealing with rodent susceptibility to various drugs, including several anesthetics, at various times of the day-night cycle.

Few experimenters have compared different behavior testing
schedules with retrograde amnesia paradigms. The extent to which
testing at different periods of the day-night cycle accounts for
inconsistencies in the literature is unknown because these data are
reported infrequently. Aside from the influence of circadian
rhythm on susceptibility to anesthetics, considerable behavior

variation has been noted for a variety of species at various periods of the day-night cycle (Elias & Elias, in press a; Jakubczak, 1970). Circadian variations in baseline levels of performance may interact with circadian variations in susceptibility to anesthesia in a very complex manner. Aside from methodological issues, the question of circadian variation in behavioral responses to anesthetics is quite important from a clinical standpoint.

Premedication

Premedication is an obvious factor of importance in evaluating the effectiveness of anesthetics, and it can be used as a research tool (Wimer, 1968). It will be discussed more fully in a later section. Animal studies generally do not need to be concerned with unavoidable confounding of premedication schedules and posttrial anesthetic treatments. It is interesting to note that few animal studies indicate the use of routine procedures to prevent respiratory, gastrointestinal or upper respiratory complications during retrograde amnesia experiments.

Training-Retention Interval

There was such a high concentration of data at the 24 hour retention testing interval that it was not possible for Porter (1972) to undertake a comparative analysis of this factor. However, he calls attention to the importance of this variable in terms of the estimation of the time course of memory formation and decay. He cites studies indicating an increase or decrease in retention with time, depending on the range of test periods (McGaugh, 1966; Irwin, Banuazizi, Kalsner & Curtis, 1968; Cherkin, 1971).

It is somewhat unfortunate that so few studies have employed intervals other than 24 hr. If memory consolidation has been affected by the amnestic treatment then intervals greater than 24 hours should also show a decrement in memory retention. The confounding of residual anesthetic effects on physiological mechanisms other than memory and the effects of the anesthetic on memory consolidation can be evaluated by retesting at intervals considerably greater than 24 hr. The case for disruption of memory consolidation would be much stronger if a number of studies indicated impaired retention for a number of days or weeks after posttrial or post-learning treatments.

Table 7

Effects of Halothane on Induction and Recovery Times[1] for Bailey's
(1971) RI Strains, the Progenitor Strains and the Reciprocal F_1
Hybrids. Means (sec) and Standard Deviations for all Groups with
Solid Lines Indicating Means which are Nonsignificantly Different
from each Other.

Induction Scores

	2 percent		3 percent		4 percent
G	110 (33)	C	44 (22)	D	27 (05)
J	109 (44)	H	43 (09)	BCF_1	27 (05)
CBF_1	106 (38)	CBF_1	42 (09)	H	26 (05)
C	106 (26)	J	41 (07)	C	26 (03)
BCF_1	94 (33)	D	41 (07)	CBF_1	25 (06)
E	90 (33)	G	41 (07)	G	25 (04)
D	86 (22)	BCF_1	41 (09)	I	25 (03)
K	86 (19)	E	41 (07)	K	24 (04)
I	80 (44)	K	39 (07)	J	24 (04)
H	67 (13)	I	38 (07)	E	24 (05)
B6	62 (18)	B6	32 (06)	B6	18 (04)

Eduction Scores

	2 percent		3 percent		4 percent
H	28 (18)	D	47 (08)	H	41 (08)
D	24 (06)	H	32 (17)	I	36 (16)
CBF_1	24 (09)	B6	29 (05)	J	35 (12)
B6	22 (16)	CBF_1	28 (13)	B6	33 (06)
BCF_1	22 (09)	I	28 (11)	D	33 (05)
E	21 (09)	K	26 (16)	CBF_1	31 (07)
K	20 (08)	J	25 (13)	G	31 (08)
I	20 (06)	E	24 (11)	BCF_1	30 (06)
C	17 (07)	BCF_1	24 (08)	E	29 (07)
G	16 (07)	G	22 (09)	K	28 (07)
J	15 (11)	C	18 (09)	C	25 (07)

[1] Taken from M. F. Elias and B. E. Eleftheriou, A genetic investigation of induction
and recovery times for halothane anesthesia. Behavior Methods and Research
Instrumentation.

Environmental and Other Variables

Many variables, in addition to those reviewed here, have important influences on the organism's response to anesthesia. Temperature, humidity, handling, prior experience, disease, diet, season, lighting and so on all have important influences on response to drug treatments. Most important, each of these variables, and each of the variables reviewed in this section, is a potential source of interaction with genotype.

GENOTYPE × TREATMENT INTERACTIONS

Induction and Recovery

In the previous section we reviewed studies which indicate that the behavioral effects of anesthetics are dose-dependent and that induction and recovery (eduction) times vary with age. Studies with halothane, conducted in our laboratory and at the Jackson Laboratory with B. E. Eleftheriou, suggest that induction and eduction times for halothane anesthesia are dose-dependent (as would be expected), but the relationship between induction and eduction at each dosage level seems to be related to similar and dissimilar sets of polygenes.

Tables 7 and 8 summarize the results of a study with Bailey's (1971) RI strains (see Chapter 1 of this text) in which induction (loss of righting reflexes) and eduction times (regaining of righting reflexes) were measured for three dosages of halothane represented as percent concentrations in the anesthetic chamber atmosphere: $2 \pm .5$; $3 \pm .5$, and $4 \pm .5$. In this study, halothane was delivered to a ventilated chamber via a Fluometric Mark IV halothane vaporizer and monitored with a Nack Vondershmitt MT/672-2 infrared analyzer. Details of the anesthetic apparatus and the procedures of anesthetization are presented in detail in a previous publication (Elias & Eleftheriou, in press a).

Data for the two sexes are combined in Tables 7 and 8 because interactions with sex were nonsignificant with and without adjustment of induction scores for age and body weight by means of covariance analyses. However, it is apparent from inspection of these tables that the strain × dose (% concentration) interaction was significant for induction and eduction scores. Induction times decreased and eduction (recovery) times increased with increasing concentrations of halothane vapor for all groups compared, but

Table 8

Effects of Halothane on Induction and Recovery Times[1] for Bailey's (1971) RI Strains, the Progenitor Strains and the Reciprocal F_1 Hybrids. Group Correlations between Induction Times and Eduction Times and between Percent Halothane Concentration for Induction and Eduction.

Between Doses Induction	r	Between Doses Eduction	r	Between Induction & Eduction r_s	
2% – 3%	.55*	2% – 3%	.58*	2%	$r = -.62$**
2% – 4%	.46	2% – 4%	.46	3%	$r = -.17$
3% – 4%	.75**	3% – 4%	.49	4%	$r = -.04$

* $P < .05$ one tailed test.

** $P < .01$ one tailed test.

[1]Taken from M. F. Elias and B. E. Eleftheriou, A genetic investigation of induction and recovery times for halothane anesthesia. Behavior Methods and Research Instrumentation. Taken by permission of the editor.

these induction and eduction scores were significantly different
for the different strains and the F_1 hybrids when multiple comparisons were done (Newman-Keuls test) within levels of concentration.
The results of multiple contrasts are summarized by connecting lines
for means which do not differ significantly ($\underline{p} > .05$). Several overlapping groupings of means, nonsignificantly different from each
other, were observed for contrasts at 2 percent halothane. Similar
results were obtained for induction and eduction times at the 4
percent concentration condition. Results were less complex at the
3 percent condition. Here, progenitor strain C57BL/6By (B6) exhibited a significantly shorter induction time than either of the F_1
hybrids and all other strains with the exception of CXBK and CXBI.
Strain CXBD exhibited significantly longer eduction times than all
other strains and both hybrids. In general, comparisons of strain
patterns for induction and eduction and for all dose levels reveal
that the pattern of strain means differed significantly, although
strain B6 (C57BL/6By) exhibited the longest induction scores consistently.

The relationship between induction times for different dose
levels, eduction times for different dose levels, and induction
and eduction times at each dose level were examined by calculating
Pearson product-moment correlations for the 11 means representing
each group and by calculating within group correlations. Within
cell (group) correlations were low and nonsignificant (r_s range
= 0.01 to -0.04). Table 8 summarizes results of correlations for
the 11 group means representing the RI strains, progenitor strains
and the reciprocal F_1 hybrids. Correlations between successively
increasing dose levels were generally significant. Thus, some
amount of variance among means at one dose level can be predicted
by inspection of variance among means at another dose level. Moreover, low and nonsignificant within-group correlations in the presence of significant between-group correlations suggests that some
sets of common genes affect induction time at 2% and 3% and at 2%
and 4% dose levels, and eduction times for 2% and 3% dose levels.

Correlations between induction and eduction were not significant for the 3 and 4 percent halothane concentrations. However,
the significant negative correlation between induction and eduction
scores for the 2 percent halothane condition (Table 8) indicates
that strain distribution patterns for induction times tend to be
the inverse of those observed for eduction times. Close examination of the strain distribution patterns (Table 7) and the magni-

tude of the correlation (Table 8) indicates that the inverse relationship is considerably less than perfect (38 percent common
variance). The presence of this low significant negative correlation suggests that several of the same genes affect induction and
eduction at 2 percent. The range of induction and eduction means
was more restricted at the 3 and 4 percent halothane conditions.
This phenomenon may account for the low and nonsignificant induction-
-eduction correlations at these higher dose (concentration) levels.
Thus, it is not possible to conclude that sets of common genes do
not affect induction and eduction times at these higher doses. It
is clear, however, that prediction of the strain distribution pattern for eduction times from examination of induction times is not
possible for the 3% and 4% concentrations.

The fact that different strain (and hybrid) distribution
patterns are obtained for different concentrations of halothane
vapor suggests that induction and eduction times in response to
various concentrations of halothane in the anesthetic chamber are
merely end points of a complex multigenic system which interacts
with anesthetic dose levels. Complex genotype-environment interactions such as these for simple behavioral responses (induction
and recovery) suggest that it may be exceedingly difficult to arrive
at simple genetic models for more complex behavioral responses to
halothane. Most important, these data illustrate the fact that the
results of experiments with a single strain of rodent or a hybrid
stock may not be expected to generalize to findings for other
strains and stocks. This is particularly true under circumstances
in which differences in strains employed from study to study are
confounded by interstudy variations in "effective" levels of anesthesia. Inadvertent variations in effective dosage levels may contribute to inconsistent findings from study to study. They result
from (1) inconsistencies in the ways in which specific anesthetic
doses are reported in the literature; (2) failure to specify dose
levels; and (3) frequent failure to report induction and eduction
times as one index of effective dosage level. These seem to be
critical parameters in view of the fact that observations of memory
facilitation or amnesia and the time course of these phenomena are
dose-related.

The fact that genotype influences responses to anesthesia, in
interaction with dose level, further emphasizes the importance of
determining drug-dose relationships prior to experimentation and
the utilization of more than one concentration of anesthetic vapor
in a single study or related studies. The doubtful value of using
only a single dose of any drug in a psycho-pharmacological study

Table 9 (a through g)

Effects of a Surgical Level of Diethyl Ether Anesthesia on Heart
Rate, Systolic Blood Pressure and Respiration for Several Groups
of Animals from the RI Strains, the Reciprocal F_1 Hybrids, and the
Two Progenitor Strains[1]. Means not differing significantly from
each other (Newman Keuls Multiple Contrasts)[2] are underlined
(Elias, Elias & Eleftheriou, unpublished).[3] (The footnotes to this
table appear on page 276.)

Table key with number of subjects per group

(10 observations/S̲)

I = CXBI (14)   CB6F$_1$ = C × B6 (19)

C = BALBc/6By (28)   H = CXBH (14)

G = CXBG (14)   B6 = C57BL/6By (26)

Table 9a-9c

Main Effect Contrasts for Blood Pressure[4,5]

Group	I	C	G	CB6F$_1$	H	B6
BP (mm Hg)	97	96	96	88	83	80

Main Effect Contrasts for Respiration

Group	G	I	CB6F$_1$	C	H	B6
Frequency/ Min	186	180	177	174	163	163

Main Effect Contrasts for Heart Rate[7]

Group	B6	I	G	CB6F$_1$	H	C
Rate/Min	546	549	547	529	477	453

Table 9-d

Main Effect (Age) Contrasts for Blood Pressure

Age	40-70 days	70-90 days	90-180 days
BP (mm Hg)	84	91	98

Table 9-e

Main Effect (Age) Contrasts for Respiration

Age	40-70 days	70-90 days	90-180 days
Frequency/Min	166	175	179

Table 9-f

Main Effect (Age) Contrasts for Heart Rate

Age	40-70 days	70-90 days	90-180 days
Rate/Min	522	512	513

Table 9-g

Means Depicting the Nature of the Significant

Age and Genotype Groups Interaction for Blood Pressure

	40-70 days	70-90 days	90-180 days
C (N = 28)	90 ± 3.2	102 ± 4.6	106 ± 9.7
B6 (N = 26)	80 ± 3.5	79 ± 1.6	85 ± 3.8
CB6F$_1$ (N = 19)	80 ± 1.2	90 ± 4.6	98 ± 2.8
G (N = 14)	78 ± 0.8	104 ± 1.8	111 ± 3.7
H (N = 14)	74 ± 1.8	85 ± 3.6	92 ± 4.7
I (N = 14)	94 ± 3.7	97 ± 4.9	100 ± 2.9

Notes to Table 9

[1]These results are preliminary in nature. Data are not yet analyzed for nonetherized controls and all RI line data has not been reduced. Thus these relationships among age and genotype may be unique to ether anesthesia. Regardless of whether they are unique to ether anesthesia, they exist under ether anesthesia, thus complicating interpretations of complex behavioral data which may be influenced by the physiological changes which are reflected in blood pressure values. If one were to equate anesthetic depth in terms of effects on blood pressure, separate equations would have to be developed for different strains at different age groups. This would not however permit similar equations for different vital signs such as heart rate, EEG, and respiration.

[2]A detailed report of this experiment with all the RI strains, nonetherized controls, and different levels of anesthesia is in preparation (P. K. Elias, M. F. Elias and B. E. Eleftheriou). Subjects were divided into age groups. Measurements were not repeated at different ages. Blood pressure recording procedures are described by Elias and Schlager (1974) and anesthesia apparatus is described by Elias, Blenkarn, Simmerman and Marsh (1971). A nose cone was used to maintain anesthetic depth when the animal was removed from the chamber for measurements.

[3]Must be interpreted with extreme caution in view of the Blood Pressure × Genotype interaction (Table 10-g).

[4]Within cell (age × genotype) SEMs range = 0.8 to 9.7.

[5]Within cell (age × genotype) SEMs range = 3.6 to 10.6.

[6]Within cell (age × genotype) SEMs range = 9.2 to 31.8.

has been emphasized by McGaugh and Petrinovitch (1965). The same logic leads to a questioning of the value of single strain studies.

Age

We have not performed diethyl ether induction and eduction time studies with the RI strains. However, several studies conducted at the Jackson Laboratory (Elias, Elias & Eleftheriou, unpublished)[5] may be of interest in view of Buchsbaum and Buchsbaum's (1962) discussion of irregular respiration as a factor in the U-shaped curve which described the relationship between age and recovery from diethyl ether. Table 9 shows RI strain differences in blood pressure, respiration, and heart rate as a function of age. All the other data from this study have not been analyzed and thus data for all RI strains are not shown. However, it may be seen that strain variations in each of these measures are observed and that a different pattern of strain differences is observed for the three age groups (Table 9). Thus, generalizations concerning the relationship between age and physiological responses to diethyl ether must take into consideration the influences of genotype on each of these variables and their relationship to each other.

Temperature and Behavioral Responses

We have already noted that the probability of obtaining decrements in performance with posttrial etherization is increased when (1) temperature in the anesthetic environment is in excess of 29°C (Alpern & Kimble, 1967; Herz et al.,1966; (2) the anesthetization chamber is saturated with ether, and (3) ether treatment is prolonged (Cherkin, 1968b; Elias, Blenkarn, Simmerman & Marsh, 1971). Increased temperature in the chamber leads to higher partial pressures of ether in its vapor phase, and thus in the inspired air (Cherkin, 1968b; Elias, Blenkarn, Simmerman & Marsh, 1971). Increased duration leads to longer periods of elevated partial pressure and thus increases "effective" dosage levels.

We have not compared behavioral responses to differing dose levels of ether anesthesia in our laboratory, but we (Simmerman, Ful-

---

[5]Elias, P. K., Elias, M. F. and Eleftheriou, B. E. A genetic investigation of systolic blood pressure in the RI strains; an unpublished study performed at the Jackson Laboratory (in preparation).

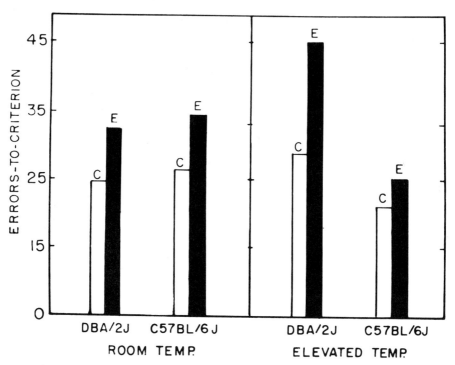

Figure 1.   Effects of temperature on behavioral response to anesthesia in two inbred strains of mice (DBA/2J) and (C57BL/6J).   Mice
were given anesthesia after daily water maze discrimination trials.
Elias, M. F. and Simmerman, S. J.   Proactive and retroactive effects
of diethyl ether on spatial discrimination learning for two inbred
mouse strains.   (A paper presented at the Eastern Psychological
Association Meetings, Atlantic City, N.J., 1971.)

ton & Elias,unpublished[6]) have data indicating that the relationship between performance decrement and temperature is affected by genotype. We were interested in determining the extent to which Wimer et al.'s (1968) findings of ether-facilitated learning in mouse strain DBA/2J but not C57BL/6J would generalize to a different kind of task and would be affected by temperature-potentiated ether. Thus, with the exception of the ether-potentiation portion of the experiment, ether was administered in the same manner as that reported by Wimer et al.(1968) and animals of the same age and sex were used. There was a major difference between our study and Wimer et al's. We used a water discrimination task. The apparatus and procedure have been described in detail in a number of publications (e.g. Elias & Simmerman, 1971a, b).

Figure 1 shows the results of this study in terms of mean errors prior to reaching a criterion of 13 out of 14 correct responses on 14 consecutive trials. At room temperature (23°C) there was no significant strain × anesthetic interaction, although performance was inferior for the posttrial etherization condition when scores were averaged for both strains (strain main effect). However, when the temperature in the testing chamber was elevated to approximately 30°C, there was a significant strain × anesthetic interaction with the DBA/2J mice exhibiting notably inferior performance (relative to C57BL/6J) under the posttrial etherization condition (Fig. 1).

While an interaction was observed for the elevated temperature condition (Fig. 1), decrements in performance were observed at both temperatures, a finding which may be related to the nature of the task and incentive to swim. Suboski et al.(1968) and Elias and Simmerman (1971a, b) have suggested that aversive properties of diethyl ether may negatively reinforce behavior responses. In our maze discrimination procedure, a correction method was used. Thus, a correct response was always followed by the anesthetic. Elias and Simmerman (unpublished) found that diethyl ether diminished incentive to respond for strains DBA/2J and C57BL/6J. Thus, it is possible that room temperature concentrations depressed performance of both strains via ether effects on performance incentive while at the higher ether temperature (Fig. 1), performance decrement was related to amnesic effects and incentive effects, but amnesic effects were more pronounced for DBA/2J than for C57BL/6J mice.

---

[6]Elias, M. F. and Simmerman, S. J. Proactive and retroactive effects of diethyl ether on spatial discrimination learning for two inbred mouse strains. A paper presented at the Eastern Psychological Association Meetings, Atlantic City, N.J., 1971.

Memory Facilitation

Wimer and his colleagues have been among the few investigators
to engage in a systematic investigation of strain differences in
behavioral response to diethyl ether anesthesia. These experiments
are summarized in Table 4 along with results of other studies of
strain differences in response to ether and halothane. The first
experiment (Wimer, Symington, Farmer & Schwartzkroin, 1968) indicated that a brief administration of ether immediately after a daily
passive or active avoidance learning trial resulted in enhanced
learning performance for mouse strain DBA/2J, but neither facilitation or decrement for mouse strain C57BL/6J. No facilitative or
decremental effects on behavior were observed when anesthetic
treatment was delayed for 2 hours, 4 hours, and 72 hours or more.

Wimer et al.'s findings were not in agreement with a large
number of studies. We (Elias & Simmerman, in press, 1971) found
decrements in performance when ether was given to C57BL/6J and
DBA/2J mice after daily learning trials. Heinze (1974) found that
light posttrial ether anesthesia resulted in avoidance learning
decrements for inbred strains (Table 4) and F_1 hybrid progeny resulting from the intercrossing of these strains. However, for each
of these contradictory studies the nature of the task was different.
We utilized a discrimination learning task in which aversive properties of the anesthetic may have influenced incentive to respond.
Heinze (1974) used a 1 trial passive avoidance task. Thus, animals
were not repeatedly exposed to ether anesthesia for a number of
days as they were in Wimer et al.'s (1968) study. Many of the
studies in which retrograde amnesia have been reported used longer
periods of anesthetization and temperature-potentiated ether. It
is interesting to note that in our study with potentiated ether,
the DBA/2J mice exhibited inferior learning relative to controls
but the C57BL/6J mice did not (Fig. 1). Thus, it appears that
differences in results between Wimer et al's findings and other
studies are related to a complex set of interactions among genotype,
task parameters, and anesthetic level. The replicability of Wimer
et al.'s findings has been established in a number of subsequent
experiment including a recent study (Wimer & Houston, 1974) in
which "light doses" of diethyl ether (9 sec. duration) given immediately after a trial resulted in learning facilitation for strain
DBA/2J, but no effect on strain C57BL/6J. Thus, one cannot dismiss
Wimer et al.'s findings easily and the question of why facilitation
occurs in one strain and not another deserves careful consideration.

Neurotransmitter activity. Wimer (1968) hypothesized that
ether-stimulation of transmitter activity was the major reason for
learning facilitation for inbred mouse strain DBA/2J. Failure of
C57BL/6J mice to show ether-facilitated learning was handled by
hypothesizing that their central transmitter release levels were
already at some optimum level. These hypotheses were tested by
pretreating the C57BL/6J mice with reserpine. Reserpine produces
a reduction in transmitter levels of norepinephrine (Glowinski &
Axelrod, 1965; Green & Sawyer, 1960), dopamine and serotonin
(Carlsson, Falck & Hillarp, 1962) and γ-aminobutyric acid (Singh &
Malhotra, 1974). Pretreated and ether-treated C57BL/6J mice exhibited performance scores indicating an improved level of learning
performance relative to the non-treated control group. Wimer concluded that of the four transmitter substances known to be affected
by reserpine, norepinephrine seemed to be the best single candidate
as the source of reserpine-induced, ether-facilitated learning. In
addition to his data, Wimer presented the following evidence in
support of the norepinephrine hypothesis: (1) ether treatments
stimulate release of norepinephrine in various brain structures
(Brewster, Bunker & Beecher, 1952; Rosenberg & DiStefano, 1962;
Voght, 1954), and (2) regional distribution of norepinephrine indicates greater activity in areas likely to be involved in learning,
i.e., the hypothalamus (Bertler & Rosengren, 1959; Carlsson et al,
1962; Voght, 1954) and the hippocampus and neocortex (Csillik &
Erulkar, 1964).

The argument in favor of ether-stimulation of increased norepinephrine activity in parts of the brain critical to learning is
interesting in view of more recent work by Eleftheriou (1974) which
has established a relationship between a single gene and hypothal-
mic norepinephrine levels in mice. Following a survey with the RI
strains (see Chapter by Eleftheriou and Elias, this text), the
gene-phenotype link was established by comparison of congenic line
B6.C-H-23^c with the two progenitor strains BALB/cBy and C57BL/By.
B6.C-H-23^c is genetically identical to inbred strain C57BL/6By
except for a short segment of the BALB/cBy chromosome which includes
the BALB/cBy allele at the H-23 locus.

Utilization of the C57BL/6By strain, the BALB/cBy strain in
conjunction with congenic line B6.C-H-23^c may provide a useful
genetic tool for exploring the norepinephrine hypothesis with
Wimer's (1968) avoidance paradigms. This may be a particularly
promising approach in view of the fact that a growing body of evidence suggests that avoidance learning, is also influenced by a

single gene (Sprott, 1974; Oliverio, Eleftheriou & Bailey, 1973;
Royce, Yeudall & Poley, 1971).

Norepinephrine or serotonin? While the results of pretreatment
of strain C57BL/6J with ether were consistent with Wimer's (1968)
norepinephrine hypothesis, a later finding by Wimer, Norman and
Eleftheriou (1973) revealed that norepinephrine levels in the hippocampus and other brain structures of DBA/2J and C57BL/6J mice were
unaltered by a combination of ether and footstock, footstock alone,
or ether alone. These data weaken seriously the hypothesis that
ether stimulated alterations in norepinephrine were responsible for
ether-stimulated memory facilitation in shock avoidance learning.
On the other hand, the Wimer, Norman and Eleftheriou's (1973) investigation indicates that serotonin may play a role in the ether-
-facilitation phenomenon. For C57BL/6J mice, a combination of
footshock and ether, similar to that used in Wimer's (1968) avoidance task, resulted in a significant increase in hippocampal serotonin (5-Ht) for treated C57BL/6J mice relative to C57BL/6J controls
(226%). In contrast, the increase in serotonin for DBA/2J mice was
only 20 percent. Fortunately, a single gene model exists for serotonin. Eleftheriou and Bailey (1972) have provided evidence for a
gene-phenotype link for serotonin levels. In this instance, the
link was established with congenic line B6.C-H-(w56). Use of the
model provided by this finding may be an important aspect of studies
designed to characterize any relationship which may exist between
ether facilitated learning and plasma serotonin levels.

Task Parameters: Massed versus Distributed Practice

While it is important to determine the physiological characteristics of an inbred strain which may account for learning facilitation in response to diethyl ether, it is also important to determine the extent to which baseline levels of performance unique to a
particular strain may influence the results of ether treatment or
treatment with any anesthetic agent. This is particularly important
for genetic studies since physiological phenotype and behavioral
response to anesthesia may be correlated only by virtue of the fact
that they are unique characteristics of a strain or strains of mice
or rats that differ in many other respects.

Based on observations that C57BL/6J mice exhibit superior performance under distributed practice schedule and did not exhibit
the ether-facilitated learning phenomenon, Wimer (1973) hypothesized
that mouse strains exhibiting superior distributed learning would

not show an ether-facilitation effect. Presumably, superior learning under distributed practice conditions is reflective of superior
memory prior to posttrial anesthetic treatment. In order to test
the generality of this hypothesis, Wimer (1973) applied his ether-
-learning paradigm to inbred mouse strains BDP/J and SJL/J.

The massed-distributed practice hypothesis was not confirmed
because mice of both strains exhibited ether-facilitated performance for distributed practice avoidance tasks for which they also
exhibited superior baseline levels of performance under the non-
-ether control condition. Based on this finding, Wimer (1973)
quite correctly pointed out the necessity for caution in inferring
relations between phenotypes from observations made on a limited
number of inbred strains as these strains differ with respect to a
wide range of behaviors which may influence the phenotype in question. In other words, ether-facilitated learning for DBA/2J and
inferior baseline levels of performance on distributed practice
schedules appear to have been associated fortuitously.

Other Task Parameters

While both strains in Wimer's (1973) experiment exhibited the
learning facilitation phenomenon, the SJL/J mice performed in a
superior manner for passive shock avoidance and strain BDP/J performed in a superior manner for active shock avoidance. This task
× genotype interaction has been found in so many experiments that
they are too numerous to cite. Several experiments in our laboratory (Simmerman, Fulton & Elias, unpublished[7]; Elias & Simmerman,
1971b) illustrate the extent to which task parameters may determine
whether or not facilitation or behavioral decrement is observed in
response to ether anesthesia. In each experiment, Wimer's (1968)
anesthetization and handling procedures were employed and mice were
of the same age. However, a spatial water maze discrimination task
was used. For this unpublished experiment, 14 male DBA/2J and 14
male C57BL/6J mice were given five trials a day with 15 minutes
between trials. Treated animals received ether immediately after
each discrimination learning trial. Control animals were handled
in the same manner but received no ether. A significant strain ×
ether treatment interaction was observed and it may be seen in

---

[7]Simmerman, S. J., Fulton, W., & Elias, M. F. Effects of task
parameters on performance following exposure to ether in C57BL/6J
and DBA/2J mice, unpublished manuscript.

Figure 2 that only the DBA/2J mice exhibited significantly fewer
errors relative to controls, and both DBA/2J and C57BL/6J control
groups exhibited similar levels of performance. Findings of ether-
-facilitated learning in strain DBA/2J mice were replicated several
months later by an experimenter unfamiliar with the literature on
ether facilitation (Rep. Exp. 1, Figure 2). A question was raised
as to whether the facilitation in learning might not relate to the
fact that ether was presented between trials, and thus could have
proactive and retroactive effects. However, posttrial etherization
after two successive trials per day (right hand graph in Figure 2)
resulted in no significant difference for either DBA/2J or C57BL/6J
mice. Moreover, Elias and Simmerman (1971b) found no facilitation
in learning when one trial was presented each day and ether was
presented prior to each trial. When ether was presented after a
single daily trial there was a main effect for ether treatment, but
no strain × treatment interaction (see Figure 1, left hand side,
this chapter). A significant strain × ether treatment interaction
was obtained when effective ether dosage was increased by testing
in an experimental chamber in which the temperature was approximately 30°C. In this case, the etherized DBA/2J mice performed more
poorly than controls (Fig. 1).

Data with regard to ether facilitation when the anesthetic
treatment was presented between trials raise additional questions
and answers none. It is possible that performance was facilitated
because each animal was exposed to five times as many ether exposures each day as compared to studies in which ether was presented
once a day either before or after one or two trials. If nothing
else, these data serve to illustrate the influence of task parameters on the direction (facilitation, no effect, or decrement)
of the anesthetic effect and its interaction with genotype. Unfortunately, little more can be said for the other studies involving
genotype comparisons and diethyl ether administration. This situation is partly related to less than adequate ether-administration
techniques which have been used in almost all studies, including
those done in the authors' laboratory[8]. A second problem is related to the fact that drug-dose relationships have not been determined in the majority of studies. Thus, effects of dosages varying
along a continuum have not been examined within a single study.
This is not easily accomplished as concentration and duration
factors are correlated.

---

[8]Subsequently, we have used halothane under more carefully controlled conditions of administration and measurement.

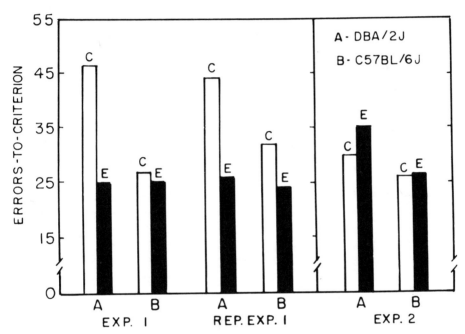

Figure 2. Effects of task parameters on behavioral responses to diethyl ether. DBA/2J and C57BL/6J mice were given ether immediately after each trial. In study 1 and the replication ether was given between trials (5/day) while in a second study (right hand side) ether was given after two successive trials each day. (Simmerman, S. J., Fulton, W., and Elias, M. F., unpublished.)

Facilitation with Heavy Doses

The extent to which simultaneous variation in many task variables and methods of procedure from study to study precludes resolution of discrepancies between studies is illustrated by comparison
of findings by Wimer and his colleagues (Table 4) and others (Table
1) with those of Suboski et al. (1968) and Black et al. (1967).
Suboski et al. and Black et al. reported ether-facilitated retention
when "effectively" heavy doses were given for long durations, relative to Wimer's procedure.

Suboski et al.'s (1968) and Black et al.'s (1967) findings are
inconsistent with the majority of studies which have reported retrograde amnesia with heavy doses of ether. Moreover, they run counter
to the general notion that light ether doses are a necessary condition for facilitation to occur for any strain or species. This
unusual finding may have been related to the use of the
Long-Evans strain of rats. On the other hand it could have been
related to a combination of factors which differed from experiment
to experiment, e.g. the learning task and the retrograde amnesia
was different than that employed by Wimer et al. (1968). The fact
that facilitation occurred only after a 3,160 second interval in
the Suboski et al. (1968) study suggests that heavy doses of ether
may not have influence memory consolidation, but rather that it
affected some other intervening variable related to recall of a
discriminated avoidance learning-habit. The influence of subject's
age on the results of this study cannot be evaluated as this information was not presented.

It is quite clear that genotype plays a major role in the results of anesthetic-behavior studies and that this influence may be
felt in several ways: (1) as it relates to task and experimental
design parameters under baseline control conditions; (2) as it
relates to the influence of the anesthetic on physiological mechanisms; (3) as it relates to the interaction of the first two
factors. Strain differences studies illustrate these points but
they do not really permit an understanding of the genetical basis
of anesthetic effects on learning. A variety of behavior genetic
methods may be used to address this latter question. Before these
are considered in any detail, it is important to review the most
important methodological factors with regard to inconsistent findings in the literature.

METHODOLOGICAL CONSIDERATIONS

The "Ether Jar"

In many experiments, animals have been anesthetized in glass beakers, or in jars containing a sponge or cotton soaked with the liquid anesthetic agent. There are a number of problems inherent in the administration of anesthetics in this manner. Generally, they are related to the vaporization of anesthetic agents (Adriani, 1962). Very high partial pressures of anesthetics are created in the ether jar or beaker. The sudden inhalation of high concentrations of ether (and many other volatile agents) is irritating to the upper respiratory tract. Respiratory irritation may lead to induction of anesthesia which is characterized by coughing, bronchial spasm, excessive respiratory tract secretions, behavior excitement and concomitant sympatho-adrenal hyperactivity. Repeated exposures to anesthetics under these circumstances may influence changes in performance which mimic changes in learning or retention.

When the anesthetic chamber becomes anesthetic-saturated, it causes excessive anesthetic depth. Excessive depth causes severe depression of the respiratory and cardiovascular systems so that acidosis and hypoxia may be superimposed on the effects of general anesthesia. Moreover, when air in a closed chamber is used as the carrier gas for the anesthetic vapor, additional derangement of respiratory gas exchange occurs as high partial pressure of the anesthetic agent encrouches on the fractional concentration of oxygen in the air. This hypoxia-inducing effect is more pronounced toward the bottom of the jar or container due to the stratification of the denser anesthetic vapor. In addition, the utilization of oxygen and excretion of carbon dioxide within a small closed chamber further reduces the partial pressure of oxygen in the environment.

Several studies indicate that hypoxia does not affect memory consolidation (Jarvik, 1964; Taber & Banuazizi, 1966) while others indicate that it does (Galluscio & Grant, 1979). However, the question of whether or not amnesic effects are produced by hypoxia seems irrelevant when one considers that sustained hypoxia produces brain damage.

The extent to which brain damage may explain results of studies in which animals have been place in saturated ether environments for extended periods of time is unknown because mortality rates

are not routinely reported. Herz, Peeke and Wyers (1966) reported
a mortality rate of 25%. Cherkin (1968b) has questioned the extent
to which "residual brain damage" may have existed in the surviving
animals, and points out that the high partial pressure of saturated
ether vapor necessitates short exposure times to prevent excessive
mortality. He argues that partial pressure at 31°C in a saturated
environment is approximately 11 times lethal partial pressure, and
that an exposure of less than 2 minutes is necessary to prevent a
100% mortality rate.

The possibility of residual brain damage and consequent effects
on behavior cannot be dismissed lightly. Many anesthesiologists
feel that neurological and behavioral side effects of hyperventilation during surgical anesthesia are related to changes in arterial
carbon dioxide tension (Pa_{CO_2}). Some believe that these effects
are reversible. Others consider that the neurological effects are
the result of cerebral ischaemia due to reduction in cerebral blood
flow accompanying lowering of the Pa_{CO_2}, and that hyperventilation
may be a potential cause of permanent brain impairment (see Whitwam,
Boettner, Gilger & Littell, 1966). A number of experiments with
human subjects have been designed to resolve this issue, but at
present the question of permanent brain damage and long term behavioral decrements remains open (Whitwam et al, 1966; Sugioka & Davis,
1960; Wollman & Orkin, 1968; Blenkarn, Briggs, Bell & Sugioka, 1972).
However, the presence of mortality, or any significant weight loss
in experimental animals is sufficient to indicate the anesthetic
technique. Furthermore, it casts serious doubts upon interpretations of retrograde amnesia effects in terms of memory consolidation because the effect of brain damage or general deficit in health
cannot be precluded.

Another major problem which is encountered when small animals
are anesthetized within closed unventilated containers is the
unpredictable and extremely variable vapor tensions of the anesthetics produced. As volatile anesthetics are vaporized, a large amount
of heat is extracted from the immediate environment. This latent
heat of vaporization results in undesirable cooling of the chamber
and the experimental animal. The drop in temperature reduces the
rate of vaporization, and consequently leads to a variable and ever-
changing concentration of anesthetic vapor in the respiratory environment.

Cherkin (1968b) and Elias, Blenkarn, Simmerman and Marsh (1971)
have pointed out that many of these methodological difficulties can

be avoided by employing well-defined gaseous mixtures of ether or a
less flammable anesthetic such as halothane. A number of references to proper techniques for anesthetizing various laboratory animals are available (e.g. Taber & Irwin, 1969; Lumb, 1963).   These
references include the volatile and nonvolatile anesthetics as well
as a discussion of hypothermia as an anesthetic technique (Taber &
Irwin, 1969). A variety of apparatus have been described for the
delivery of inhalation anesthetics ranging from inexpensive systems
(Elias, Blenkarn, Simmerman & Marsh, 1971) to highly sophisticated
apparatus (Ravento, 1956; Stiles, 1959; Woods, Haggart, 1957;
Zauder & Orkin, 1959). A publication by Ayerst Laboratories (1957)
provides a list of companies which produce clinical anesthesia apparatus.

Other review papers have placed an equally heavy emphasis on
anesthetic technique as a significant influence on conflictual data
in the literature. Cherkin (1968b) notes that

> "The results of memory consolidation research will con-
> tinue to be ambiguous and controversial until experimen-
> tal methodology takes into strict account the role of
> dose-dependence and duration-dependence of amnesia
> treatments...The confounding variables introduced by non-
> optimal amnesic methodology provide a plausible parsim-
> onious interpretation of conflicting interpretations of
> retrograde amnesia experiments." (p. 256).

Effective Anesthetic Depth

Measurement of effective anesthetic depth is no less important
than measurement and specification of concentrations of inhalation
anesthetic in the inspired air. Faulconer (1952) has noted that
even the commonly accepted signs by which depth of anesthesia is
assessed clinically are not a totally reliable index of anesthetic
depth.

Dr. Maynard B. Chenoweth elegantly and precisely summarized
the extent and exact nature of the measurement problem at a work-
shop on "Effects of anesthesia on metabolism and cellular functions"
held under the auspices of the Committee on Anesthesia of the
National Academy of Sciences-National Research Council (Bunker &
Vandam, 1965).

> "Now turning toward the design of the experiment, let us
> consider the dose response curve which exists for

anesthetics, as for all other drugs, in the typical sig-
moid shape. It simply tells us that the response is
related to the dose in a predictable fashion. Of more
importance is the curve showing the response to an anesthetic at some constant dose with time. There is both a
beginning and an end which are well defined and a constant plateau which is, in practice, laboriously maintained. This is a situation rather uncommonly met with
in drug actions, even though it may be the aim. It leads
to special problems: a) when and what is the response?
We may define the response in this case by the clinical
behavior of the patient, or, if you prefer, by a more
precise examination of the electroencephalographic pattern or, under special conditions, circulatory, respiratory, or biochemical criteria. The anesthesiologists and
pharmacologists will recognize immediately that I have
passed over the hardest part of the problem for the exact
definition of how deeply anesthetized a patient is at any
given time could well be the topic of an entire conference...

   Another aspect of determining the dose-response is
knowing the dose that has been employed. Here again we
run into particular difficulty in our special situation.
With the barbituates, we can use a gravimetric expression,
that is to say, give the number of milligrams per kilogram
that is given intravenously, but with volatile anesthetics,
except for emulsions of methoxyflurane or roflurane given
intravenously, this is not a very practical method. The
alternative, the analytical expression, simply the milligrams per milliliter of arterial blood or of central nervous system tissue or other tissue under study sounds
very elegant, but requires something more in the way of
analytical facilities and help than is always available,
although it may ultimately be the final way to get at the
important information.

   I will gloss over individual variation among patients
as a problem because it is common to every drug and presents no unique character here, to leap to the final and
one of the most difficult problems. That is the problem
of the control observations. It is necessary to differentiate effects of anesthesia from effects of anesthetics." (p. 186-187).

Bunker and Vandam's (1965) report on this conference should be

required reading for all investigators who would use inhalation
anesthetics as a tool to investigate the interaction of genotype
and anesthetic effects on behavior. Most likely, some portion of
the individual variance in individual responses to anesthesia referred to by Dr. Chenoweth is based on unique individual genetic
makeup and very possibly effects of unknown mutant genes influencing metabolic pathways.

   It is quite clear that most psychopharmacogeneticists will not
be able to achieve the degree of sophistication suggested in Dr.
Chenoweth's remarks, but certainly any attempts to more precisely
deliver and specify anesthetic concentrations than have been widely
employed in the literature would be a step in the right direction.
It is not an easy matter to design experiments with inhalation anesthetics. The fact that individual variation and paradoxical responses to inhalation anesthetics are so often referred to in the human
literature indicates that genotype differences and mutagenic effects
may well explain what have been referred to as paradoxical anesthetic effects[9], and thus the eventual payoff in an applied clinical
sense may justify the effort.

                              Age and Sex

   Other methodological issues include the neglect of age as a
factor in the design of experiments and the frequently observed
failure to specify age and/or sex in experimental reports. These
problems and special design considerations for aging and developmental studies have been summarized in a previous chapter (Elias
& Elias, in press b) dealing with behavioral endocrinology and
aging.

       BEHAVIOR GENETIC APPROACHES VERSUS COMPARATIVE STUDIES

   We have emphasized the importance of genetic factors in anesthetic effects on behavior. Many behavior genetic reviews leave
no doubt that genotype influences memory consolidation and other
aspects of behavior that are susceptible to the influence of anesthetics. Strain differences studies have contributed to this literature because they provide a model for genotype which may be used
in experiments designed to characterize genotype × treatment interactions. However, strain comparisons provide very little informa-

---

[9] B. E. Eleftheriou suggested the possibility of a genetical basis
for so-called paradoxical effects to M. F. Elias in June of 1974.

tion beyond the demonstration that genotype and environment interactions determine behavioral responses to anesthetics and that behavior has a genetic component. As Sprott (1974), Eleftheriou and
Elias (this volume), Henderson (1969) and others have pointed out
more information is required if behavioral-genetic analyses are to
contribute to the understanding of how genotype influences behavioral response to anesthetics.

Manosevitz, Lindzey and Thiessen (1969) have provided a book of
published research papers which provides examples of a variety of
behavior-genetic approaches which take advantage of Mendelian
genetics, biometric approaches and the synthesis of the two. These
techniques include the diallel cross method, the use of mutants,
and selection. In addition, there are research reports and reviews
which provide examples of the use of mutant stocks (Thiessen, 1970;
Oliverio & Messeri, 1973; Elias & Eleftheriou, 1972), and the limitations of studies with mutants (Elias & Eleftheriou, in press b;
Wilcock, 1969). Sprott (1974) has provided an excellent example of
the use of classical testcross procedures which may be used to test
single gene hypotheses. Many texts describe methods of behavioral
genetic analyses (e.g. Fuller & Thompson, 1960). None of these
approaches have been used in the study of anesthetic effects on
behavior to any significant extent.

The diallel cross. The diallel cross method appears to be a
particularly useful approach (Broadhurst, 1969) for psychopharmacogenetic research with mammals because it provides information
about polygene systems in a single generation (the F_1) so that
investigators need not wait for the results of breeding the F_2
backcrosses on the double backcrosses necessary for complete biometric analyses. Broadhurst (1969) suggests that diallel crossing,
or the method of complete intercrossing (Schmidt, 1919) represents
an extensive method of analysis rather than intensive procedure
because it surveys the genetical basis of behavior in a sizable
number of strains at once, rather than concentrating on a more
exhaustive analysis utilizing two or three strains.

Selection. We have found selection to be a particularly
useful tool for the development of physiological phenotypes of
interest to behaviorists (Elias & Schlager, 1974). Early selection
experiments in behavior genetics were primarily directed toward
selection for behavior phenotype and were beset by a number of
methodological errors (Wahlsten, 1972). When used correctly, selection can be a particularly useful tool for the development of

behavioral and physiological models (Schlager, 1974). For example, the work of Wimer and his colleagues (Wimer et al.,1968; Wimer, 1968; Wimer, 1970) suggests that different levels of neurohumors and neurotransmitter substances play a role in whether or not facilitation in learning is observed for a particular strain of mice. One might attempt to select for high and low levels of neurotransmitters in whole brain or various parts of the brain and then to compare these high and low selection lines within the context of the posttrial anesthetic paradigm. Alternatively, or in a parallel set of selection studies, one might select for resistance and/or susceptibility to anesthetic effects for a particular response index. The next step would be to explore corresponding changes in neurotransmitter levels and other potentially relevant physiological variables. Appropriate controls such as randomly bred control lines, and the testing of generations formed by an initial cross of selected lines would be essential to determine the genetical basis of the emergence of phenotypic traits associated with selection, e.g. linked gene effects, and to preclude accidents of selection which result in a fortuitous relationship between genotype and phenotype. The major limitation of the application of selection to the development of physiological or behavioral phenotype is related to the fact that many physiological and behavioral interactions determine whether or not inhibition or facilitation will be observed, and thus it is most difficult to select for a specific physiological phenotype (e.g. level of serotonin or norepinephrine in the hippocampus) without selecting for a variety of correlated physiological and behavioral characteristics.

Single Gene Studies

The Recombinant Inbred strains and congenic lines developed by Bailey (1971) may be useful in testing single gene hypotheses with regard to behavior responses to anesthesia. This is not to suggest, a priori, that a single locus influences the many complex physiological and concomitant behavioral changes that may take place in response to anesthesia, but rather that one should not overlook the possibility of a major locus effecting or modulating some critical intervening variable, e.g. serotonin levels or changes in a key neurotransmitter in a specific region of the brain under conditions of footshock or ether treatment. If one could link this critical intervening variable to a single gene, at a particular locus on a given chromosome, the end result would be a rather powerful and precise genetic model for studying the relationship of that gene to behavioral responses to a given anesthetic. On the other hand,

one might establish a link between a single gene at a given locus
and facilitation or impairment in learning as a function of specific
drug-dose and posttrial etherization parameters. The next step
would be to examine physiological characteristics intervening between the gene and behavior. Of course, baseline levels of performance on the task in question and its relationship to this single
gene would have to be taken into consideration. A given gene may
be related (via intervening physiological mechanisms) to performance
differences between a control and treatment condition, and yet
another gene may influence baseline (control performance).

To our knowledge, no investigator has attempted to relate a
single locus to anesthetic treatment effects on specific behaviors,
although Eleftheriou and his colleagues (Eleftheriou, 1974;
Eleftheriou & Bailey, 1972; Oliverio, Eleftheriou & Bailey, 1973)
have utilized the Recombinant Inbred strains to obtain gene-phenotype linkage for several biochemical and behavioral phenomena that
have been identified as important to diethyl ether effects on learning. Similarly, via backcross techniques, Sprott (1974) has presented evidence for a single locus influence on passive avoidance
learning, a key task in retrograde amnesia and behavior facilitation
studies with diethyl ether.

One objection to the single gene approach to understanding the
way in which genes influence anesthetic effects on learning and
other aspects of behavior is that it is "like looking for a needle
in a haystack." In other words, a question may be raised as to
whether it is reasonable to expect that behaviors as complex as
retrograde amnesia are influenced by a single gene. We feel that
this is more a question of research strategy than it is a challenge
to the use of Recombinant Inbred (RI) strains or any other single
gene research method. We are encouraged with regard to the potential usefulness of this approach by the neurohumoral responses (presumably related to ether effects on behavior) which have been linked
to specific genes.

Effects of Halothane on the RI Strains

Investigations in our laboratory and in collaboration with
B. E. Eleftheriou do not include studies of the effects of diethyl
ether on behavior for the RI strains, although we have completed a
survey of the behavioral response of the RI strains to halothane
anesthesia using the 1 trial-per-day spatial discrimination task
described previously in this chapter. The RI strains, one of the

reciprocal F_1 hybrids, and the two progenitor strains were subjected to posttrial halothane treatments (6% in the inspired air) using a modification of clinical anesthesia apparatus described previously (Elias & Eleftheriou, in press a). Examination of Figure 3 (top) indicates that inbred progenitor strains BALB/cBy and RI strain CXBD exhibited impaired learning ability as the result of immediate posttrial halothane administration. Significant differences between treated and control mice were observed for the BALB/cBy and CXBD strains. Lower dosage levels and longer intervals between trials and treatment (30 min.) revealed no deleterious effects on performance for strains BALB/cBy and CXBD.

Based on the observed pattern of group means in Figure 3, a dominant allele for resistance to halothane was postulated and a parsimonious model for the relationship between genotype and behavior under halothane was generated. This hypothetical single locus model was as follows: BALB/cBy ($\underline{a}/\underline{a}$), CXBD ($\underline{a}/\underline{a}$), CBF_1 ($\underline{A}/\underline{a}$) and the remaining strains (all $\underline{A}/\underline{A}$). In this instance A is a hypothetical dominant allele for resistance to halothane effects. The model was tested by performing a variety of backcrosses. The distribution of scores was inconsistent with a single locus hypothesis and thus the single gene model was rejected and a congenic line was not selected for gene-behavior link testing. Subsequent and more detailed analyses of speed of response and various kinds of errors for the control animals indicated that polygenes influence the performance of the control group for our discrimination task (Elias & Eleftheriou, in press b). While we were not able to establish a major gene-behavior link in this preliminary study, it is presented here as an example of the steps which may be taken to explore the possibility of behavior-gene linkage.

An interesting relationship between F_1 hybrid $CB6F_1$ and the inbred strains did emerge when induction and eduction times were examined. There was very little relationship between either induction times and trials-to-criterion or eduction times and trials-to--criterion when strain distribution patterns were compared for these measures. However, the $CB6F_1$ hybrids differed from all other groups in the direction of statistically, significantly greater resistance to halothane induction. This finding suggests a heterotic effect for the $CB6F_1$ hybrids as their induction scores exceeded those observed for both parents. The basis of this finding was not explored, and the reciprocal $BC6F_1$ hybrids (C57BL/6By mothers and BALB/cBy fathers) were not tested. Thus, the possible role of maternal (sex linked) effects was not examined. Cross-fostering

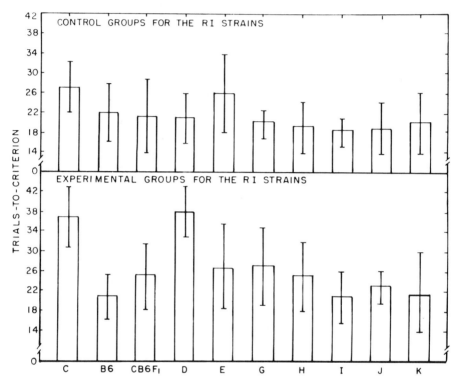

Figure 3. Effects of posttrial treatment with halothane (6% concentration) on discrimination learning (errors-to-criterion) for the
Recombinant Inbred Strains, (Bailey, 1971). Decrements observed for
treated strains BALB/cBy (C) and CXBD (D) were for immediate posttrial anesthetization. Delayed administration and lower concentrations resulted in no behavioral effects on BALB/cBy or CXBD mice
(Elias, M. F. & Eleftheriou, B. E., unpublished.)

experiments which would permit the separation of environmental from
genetic effects on F_1 response to halothane were not performed, and
each induction time was measured immediately after the animal had
completed a trial in the water maze. Thus, heterosis in response
to high and potentially lethal dosages of halothane remains an
interesting hypothesis for further testing. We mention this result
to illustrate the fact that the RI strains may be used in contexts
other than as a preliminary step in the testing of a single gene
hypothesis.

     Regardless of the genetic approach used in anesthetic studies,
the interaction of genotype and developmental factors will undoubtedly be of importance. Few retrograde amnesia studies have been
concerned with developmental stages or age. There has been one
important study dealing with chronic exposure to halothane during
and after important periods of early development. This study did
not deal with the descriptive questions regarding genotype × treatment interactions. However, the results of this experiment indicate
that developmental genetics studies constitute an important area
for future research with inhalation anesthetics such as halothane.

CHRONIC EXPOSURE TO HALOTHANE: A DEVELOPMENTAL STUDY

Learning Deficits and Cerebral Synaptic Malformation

     In a very well controlled study, Quimby, Aschkinase, Bowman,
Katz, and Chang (1974) examined the effects of chronic exposure of rats
to 10 ppm halothane during early life. The study was stimulated by
a concern with regard to the possibly toxic effects of anesthetics
on surgical personnel who have been chronically exposed to anesthetic vapors (Nikky, 1972). Choice of halothane was based on two
factors: (1) halothane, used in conjunction with nitrous oxide, is
the most popular inhalation anesthetic in this country, and (2)
there are data which suggest that behavioral deficits occur as a
result of chronic exposure to halothane in the operating theater.
Quimby et al. (1974) make reference to data which indicate that
halothane concentrations average 10 parts per million (ppm) in the
operating theater, and that anesthesiologists stationed near the
exhaust of the patient's breathing circuit, may be exposed to a
considerably greater concentrations (Linde & Bruce, 1969; Whitcher,
Cohen & Trudell, 1971). Bruce, Bach and Arbit (1974) reported that
4 hours of exposure to 15 ppm halothane with 500 ppm nitrous oxide
produce deficits in cognition, motor response, and perception.
Quimby et al. (1974) note that a decline in capacity during surgery

is of obvious concern, and cite several studies indicating that
operating room nurses and anesthesiologists may possibly suffer
long-term physiological effects resulting from chronic exposure to
halothane (Bruce, Eide, Linde & Eckenhoff, 1968; Cohen, Bellville &
Brown, 1971), although data do not exist that would support unequivocally a hypothesis of performance impairment resulting from
chronic exposure. The purpose of the Quimby et al. study was to
examine the hypothesis of deficit from chronic exposure at critical periods of the life span.

Sprague-Dawley rats were assigned to a control group and three
treatment groups were exposed to a range of 8 to 12 ppm concentration of halothane inspired air for eight hours a day, five days a
week. One treatment group (early development) was exposed from
conception to 60 days of age. A second treatment group (later
development) was exposed from day 60 through the behavioral testing
period of 60 days, and a third treatment group was exposed through
both early and late developmental periods. Half the subjects in
each group were tested at 130 days; half were tested beginning at
150 days. The behavioral task was a light-dark discrimination
with footshock escape incentive. There was a 30 percent increase
in errors (relative to the non-treated control group) for the groups
exposed to halothane early in development and throughout both early
and late development. Similar results were obtained for a spatial
discrimination task performed for appetitive reinforcement.

It is fairly certain that the learning decrements observed
were not transitory, since they occurred for rats that were last
exposed to trace amounts of halothane 75 to 90 days prior to behavioral testing. The critical exposure period appeared to be early
in development as no behavioral deficits were observed for the
animals first exposed to the anesthetic treatment after 60 days of
age. Moreover, electronmicroscopic examination of tissue samples
from the "superior parasagittal cerebral cortex" of the rats exposed
to halothane from conception to parturition showed evidence of neuronal degeneration. Furthermore, there was a permanent failure of
formation of the synaptic web and postsynaptic membrane density in
30 percent of the postsynaptic membranes. Only slight neuronal
damage was apparent for the rats that were chronically exposed to
halothane as adults.

Quimby and his colleagues (1974) point to the very important
implication of this study with regard to the chronic exposure of
pregnant women to halothane even when trace levels are as low as

questions may be obtained via a number of genetic techniques including the diallel cross.

RETROGRADE AMNESIA AND BEHAVIORAL DECREMENT IN HUMANS

Space does not permit a detailed review of the human literature on the effects of anesthetics on human behavior, nor does it
permit a review of the literature relating to the toxic effects of
halothane for a small percentage of patients (National Halothane
Study, 1966). Human behavior genetic techniques in the form of
biometric analyses and twin studies have not been applied to these
problems to any significant extent. We could find no behavioral
genetic studies dealing with effects of anesthetics on human learning and performance variables. Most likely, this paucity of literature is related to the fact that the complexity and time consuming
nature of human anesthetic studies does not permit the collection
of data for the very large number of cases required for biometric
genetic analyses. However, the number of clinical references to
individual differences in behavioral responses and paradoxical responses to various anesthetic agents in a small number of patients
is impressive. Examples include the isolated reports of massive
hepatic necrosis following halothane anesthesia (Burnap, Galla &
Vandam, 1958) and ether-induced convulsions for small numbers of
previously normal individuals (Owens, 1958).

Table 10 summarizes the results of studies of retrograde amnesia in humans. Many of these studies are summarized in a more
extensive form in Porter's (1972) review paper. The literature on
human behavioral response to anesthetics is difficult to relate to
the animal literature (Tables 1 to 4) because most of the studies
on retrograde amnesic effects have been done with Nitrous Oxide
(N_2O). When nitrous oxide is administered immediately after a
series of nonsense syllables, facilitation of recall is observed
(Steinberg et al., 1957b; Summerfield et al., 1959). Impairment of
recall is frequently observed when N_2O is administered through the
training period, although these studies are not designed in such a
way that effects of the anesthetic on acquisition and memory processes can be separated. Thus, human studies with anesthetics have
contributed relatively little to an understanding of memory processes, although they are important from a descriptive clinical standpoint. Aside from the question of retroactive amnesia for events
during surgery, there are several other questions of practical
importance that have not been fully resolved. These questions may
be amenable to at least partial resolution via effective utiliza-

Table I. Rating Scale for the Behavioral Effects of Psychomotor Stimulants in Rats

Table Explanation

Duration: NS = not specified; throughout = treatment given throughout behavior testing procedure;

immediate = treatment immediately after a trial, training, or sensory experience.

Dosage: %I.A. = percent inspired air.

Results: results as compared to controls as given by Porter (1972).

Author	Task	Duration (sec)	Dosage %I.A.	TTI	Results
Choy et al (1969)	Series of nonsense syllables	1800	40%	5 min	Amnesia
Steinberg (1954)	Digit span	300+	30%	throughout	Impairment

Steinberg et al (1957a)	Series of nonsense syllables	300[+]	30%	throughout	Impairment
Steinberg et al (1957b)	Series of nonsense syllables	750	30%	immediate	Facilitation
Summerfield et al (1959)	Series of nonsense syllables	750	30%	immediate	Facilitation
Henrie et al (1961)	Series of nonsense syllables	600	30%	throughout	Impairment
Parkhouse et al (1960)	Nonsense syllables	NS	20,30,40%	throughout	Increasing impairment with increasing concentration
Berry (1965)	Missing digit short term recall	NS	"sub-anesthetic"	throughout	Impairment
Berry (1968)	Missing digit short term recall	NS	15,25,35%	throughout	No effect
Robson et al (1960)	Number recall	300	5% below level that impairs consciousness	throughout	Impairment
McKinney (1932)	Series of nonsense syllables	NS	25%	throughout	Impairment

tion of animal models. The reader may wish to consult a paper by
Cherkin and Harroun (1971) in which human studies are discussed in
the context of the retrograde amnesia literature and the various
models for memory consolidation.

Cherkin and Harroun review a number of studies which document
the fact that postoperative recall of events during surgery can be
prevented by light anesthesia (e.g. Artusio, 1955; Brice,
Hetherington & Utting, 1970) and that the probability of incomplete
amnesia after surgical operations is low (Hutchinson, 1960).
However, they point out that recall is not always prevented by seemingly adequate anesthesia (e.g., Alment, 1959; Erickson, 1963).
Apparently individual patient variation and variations in information content play a role in conflicting results (Hutchinson, 1960).
Results of a number of studies reviewed by Cherkin and Harroun
(1971) indicate that information of a highly emotional nature results in unpleasant recall for some patients. The question of
memory for psychologically traumatic events during surgery is of
considerable practical importance due to the use of light anesthesia for high risk patients, e.g., heart surgery or surgery with
elderly patients.

Hyperventilation

Controlled ventilation is freqently employed in surgical operations in order to reduce the amount of an anesthetic required and
in order to suppress spontaneous respiratory movements (Geddes &
Gray, 1959). However, there is evidence that cerebral hypoxia may
be introduced as the result of this procedure. Cerebral hypoxia
results from diminished blood flow caused by vasoconstriction which
is, in turn, caused by the hypocapnia resulting from hyperventilation (Sugioka & Davis, 1960). This evidence has contributed to a
debate as to whether or not harmful behavioral effects result from
the practice of controlled ventilation of surgical patients, and,
if so, whether the behavioral effects are transitory or permanent
manifestations of brain damage. Positive and negative evidence for
behavior impairment exists, although the weight of the evidence,
particularly from well controlled studies (Blenkarn, Briggs, Bell
& Sugioka, 1972) indicates that (1) a wide variety of higher order
cognitive functions and reaction time are unaffected by hypocapnic
hyperventilation, and (2) slowing of response in a previous study
(Wollman & Orkin, 1968) may have been due to failure to practice
subjects for a sufficient period of time to permit response stabi-
lization prior to the anesthetic and hyperventilation procedures.

However, differences in other features of the Blenkarn et al. (1972)
and the Wollman and Orkin (1968) studies, such as the various combinations of anesthetic drugs employed during ventilation procedures, may account for differences in results.

Blenkarn et al. (1972) point out that absence of behavioral
effects in their study and with their particular battery of tests
does not exonerate hyperventilation. This cautious interpretation
of negative results seems quite appropriate in view of the fact
that the experiment was done with healthy young subjects and was
not complicated by surgical trauma or pre-existing disease. Each
of these latter variables are of critical importance in applied
clinical practice.

If an animal model were to be employed to study the behavioral
effect of hyperventilation, the relationship between behavior and
ultrastructural changes could be examined in the same manner as
they were in the halothane study by Quimby and his associates (1974).
Degree of surgical trauma could be manipulated, and the factor of
pre-existing health conditions could be studied using animal models
for the various disease processes such as diabetes or hypertension.
Developmental studies could be done over a large segment of the
life-span. This kind of research may not be impractical with small
animals. Siegler and Rich (1973) have described a device which can
be used to ventilate mice during surgery.

Premedication

The necessity for preoperative medication of surgical patients
has created difficulties in determining whether or not post-amnestic
symptoms are related to preoperative medication (e.g. atropine,
ethidine, pentibarbitone), combinations of anesthetics administered
prior to and during surgery (e.g. thiopentone, halothane, and nitrous oxide) or combinations of effects produced by preoperative
medication and anesthesia. A study by Gruber and Reed (1968)
suggests that amnestic effects are related primarily to the general
anesthetic rather than preoperative medication, although there is
by no means universal agreement that this is true. Utilization of
animal models in this context may be particularly useful in determining whether preoperative medication and anesthetic interactions
are influenced by genotype, age, and a variety of environmental and
disease and stress factors which may be experimentally manipulated
at various periods of the life-span.

10 ppm. It is possible that such exposure could result in enduring damage to the brain of the fetus. While one cannot eliminate the possibility that the effect on the developing brain of the rat was species-specific or possibly even strain-specific, the implications of the finding emphasize the importance of conducting studies at the primate level. Furthermore, a search for gene-phenotype linkage with Mus musculus as a model may ultimately determine the underlying mechanisms of brain impairment resulting from chronic halothane exposure.

Quimby et al. (1974) point out that while the behavioral data provided no indication of damage in the adult rat exposed to trace doses of halothane, the exposure period was limited and that increased halothane concentrations or behavioral tasks, more specifically related to memory registration, might reveal deficits. They also make a point which is particularly encouraging to the behavioral scientist. Morphological damage became manifest only at the ultrastructural level. The various organs, including the brain, appeared normal under light microscopy. However, the behavioral tests appeared to be as sensitive as electronmicroscopy for the detection of damage from exposure to the trace levels of halothane. We add a note of caution. The presence of both behavioral and ultrastructural deficits in one inbred strain of a species, as the result of a given experimental treatment, may not necessarily indicate a direct cause and effect relationship. There is the possibility, remote as it may be in this case, that behavioral and structural impairment are correlated as a result of linked genes, one or more influencing structure and the other(s) behavior, or as a result of the fortuitous association of genes influencing structural change and behavioral changes in the same inbred strain.

The testing of a number of inbred strains might help to dissociate structural and behavioral effects. However, the issue may be resolved in a more conclusive manner by means of behavior genetic analyses techniques such as (1) selection (see Elias & Schlager, 1974; Elias, Elias & Schlager, 1975), (2) testing of congenic lines (Eleftheriou & Bailey, 1972; Elias & Eleftheriou, in press b), or (3) testing of single gene mutants (see Elias & Eleftheriou, 1972; Oliverio & Messeri, 1973) which may be employed in an effort to resolve the question of gene linkage or gene-behavior associations by virtue of the influence of a major gene. Other genetic questions of interest have to do with the mode of inheritance of susceptibility to trace halothane concentrations and whether or not F_1 hybrids are resistant to effects of chronic exposure. Answers to these

SUMMARY AND IMPLICATIONS FOR NEW DIRECTIONS

It appears that understanding of the relationship between genotype and behavioral effects of anesthetics and anesthesia (the psychopharmacogenetic approach) may be facilitated by increasing utilization of behavior genetic techniques and methods that go beyond the repeated demonstration that genotype interacts with environmental factors.

There seems to be clear evidence for the fact that anesthesia results in retrograde amnesia when it is present during a critical period after information input. The critical period may reflect consolidation of an electrophysiological memory trace. However, more precise control of anesthetic dosages in combination with systematic and programatic studies will be necessary to characterize the mechanisms which intervene between genes and behavioral response to anesthesia.

One may question whether there is anything further to be gained from studying the time course of memory consolidation in a behavior genetic study employing the retrograde amnesia paradigm. This approach may reveal little about the underlying mechanisms of memory. A more profitable strategy may be to capitalize on data which implicate the neurotransmitter substances as an important link between genes and memory processes. An excellent example of this research strategy, employed in a non-behavior genetic context, is provided by the recent work of Drachman and Leavitt (1974).

Drachman and Leavitt (1974) utilized the classical psychopharmacological research paradigm. They compared a range of agents that selectively, yet reversibly, block or enhance functions of neuronal systems which have been implicated in memory and cognitive functioning. Wimer (1968) used this strategy when he injected reserpine into C57BL/6J mice to test his norepinephrine hypothesis. The purpose of Drachman and Leavitt's (1964) study was to determine the relationship of the cholinergic system of the brain to memory and cognitive function in humans. To this end they employed scopolamine, methscopolamine bromide and physostigmine.

Scopolamine is an anticholenergic agent that produces an amnestic syndrome and is often used with analgesic agents to produce twilight sleep. Methscopolamine is pharmacologically dissimilar to scopolamine, but mimics its peripheral effects. It does not influence CNS functioning directly and it is thus a useful control drug

which may be employed to separate the central and peripheral effects
of scopolamine. Physostigmine is an anticholinesterase agent that
prolongs the action of neuronally released acetycholene and thus
acts in an opposite manner to that of scopolamine.

Subjects that received scopolamine exhibited a pattern of results suggesting impairment of memory storage and other cognitive
functions. Neither methscopolamine nor physostigmine appeared to
produce any significant changes in memory or other cognitive processes. Most interesting, from a life-span developmental viewpoint,
was the finding that memory and cognitive deficits induced by scopolamine were markedly similar to deficits observed for older subjects. A number of reasons for this similarity were discussed by
the authors.

The point we wish to make is that the psychopharmacological
research strategy may represent a more productive approach to the
understandings of the behavior genetics of memory processes than
does employment of general anesthetic agents within retrograde
amnesia paradigms. Moreover, human behavior genetic analyses which
may be applied with great difficulty, if at all, to human retrograde amnesia studies may be more easily accomplished with the drug
comparison paradigm.

Drug comparison paradigms may be particularly useful in research programs designed to determine the genetical basis of memory
processes. Chlorpromazine, scopolamine, physostigmine, amphetamine,
have been related to memory learning and other aspect of performance
in mice and rats (Anisman, Whalsten & Kokkinidis, in press; Anisman,
in press; Fuller, 1970). While the action of amphetamine appears
to be modulated by polygenes (Oliverio, Eleftheriou & Bailey, 1973),
it has been possible to determine the number of location of loci
which influence some agents. For example, a locus modulating the
effects of scopolamine on activity (Oliverio, Eleftheriou, &
Bailey, 1973), a locus modulating the effects of chlorpromazine on
avoidance behavior, (Castellano, Eleftheriou, Bailey & Oliverio,
1973), and a locus modulating hypothalamic norepinephrine levels
(Eleftheriou, 1974) have been identified for mice. The association
of the action of an agent, with a single locus (a given location
on a chromosome provides) a very precise genetic model for the study
of the effects of that agent on behavior.

The recommendation that increased research efforts be directed toward the use of drugs that have been implicated in learning and memory

processes as a means of exploring the genetic basis of memory with
genetic models, does not imply that descriptive studies (strain
comparisons) have no value or that studies of effects of anesthetics on behavior should be discontinued. Studies which related
differences in genotype to behavioral and structural alterations
resulting from chronic exposure to trace doses of anesthetics would
be particularly worthwhile if they were done in a life-span context.
Strain difference studies would also be a useful first step in
studies designed to separate effects of premedication, hyperventilation, surgical stress and various combinations of anesthetics
which influence behavior.

In short, it seems unlikely that much more in the way of
understanding the genetical basis of anesthetic effects on behavior
can be accomplished by strain comparison within the context of the
tradition retrograde amnesia paradigm. Strain comparisons may be
an appropriate first step in the much needed developmental studies
with implications for clinical anesthesiology. However, increased
sophistication in the administration of inhalation anesthetics and
the specification of anesthetic doses is an absolutely essential
prerequisite to these research programs if they are not to lead to
the conflicting findings which characterize the present literature
on anesthesiology and retrograde amnesia, anesthesia and the time
course of memory consolidation.

Acknowledgements

Preparation of this chapter was supported in part by a grant
from the National Institute of Child Health and Human Development to
MFE (HD-08220). Studies cited as from "our laboratory" were conducted at Allegheny College, Duke University, and the Jackson Laboratory
in collaboration with Dr. Basil E. Eleftheriou. They were supported
in part, by grants from the National Science Foundation (GB 6710)
and the United Health Services of North Carolina to MFE, and grants
from National Institute of Child Health and Human Development (HD
05860, HD 05523 to Dr. Basil E. Eleftheriou.

Thanks are extended to Mrs. Nicole Maier for her careful editing
and typing of the manuscript submitted to the editor. We also
acknowledge the contributions of G. Douglass Blenkarn, M.D. (Duke
University, Scott Simmerman (University of North Carolina), Basil E.
Eleftheriou, Ph.D. (The Jackson Laboratory), and Donald W. Bailey,
Ph.D. (The Jackson Laboratory) for various contributions including
laboratory space, critiques of the literature, and co-authorship of
various studies cited as from our laboratory.

REFERENCES

ABEELEN, J. H. G.V. 1963, Mouse mutants studied by means of etholog-
    ical methods, Genetica 34:79.

ABT, J. P., ESSMAN, W. B., & JARVIK, M. E., 1961, Ether induced
    retrograde amnesia for one trial conditioning in mice, Science
    133:1477.

ADAM, N., 1972, Effects of general anesthetics on memory function
    in man, J. Comp. & Physiol. Psychol. 83:294.

ADRIANI, J., 1962, "The chemistry and physics of anesthesia," New
    York, Thomas.

AGRANOFF, B. W., DAVIS, R. E., & BRINK, J. J., 1965, Memory fixa-
    tion in the goldfish, Proc. Nat. Acad. Sci. 54:788.

ALPERN, H. P., & KIMBLE, D. P., 1967, Retrograde amnesic effects of
    diethyl ether and bis(trifluoroethyl) ether, J. Comp. & Physiol.
    Psychol. 63:168.

ALMENT, E. A. J., 1959, Consciousness during surgical operations,
    Brit. Med. Jour. 2:1258.

A.M.A. Fundamentals of Anesthetic, 1954, W. B. Saunders Company,
    Philadelphia, 3rd edition.

ANISMAN, H., WAHLSTEN, D., & KOKKINIDIS, L., in press, Effects of
    d-amphetamine and scopolamine on activity before and after
    shock in three mouse strains, Pharmacol. Biochem. & Behav.

ANISMAN, H., in press, Differential effects of scopolamine and
    d-amphetamine on avoidance: Strain interactions, Pharmacol.
    Biochem. & Behav.

ARDUINI, A., & ARDUINI, M. G., 1954, Effects of drugs and metabolic
    alterations on brain stem arousal mechanism, J. Pharmacol. &
    Exp. Thera. 110:76.

ARTUSIO, J. F. JR., 1955, Ether analgesia during major surgery,
    J. Amer. Med. Assoc. 157:33.

AYERST LABORATORIES, 1967, Fluothane (halothane). For precision
    inhalation anesthesia. A guide to its use based on decade of
    clinical experiment, Ayerst Laboratories, New York, New York.

BAILEY, D. W., 1971, Recombinant-inbred strains, Transplantation
    11:325.

BARONDES, S. H., & COHEN, H. D., 1968, Arousal and the conversion
    of "short-term" to "long-term" memory, Proc. Nat. Acad. Sci.
    61:923.

BERGER, B. D., 1970, Learning in the anesthetized rat, Fed. Proc. 29:749 (Abs.)

BERRY, C., 1965, Effects of a drug on immediate memory, Nature (London). 207:1012.

BERRY, C., 1968, Individual differences in short-term memory, Nature (London). 220:302.

BERTLER, A., & ROSENGREN, E., 1959, Occurrence and distribution of catechol amines in brain, Acta. Physiol. Scand. 47:350.

BLACK, M., SUBOSKI, M. D., & FREEDMAN, N. L., 1967. Effects of cortical spreading depression and ether following one-trial discriminated avoidance learning, Psychon. Sci. 9:597.

BLENKARN, G. D., BRIGGS, G., BELL, J., & SUGIOKA, K., 1972, Cognitive function after hypocapnic hyperventilation, Anesthesiology 37:381.

BLOCH, V., 1970, Facts and hypothesis concerning memory consolidation processes, Brain Res. 24:561.

BOHDANECKY, Z., KOPP, R., & JARVIK, M. E., 1968, Comparison of ECS and flurothyl-induced retrograde amnesia in mice, Psychopharmacol. 12:91.

BREWSTER, W. R. JR., BUNKER, J. P., & BEECHER, H. K., 1952, Metabolic effects of anesthesia. VI. Mechanism of metabolic acidosis and hyperglycemia during ether anesthesia, Amer. J. Physiol. 171:37.

BROADHURST, P. L., 1969, The diallel cross method, in, "Behavioral genetics: Method and research," (M. Manosevitz, G. Lindzey and D. D. Thiessen, eds.), Appleton-Century, New York,   p. 142.

BRICE, D. D., HETHERINGTON, R. R., & UTTING, J. E., 1970, A simple study of awareness and dreaming during anesthesia, Brit. J. Anaes. 42:535.

BRUCE, D. L., BACH, M. J., & ARBIT, J., 1974, Trace anesthetic: Effects on perceptual cognitive and motor skills, Anesthesiology 35:348.

BRUCE, D. L., EIDE, K. A., LINDE, H. W., & ECKENHOFF, J. E., 1968, Cause of death among anesthesiologists: A twenty year survey, Anesthesiology 29:565.

BUCHSBAUM, M., & BUCHSBAUM, R., 1962, Age and ether anesthesia in mice, Proc. Soc. Exper. Biol & Med. 109:68.

BUNKER, J. P., & VANDAM, L. D., 1965, Effects of anesthesia on metabolism and cellular functions, Pharmacol. Rev. 17:183.

BUREŠ, J., 1959, Reversible decortication and behavior, in, "Second conference on the CNS and behavior," (M. B. A. Brazier, ed.), Josiah Macy, Jr., Foundation, New York, p. 207.

BUREŠ, J., & BUREŠOVA, O., 1963, Cortical spreading depression as a memory disturbing factor, J. Comp. & Physiol. Psych. 56:268.

BURNAP, T. K., GALLA, S. J., & VANDAM, L. D., 1958, Anesthetic circulatory and respiratory effects of fluothane, Anesthesiology 19:307.

BURNHAM, W. H., 1903, Retroactive amnesia: Illustrative cases and a tentative explanation, Amer. J. Psychol. 14:382.

CARLSSON, A., FALCK, B., & HILLARP, N. A., 1962, Cellular localization of brain monoamines, Acta. Physiol. Scand. 56, Suppl. 196

CASTELLANO, C., ELEFTHERIOU, B. E., BAILEY, D. W., & OLIVERIO, A., 1973, Chlorpromazine and avoidance: A genetic analysis, Psycho pharmacol. 34:309.

CHERKIN, A., 1966, Memory consolidation: Probit analysis of retrograde-amnesia data, Psychon. Sci. 4:169.

CHERKIN, A., 1968a, Molecules, anesthesia, and memory, in, "Structural chemistry and molecular biology," (A. Rich and N. Davidson- eds.), W. H. Freeman, San Francisco, p. 325.

CHERKIN, A., 1968b, Retrograde amnesia: Role of temperature, dose, and duration of amnesic agent, Psychon. Sci. 13:255.

CHERKIN, A., 1969, Flurothyl toxicity: a remarkable species difference between chick and mouse, Psychopharmacologia 15:404.

CHERKIN, A., 1971, Biphasic time course of performance after one--trial avoidance training in the chick, Commun. in Behav. Biol. 5:183.

CHERKIN, A., & HARROUN, P., 1971, Anesthesia and memory processes, Anesthesiology 34:469.

CHERKIN, A., & LEE-TENG, E., 1965, Interruption by halothane of memory consolidation in chicks, Fed. Proc. 24:328 (Abs.).

CHOROVER, S. L., & SCHILLER, P. H., 1966, Reexamination of prolonged retrograde amnesia in one-trial learning. J. Comp. & Physiol. Psychol. 61:34.

CHOY, T., & PARKHOUSE, J., 1969, Laboratory studies of inhalation anaesthetics, Brit. J. Anaes. 41:827.

COHEN, E. N., BELLVILLE, J. W., & BROWN, B. W., 1971, Anesthesia, pregnancy and miscarriage, Anesthesiology 35:343.

CRAIK, F. I. M., 1968, Short term memory and aging process,in "Human aging and behavior," (George A. Talland, ed.), New York, Academic Press, p. 131.

CROSSLAND, J., & MERRICK, A. J., 1954, The effect of anesthesia on the acetylcholine content of brain, J. Physiol. London. 125:56.

CSILLIK, B., & ERULKAR, S. D., 1964, Labile stores of monoamines in the central nervous system: A histochemical study, J. Pharmacol & Exp. Thera. 146:186.

DAVIS, H. S., DILLON, W. H., COLLINS, W. F., & RANDT, C. T., 1958, The effects of anesthetic agents on evoked central nervous system responses: muscle relaxants and volatile agents, Anesthesiology 19:441.

DEUTSCH, J. A., 1962, Higher nervous function: The physiological bases of memory, Ann. Rev. Psychol. 24:259.

DOMINO, E. F., 1967, Effects of preanesthetic and anesthetic drugs on visually evoked responses, Anesthesiology 28:184.

DRACHMAN, D. A., & LEAVITT, J., 1974, Human memory and the cholinergic system, Arch. Neurol. 30:113.

DYE, C. J., 1969, Effects of interruption of initial learning upon retention in young, mature and old rats. J. Gerontol. 24:12.

ELEFTHERIOU, B. E., 1974, A gene influencing hypothalamic norepinephrine levels in mice, Brain Res. 70:538.

ELEFTHERIOU, B. E., & BAILEY,D. W., 1972, A gene controlling plasma serotonin levels in mice, J. Endocrinol. 55:225.

ELIAS, M. F., BLENKARN, G. D., SIMMERMAN, S. J., & MARSH, G. R., 1971, Administration of inhalation anesthetics to small animals Some problems and solutions, Behav. Res. Meth. & Instrumen. 3:70.

312   M. F. ELIAS & C. A. PENTZ

ELIAS, M. F., & ELEFTHERIOU, B. E., 1972, Reversal learning and RNA labeling in neurological mutant mice and normal littermates, Physiol. & Behav. 9:27.

ELIAS, M. F., & ELEFTHERIOU, B. E., in press a, A genetic investigation of induction and eduction times for halothane anesthesia, Behav. Res. Meth. & Instrumen.

ELIAS, M. F., & ELEFTHERIOU, B. E., in press b, A genetic analysis of water maze discrimination learning for Mus musculus: Polygenes and albinism, Physiol. & Behav.

ELIAS, M. F., & ELIAS, P. K., in press a, Motivation and activity, in, "Handbook of the Psychology of Aging," (J. E. Birren and K. W. Schaie, eds.), Van Nostrand Reinhold Company, New York.

ELIAS, M. F., & ELIAS, P. K., in press b, Hormones aging and behavior in mammals, in, "Hormonal correlates of behavior," (B. E. Eleftheriou and R. L. Sprott, eds.), Plenum Press, New York.

ELIAS, J.W., ELIAS, M. F., & SCHLAGER, G., 1975, Aggressive social interaction in mice genetically selected for blood pressure extremes, Behav. Biol. 13:155.

ELIAS, M. F., & KINSBOURNE, M., 1974, Age and sex differences in the processing of verbal and nonverbal stimuli, J. Gerontol. 29:162.

ELIAS, M. F., & SCHLAGER, G., 1974, Discrimination learning in mice genetically selected for high and low blood pressure: Initial findings and methodological implications, Physiol. & Behav. 13:261.

ELIAS, M. F., & SIMMERMAN, S. J., 1971a, Strain differences in memory and incentive as a function of external stimulation. Psychon. Sci. 22:189.

ELIAS, M. F., & SIMMERMAN, S. J., 1971b, Proactive and retroactive effects of diethyl ether on spatial discrimination learning in inbred mouse strains DBA/2J and C57BL/6J, Psychon. Sci. 22:299.

ELLIOTT, K. A. C., SWANK, R. L., & HENDERSON, D., 1950, Effects of anesthetics and convulsants on acetylcholine content of brain, Amer. J. Physiol. 162:469.

ERICKSON, M. H., 1963, Chemo-anesthesia in relation to hearing and memory, Amer. J. Clin. Hyp. 6:31.

ESSMAN, W. B., & JARVIK, M. E., 1961, Impairment of retention for a conditioned response by ether anesthesia in mice, Psychopharmacologia 2:172.

FAULCONER, A., 1952, Correlation of concentrations of ether in arterial blood with electro-encephalographic patterns occurring during ether-oxygen and during nitrous oxide, oxygen and ether anesthesia of human surgical patients, Anesthesiology 13:361.

FRECKLETON, W. C., & WAHLSTEIN, D., 1968, CO_2-inducted amnesia in the cockroach, Psychon. Sci. 12:179.

FREIDMAN, R. C., RICHART, R. M., & VANDE WIELE, R. L., 1974, "Sex differences in behavior," John Wiley&Sons, New York.

FRENCH, J. D., VERZEANS, M., & MARGOUN, H. W., 1953, A neural basis of the anesthetic state, A.M.A., Arch. Neurol. & Psychiat. 69:519.

FULLER, J. L., 1970, Strain differences in the effects of chlorpromazine and chlordiazepoxide upon active and passive avoidance in mice, Psychopharmacologia 16:261.

FULLER, J. L., & THOMPSON, W. R., 1960, "Behavior genetics," Wiley & Sons, New York.

GALAMBOS, R., 1967, Introduction: Brain correlates of learning, in, "The neurosciences, a study program," (G. C. Quarton, T. Melnecluk and F. O. Schmitt, eds.), Rockefeller University Press, New York.

GALLUSCIO, E. H., & GRANT, A., 1970, Hypoxia and retrograde amnesia, Psychon. Sci. 18:17.

GALLUSCIO, E. H., 1971, Retrograde amnesia induced by electroconvulsive shock and carbon dioxide anesthesia in rats, J. Comp. & Physiol. Psychol. 75:136.

GEDDES, I. C.,&GRAY, T. C., 1959, Hyperventilation for the maintenance of anesthesia, Lancet 2:4.

GLICKMAN, S. E., 1958, Preservative neural processes and consolidation of the memory trace, Psychol. Bull. 3:218.

GLOWINSKI, J., & AXELROD, J., 1965, Effect of drugs on the uptake, release and metabolism of H^3-norepinephrine in the rat brain, J. Pharmacol. & Exp. Thera. 149:43.

GOODMAN, L. S., & GILMAN, A., 1970, "The pharmacological basis of therapeutics," The Macmillan Company, London, 4th edition.

GRAY, T. C., & NUNN, J. F., 1971, "General anaesthesia," Butterworths Company, London, 3rd edition.

GREEN, H., & SAWYER, J. L., 1960, Intracellular distribution of norepinephrine in rat brain, I. Effect of reserpine and the monoamine oxidase inhibitors, trans-2-phenylcyclopropylamine and 1-isonicotinyl-2-isopropyl hydrazine, J. Pharmacol. & Exp. Thera. 129:243.

GRUBER, R. P., & REED, D. R., 1968, Postoperative anterograde amnesia, Brit. J. Anaes. 40:845.

GUTEKUNST, R., & YOUNISS, J., 1963, Interruption of imprinting following anesthesia, Percep. Motor Skills. 16:348.

HEBB, D. O., 1949, "The organization of behavior," Wiley and Sons, New York.

HEINZE, W. J., 1974, Genotypic influences on ether-induced retrograde amnesia in rats, Behav. Biol. 11:109.

HENDERSON, N. D., 1969, Prior treatment effects on open field behavior of mice: A genetic analysis, in, "Behavioral genetics: Method and research," (M. Manosevitz, G. Lindzey and D. Thiessen, eds.), Appleton Century Crofts, New York, p. 475.

HENRIE, J. R., PARKHOUSE, J., & BICKFORD, R. G., 1961, Alteration of human consciousness by nitrous oxide as assessed by electroencephalography and psychological tests, Anesthesiology, 22:247.

HERZ, M. J., 1969, Interference with one-trial appetitive and aversive learning by ether and ECS, J. Neurobiol. 1:111.

HERZ, M. J., 1962, The effects of ether on the retention of a one--trial avoidance response. MA thesis, San Francisco State College.

HERZ, M. J., PEEKE, H. V. S., & WYERS, E. J., 1966, Amnesic effects of ether and electroconvulsive shock in mice, Psychon. Sci. 4:375.

HOSEIN, E. A., & ARA, R., 1962, The influence of pentobarbital and ether narcosis on the brain concentration of various esters with acetylcholine activity, J. Pharmacol. & Exp. Thera. 135:230.

HUTCHINSON, R., 1960, Awareness during surgery, Brit. J. Anaes. 33:463.

HUTT, C., 1972, Sex differences in human development, Hum. Devel. 15:153.

HYDEN, H., 1967, Biochemical changes accompanying learning, in, "The neurosciences, a study program," (G. C. Quarton, T. Melnecluk and F. O. Schmitt, eds.), Rockefeller University Press, New York, p. 765.

IRWIN, S., BANUAZIZI, A., KALSNER, S., & CURTIS, A., 1968, One-trial learning in the mouse. I. Its characteristics and modification by experimental-seasonal variables, Psychopharmacologia 12:286.

JACKSON, H., 1884, The Croonian lectures on evolution and dissolution of the nervous system, Brit. Med. J. 1:591;660;703.

JAKUBCZAK, L. F., 1970, Age, food deprivation and the temporal distribution of wheel running of rats, Proc. 78th Ann. Con. Amer. Psychol. Ass. 689.

JARVIK, M. E., 1964, The influence of drugs upon memory, in, "Ciba foundation symposium on animal behavior and drug action," (H. Steinberg, H. V. S. DeReuck and J. Knights, eds.), Little-Brown, Boston, p. 44.

JARVIK, M. E., 1968, Consolidation of memory, in, "Psychopharmacology: A review of progress 1957-1967," (D. H. Efron, ed.),U.S. Govt. Printing Office, Washington, P. H. S. Publ. No. 1836, 885.

KARCZMAR, A. G., 1970, Central cholinergic pathways and their behavioral implications, in, "Principles of psychopharmacology," (W. G. Clark, K. S. Ditman, C. P. Leske, and D. X. Freedman, eds.), Academic Press, New York, p. 57.

KLEMM, W. R., 1969, ECS and estrous cycle interactions in one-trial avoidance behavior of rats, Comm. in Behav. Biol. 4:59.

LARRABEE, M. G., & POSTERNAK, J. M., 1952, Selective action of anesthesitcs on synapses and axons in mammalian sympathetic ganglia, J. Neurophysiol. 15:91.

LEUKEL, F., & QUINTON, E., 1964, Carbon dioxide effects on acquisition and extinction of avoidance behavior, J. Comp. & Physiol. Psych. 57:267.

LICO, M. C., HOFFMANN, A., & COVIAN, M. R., 1968, Autonomic conditioning in the anesthetized rabbit, Physiol. & Behav. 3:673.

LINDE, H. W., & BRUCE, D. L., 1969, Occupational exposure of anesthetists to halothane, nitrous oxide and radiation, Anesthesiology 30:363.

LUMB, W. V., 1963, "Small animal anesthesia," Lea and Febiger, Philadelphia.

MANOSEVITZ, M., LINDZEY, G., & THIESSEN, D. D., 1969, "Behavioral genetics: Method and research," Appleton-Century, New York.

MARSHALL, W. H., 1959, Spreading cortical depression of Leão, Physiol. Rev. 39:239.

MATTHEWS, J. H., MARTE, E., & HALBERG, F., 1964, A circadian susceptibility-resistance cycle to fluothane in male B1 mice, Canad. Anes. Soc. J. 118:280.

MAYMAN, C. I., GATFIELD, P. D., & BRECKENRIDGE, B. McL., 1964, The glucose content of brain in anesthesia, J. Neurochem. 11:483.

MAZZIA, V. D. B., & RANDT, C., 1966, Amnesia and eye movements in first stage anesthesia, Arch. Neurol. 14:522.

McGAUGH, J. L., 1966, Time-dependent processes in memory storage, Sci. 153:1351.

McGAUGH, J. L., & PETRINOVICH, L. F., 1965, Effects of drugs on learning and memory, Internat. Rev. Neurobiol. 8:139.

McKINNEY, F., 1932, Nitrous oxide anesthesia as an experimental technique in psychology, J. Gen. Psych. 6:195.

MEIER, G. W., & FOSHEE, D. P., 1963, Genetics, age, and the variability of learning performances, J. Genet. Psych. 102:267.

MILLER, R. R., & SPRINGER, A. D., 1973, Amnesia, consolidation, and retrieval, Psychol. Rev. 80:69.

MOORE-EDE, M. C., 1973, Circadian rhythms of drug effectiveness and toxicity, Clin. Pharmacol. & Thera. 14:925.

MORI, K., WINTERS, W. D., & SPOONER, C. E., 1968. Comparison of reticular and cochlear multiple unit activity with auditory evoked response during various stages induced by anesthetic agents. II. Electroencephal. & Clin. Neurophysiol. 24: 242.

MOSCONA, M. H., & MOSCONA, A. A., 1963, Inhibition of adhesiveness and aggregation of dissociated cells by inhibitors of protein and RNA synthesis, Science 142:1070.

MULLER, G. E., & PILZECKER, A., 1900, Experementelle Beitrage zur Lehre vom Gedachtnis, Zeit. fur Psychol. und Physiol. der Sinnersorgane. Suppl. No. 1.

MUNSON, E. S., MARTUCCI, R. W., & SMITH, R. F., 1970, Circadian variation in anesthetic requirement and toxicity in rats, Anesthesiology 32:507.

NACHMAN, M., & MEINECKE, R. O., 1969, Lack of retrograde amnesia effects of repeated electroconvulsive shock and carbon dioxide treatments, J. Comp. & Physiol. Psych. 68:631.

NAKANISHI, Y. H., KATAO, H., & IWASAKI, T., 1963, Inhibitory effects of chloramphenicol on the histogenetic aggregration of dissociated cells, Jap. J. Hum. Genet. 38:257.

NASH, J., 1970, Sex differences and their origins, in, "Developmental psychology. A psychobiological approach," (J. Nash, ed.), Prentice Hall, Englewood Cliffs, N.J.

NATIONAL HALOTHANE STUDY: Possible association between halothane anesthesia and postoperative hepatic necrosis, 1966, J. Amer. Med. Assoc. 197:121.

NELSON, W., & HALBERG, F., 1973, An evaluation of time dependent changes in susceptibility of mice to pentobarbitol injection, Neuropharmacol. 12:509.

NIKKY, P., 1972, On anesthetic gas harmful to the operating theater staff, Ann. Clin. Res. 4:247.

OLIVERIO, A., ELEFTHERIOU, B. E., & BAILEY, D. W., 1973, Exploratory activity: Genetic analysis of its modification by scopolamine and amphetamine, Physiol. & Behav. 10(5):893.

OLIVERIO, A., & MESSERI, P., 1973, An analysis of single-gene effects on avoidance, maze, wheel running, and exploratory behavior in the mouse, Behav. Biol. 8:771.

OWENS, G., 1958, Further studies on ether convulsion: Fat embolization and its association with neurologic deficits, Neurol. 8:827.

PAOLINO, R. M., QUARTERMAIN, D., & MILLER, N. E., 1966, Different temporal gradients of retrograde amnesia produced by carbon dioxide anesthesia and electroconvulsive shock, J. Comp. & Physiol. Psych. 62:270.

PARKHOUSE, J., HENRIE, J. R., DUNCAN, G. M., & ROME, H. P., 1960, Nitrous oxide analgesia in relation to mental performance, J. Pharmacol. & Exp. Ther. 128:44.

PEARLMAN, C. A., 1966, Similar retrograde amnesic effects of ether and spreading cortical depression, J. Comp. & Physiol. Psych. 61:306.

PEARLMAN, C. A., SHARPLESS, S. K., & JARVIK, M. E., 1961, Retro-
    grade amnesia produced by anesthetic and convulsive agents,
    J. Comp. Physiol. Psychol. 54:109.

PORTER, A. L., 1972. An analytical review of the effects of non-
    -hydrogen-bonding anesthetics on memory processing, Behav.
    Biol. 7:291.

PORTER, A. L., 1974, Effects of non-hydrogen bonding anesthetics on
    memory in the chick, Behav. Biol. 10:365.

QUIMBY, K. L., ASCHKINASE, L. J., BOWMAN, R. E., KATZ, J., & CHANG,
    L. W., 1974, Enduring learning deficits and cerebral synaptic
    malformation from exposure to 10 PPM halothane, Sci. 185:625.

QUINTON, E. E., 1966, Retrograde amnesia induced by carbon dioxide
    inhalation, Psychon. Sci. 5:417.

RANSMEIER, R. E., & GERARD, R. W., 1954, Effects of temperature,
    convulsion and metabolic factors on rodent memory and EEG,
    Amer. J. Physiol. 179:663.

RAVENTOS, J., 1956, The action of fluothane - a new volatile
    anaesthetic, Brit. J. Pharmacol. 11:394.

RIEGE, W. H., & CHERKIN, A., 1973, Retroactive facilitation of mem-
    ory of goldfish by flurothyl, Psychopharmacologia 30:195.

ROBSON, J. G., BURNS, B. D., & WELT, P. J. L., 1960, The effect of
    inhaling dilute nitrous oxide upon recent memory and time es-
    timation, Canad. Anaesthestists Soc. J. 7:399.

ROSEN, J., 1959, Hearing tests during anaesthesia with nitrous
    oxide and relaxants, Acta Anesthes. Scand. 3:1.

ROSENBERG, F. J., & DiSTEFANO, V., 1962, A central nervous system
    component of epinephrine hyperglycemia, Amer. J. Physiol.
    203:782.

ROYCE, J., YEUDALL, L., & POLEY, W., 1971, Diallel analysis of
    avoidance conditioning in inbred strains of mice, J. Comp. &
    Physiol. Psych. 76:353.

SCHLAGER, G., 1964, Selection for blood pressure levels in mice,
    Genetics 76:537.

SCHMID, J., 1964, Zur Frage der Störung der Sozalen Bindung durch
    Narkosemittel, Zugleich ein Beitrag zur Störung der Sozalen
    Bindung durch Narkose, Seit. für Vergleichende Physiologie
    47:559.

SCHMIDT, J., 1919, La valeur de l'individu à titre de générateur
    appreciée suivant la methode du croisement diallèle, Cancer
    Res. Lab. Carlsberg. 14:1.

SIEGLER, R., & RICH, M. A., 1963, Artificiel respiration in mice
    during thoracic surgery: A simple, inexpensive technique, Proc.
    Soc. Exp. Biol. & Med. 114:511.

SINGH, S. I., & MALHOTRA, C. L., 1964, Amino acid content of monkey
    brain. III. Effects of reserpine on some amino acids of cer-
    tain regions of monkey brain, J. Neurochem. 11:865.

SPROTT, R. L., 1974, Passive-avoidance performance in mice:
    Evidence for single-locus inheritance, Behav. Biol. 11:231.

STEINBERG, H., 1954, Selective effects of an anesthetic drug on
    cognitive behavior, Quart. J. Exp. Psych. 6:170.

STEINBERG, H., & SUMMERFIELD, A., 1957a, Influence of a depressant
    drug on acquisition in role learning, Quart. J. Exp. Psych.
    9:138.

STEINBERG, H., & SUMMERFIELD, A., 1957b, Reducing interference in
    forgetting, Quart. J. Exp. Psych. 9:146.

STEINBERG, H., & TOMKIEWICZ, M., 1968, Drugs and memory, in,
    "Psychopharmacology," (D. H. Efron, ed.), PHS Publ. 1836, U.S.
    Govt. Printing Office, Washington, D.C., p. 879.

STILES, S. W., 1959, Induction of ether anesthesia in cats, J. Amer.
    Vet. Med. Ass. 134:275.

STREICHER, E., & GARBUS, J., 1955, The effect of age and sex on the
    duration of hexobarbitol anesthesia in rats, J. Gerontol. 10:
    441.

SUBOSKI, M. D., LITNER, J., & BLACK, M., 1968, Further on the
    effects of ether anesthesia following one-trial discriminated
    avoidance learning, Psychon. Sci. 10:161.

SUGIOKA, K., & DAVIS, D. A., 1960, Hyperventilation with oxygen-
    a possible cause of cerebral hypoxia, Anesthesiology 21:135.

SUMMERFIELD, A., & STEINBERG, H., 1959, Using drugs to alter
    memory experimentally in man, in, "Neuropsychopharmacology,"
    (P. B. Bradley, P. Dencker and C. Radpuco-Thomas, eds.),
    Elsevier, New York, p. 481.

TABER, R. I., & BANUAZIZI, A., 1966, CO_2-induced retrograde amnesia
    in a one-trial learning situation, Psychopharmacologia 9:382.

TABER, R., & IRWIN, S., 1969, Anesthesia in the mouse, Fed. Proc. 28:1528.

THIESSEN, D. D., 1970, Reply to Wilcock on gene action and behavior, Psych. Bull. 75:103.

THOMPSON, R., 1957, The effect of ECS on retention in young and adult rats, J. Comp. Physiol. Psych. 50:644.

UNGAR, G., & KEATS, A. S., 1973, Inhibition of embryonic brain cell aggregration by general anesthetics, Anesthesiology 39:362.

VOGHT, M., 1954, The concentration of sympathin in different parts of the central nervous system under normal conditions and after the administration of drugs, J. Physiology, London. 123:451.

WAHLSTEN, D., 1972, Genetic experiments with animal learning: A critical review, Behav. Biol. 7:143.

WEISS, T., & FIFKOVA, E., 1961, Bioelectric activity in the thalamus and hypothalamus of rats during cortical spreading EEG depression, Electroencephal. & Clin. Neurophysiol. 24:242.

WHITCHER, C. E., COHEN, E. N., & TRUDELL, J. R., 1971, Chronic exposure to anesthetic gases in the operating room, Anesthesiology 35:348.

WHITWAM, J. G., BOETTNER, R. B., GILGER, A. P., & LITTELL, A. S., 1966, Hyperventilation, brain damage and flicker, Brit. J. Anaes. 38:846.

WILCOCK, J., 1969, Gene action and behavior: An evaluation of major gene pleiotropism, Psych. Bull. 72:1.

WIMER, R. E., 1968, Bases of a facilitative effect upon retention resulting from posttrial etherization, J. Comp. & Physiol. Psych. 65:340.

WIMER, R. E., 1973, Dissociation of a phenotypic correlation: Response to posttrial etherization and to variation in temporal distribution of practice trials, Behav. Genet. 3:379.

WIMER, R. E., & HUSTON, C., 1974, Facilitation of learning performance by posttrial etherization, Behav. Biol. 10:385.

WIMER, R. E., NORMAN, R., & ELEFTHERIOU, B. E., 1973, Serotonin levels in hippocampus: Striking variations associated with mouse strain and treatment, Brain Res. 63:397.

WIMER, R. E., SYMINGTON, L., FARMER, H., & SCHWARTZKROIN, P., 1968, Differences in memory processes between inbred mouse strains C57BL/6J and DBA/2J, J. Comp. & Physiol. Psych. 65:126.

WINTERS, W. D., & WALLACH, M. B., 1970, Drug-induced states of CNS excitation: A theory of hallucinosis, in, "Psychotomimetic Drugs," (D. H. Efron, ed.), Raven, New York, p. 193.

WOLLMAN, S. B., & ORKIN, L. R., 1968, Postoperative human reaction and hypocarbia during anaesthesia, Brit. J. Anaes. 40:920.

WOODBURY, D. M., ROLLINS, L. T., GARDNER, M. D., HIRSCHI, W. L., HOYAN, J. R., RALLISON, M. L., TANNER, A. S., & BRODIE, D. A., 1958, Effects of carbon dioxide on brain excitability and electrolytes, Amer. J. Physiol. 192: 79.

WOODS, L. A., & HAGGART, J., 1957, Apneic and hypotensive effects of local anesthetic drugs in dogs and mice under general anesthesia, Anesthesiology 18:831.

ZAUDER, H. L., & ORKIN, L. R., 1959, Chamber for anesthetization of small animals, Anesthesiology 20:707.

SPECIES DIFFERENCES IN RESPONSE TO AMPHETAMINE

Everett H. Ellinwood, Jr., M.D. and M. Marlyne Kilbey, M.D.

Behavior Neuropharmacology Section, Psychiatry Department,

Duke University, Durham, North Carolina

CONTENTS

INTRODUCTION

     Variation in response to drugs has been accepted as an una-
voidable and complicating factor by most persons who have sought
to clarify drug actions on any level: pharmacological, neurological, or psychological. Now, however, the contribution of genetic
factors to that variance is coming under investigation. There is
some evidence that pharmacological actions vary across strains of
animals, and that this differential activity may reflect mechanisms
controlled by genetic factors (Miller et al., 1968; Kilbey et al.,
1972; Richardson et al., 1972) which also systematically influence
behavioral patterns. For example, one set of investigations
(Oliverio et al., 1973; Oliverio et al., 1974) has identified single genes controlling exploratory activity and the effect of scopolamine on this response. As many drug effects are thought to be
modulated via brain amines (Cooper et al., 1974), and as lines of
evidence have suggested that variation seen in biogenic amines may
be controlled, in part, by genetic factors (Maas, 1962, 1963;
Sudak and Maas, 1964a, 1964b; Schlesinger et al., 1965; Karczmar
and Scudder, 1967; Karczmar et al., 1973; Barchas et al., 1974),
studies which administer drugs to various strains of animals and
measure the resulting behavior and the effects on brain amines have
been used to identify the relationships between drug action, biogenic amines and genetic factors.

     The purpose of this paper is to review the variation seen in
response to amphetamine. Behavioral stereotypes, thermal responses,
and several differential responses in man will be considered. It
is our hope that this will establish what is known of the variation
seen in these phenomena, clarify which response patterns are influ-

enced by genetic factors, and identify those questions which may
be answered by this experimental approach in the near future.

AMPHETAMINE-INDUCED STEREOTYPY

Amphetamine is believed to cause an increased activity of dopamine (DA) and norepinephrine (NE) at postsynaptic receptors by
stimulating release and/or blocking reuptake of endogenous catecholamines (CA) (Cooper et al., 1974). In experimental animals, the
behavrioral response consists of two primary components: (1) an
increased motor activity, including locomotion and exploring behavior, that is most characteristic of lower doses of amphetamine or
initial stages of intoxication; and (2) stereotyped behaviors
(Randrup et al., 1963; Randrup and Munkvad, 1967; Ellinwood, 1968,
1969) usually described as behavior showing little variation, that
is, a single activity, or a sequence of actions which dominates the
animal's behavior. Amphetamine-induced stereotyped behavior (AISB)
has been used as an animal model of psychoses (Wallach 1974), and
potential neuroleptics are tested for their ability to block AISB.
Because of this, stereotyped behavior has been studied extensively.
It is seen in rats, mice, guinea pigs, cats, monkeys, chickens,
pigeons, dogs, chimpanzees and man.

Amphetamine-induced stereotypies in man appear as an early component of amphetamine psychosis. In spite of a great deal of individual variability, a fully developed amphetamine psychosis usually
presents a fairly distinct syndrome characterized by delusions of
persecution, ideas of reference, visual, tactile, and auditory hallucinations, changes in body image, hyperactivity, and excitation.
The consciousness is clear; the individual is oriented in space and
time. Highly developed fixed delusions as well as compulsive behaviors are seen.

In animals, stereotyped behavior is compulsive or "Zwangsnagn."
It is seemingly nondistractible, with a "driven" rapid, repetitious
character (Janssen et al., 1965). This is represented best by the
"compulsive" gnawing and sniffing noted in rats. Alternately, AISB
appears purposeless because its significance, if any, is not obvious
to the experimenter, and once initiated it is not responsive to external stimulus contingencies (Emele et al., 1961). Animals may
perform repetitious movements associated with specific behaviors,
such as searching movements of looking and sniffing, which do not
seem related to the presence of significant visual or olfactory
stimuli in the immediate environment. Behavior also occurs that
has been described as abortive in that behavioral sequences are
initiated and are not completed (Ellinwood, 1968). Additionally,
AISB may appear dysjunctive, indicating a lack of an association
between posture and ongoing movements or between posture and movements of different regions of the body (Ellinwood, 1969). Dyskinesia, ataxia, and bizarre posture may develop with chronic ampheta-

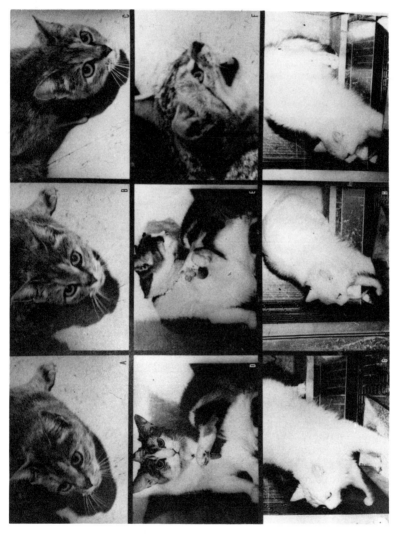

Fig. 1. Repetitive stereotyped patterns of behavior induced by chronic methedrine administration: (A–C) side-to-side head turning and looking; (D–E) abortive grooming reaction; (F) hissing on any approach; (G–I) sniffing small area in cage (from Ellinwood, 1969; reprinted by permission from Seminars in Psychiatry).

mine intoxication. Fig. 1 illustrates some of the AISB in the cat.
Stereotypies are influenced by several factors, among which are:
(1) species specific behavior patterns, (2) environmental contingencies, and (3) dose, duration, and frequency of drug administration. These factors will be discussed further.

Species Specific Behavior

The behaviors that become "locked in" to the stereotypies are
species-specific behaviors (Randrup and Munkvad, 1967; Ellinwood,
1971) and, in general, are represented in stereotypies on the basis
of their prepotencies in the animal's fundamental repertoire, although they often are modified by an interaction with the environmental contingencies present at the initiation of the amphetamine
intoxication (Ellinwood and Kilbey, 1975). One common denominator
of AISB noted across species is a high prepotency of patterns of
searching, examining and attending - at least the motor components
of these processes are noted (Ellinwood, 1971). For example, in
macronosmatic animals, the primary stereotypy is sniffing. They
also involve fundamental behaviors, such as licking and gnawing.
These are examination patterns in rodents which develop early in
ontogeny. Rudimentary grooming behavior, incorporating licking, is
detectable by Day 2 after birth, and sniffing is seen by Day 12
(Lal and Sourkes, 1973). Gnawing in the rodent is incorporated in
many behavioral sequences, including nest-building and eating, as
well as examining. Moving up the phylogenetic scale to cats, sniffing, which develops in the first postnatal week (Rosenblatt, 1972),
is seen in the AISB and looking movements become prominent. In primates, a totally new dimension is added to AISB - that of eye-hand
examination patterns (Ellinwood, 1971). In the primate, these patterns are quite specific and consist primarily of picking, probing
with the hands, and also clasping and examining them. Fitz-Gerald
(1967) described self-picking which resulted in sores in chimpanzees given amphetamine. Even in humans, one notes stereotypies of
behavior that have substrates in these motor patterns (Ellinwood,
1968, 1972a; Ellinwood and Sudilovsky, 1973b). This is illustrated
by the patient in Fig. 2 demonstrating the dermal manifestations of
delusions of parasitosis. These delusions are quite common in stimulant abusers experiencing an amphetamine-associated psychosis and
may represent an intensification of the sensations originally described by the drug user as tingling, creeping, or itching of the
skin. These patients believe they have parasites, mites, or lice
under the surface of the skin. The compulsive rubbing and digging
behaviors which are seen in these patients appear to be similar to
the grooming-examining stereotypies seen in animals. Because of
these similarities, it would seem that in these species (man, chim-
panzee, monkey, cat, and rat), intrinsic investigatory and grooming
patterns of behavior are being stimulated by amphetamine and are
subsequently incorporated in a stereotyped behavioral pattern, and,
in some cases, provide the substrate for delusion formation.

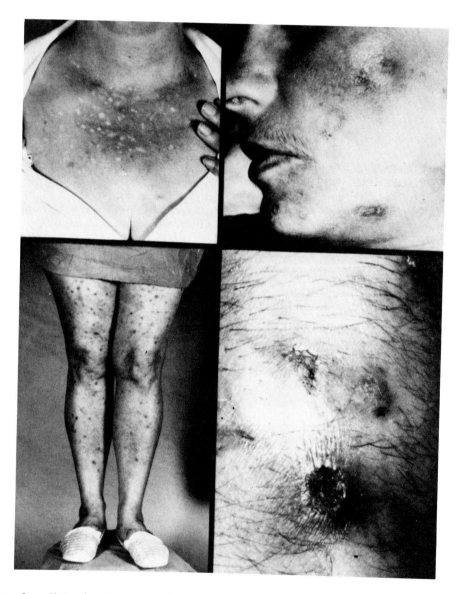

Fig. 2.   Skin lesions resulting from "grooming behavior" in patients
with delusions of parasitosis (from Ellinwood, 1972a).

Environmental contingencies. Knowledge of stimulus properties of drugs (Schuster and Balster, 1975) would predict that the
stereotypy induced by amphetamine would reflect environmental factors. Yet, very few investigations of these possible relationships
have been completed. Ellinwood and Escalante (1970a, 1970b) have
noted that cats administered methedrine and observed while in cages
tended to develop stereotyped sniffing behavior, while cats observed
in an open space develop stereotyped looking from side to side.
Operant behaviors have been reported to become incorporated in
stereotypies after drug administration. Teitlebaum and Derks (1958)
described rats in shock avoidance paradigms that turned a wheel for
hours without reward after amphetamine injections. Rats trained to
lever-press in order to avoid shock similarly developed a stereotyped bar-press (Lyon and Randrup, 1971). However, with sustained
self-administration of methamphetamine, learned bar-press response
originally incorporated in the stereotypy have been observed to be
replaced with head movement responses which appeared originally as
part of an amphetamine arousal pattern (Ellinwood and Kilbey, 1975).

Drug related factors. Drug-related factors of importance in
amphetamine-induced stereotypies include amount, duration, and frequency. Rats given 3 mg/kg l-amphetamine showed a peak at Level 5
on our rating scale, which represents hyperactivity. Rats given
12 mg/kg d-amphetamine showed constricted or reactive behaviors.
Figure 3 shows this relationship. In general, we have found that
low doses induce hyperactivity; moderate doses induce stereotyped
behavior, and high doses are associated with a constricted and/or
reactive behavior pattern. Chronic administration also changes the
response topography. Segal and Mandell (1974) report that with administration of 2.5 mg/kg amphetamine over 15 days there is an augmentation of stereotyped behavior. In our work, we have shown that
amphetamine-induced stereotypies are comprised primarily of the pos-
tural-motor components of attending and examining. From the initial
administration of amphetamine these stereotyped behaviors are more
constricted in the rat than the cat or primate, although all three
show change with duration of drug administration. In cats and
monkeys, administered amphetamine over a two-week period, grooming
and hand-eye examination stereotypies become fragmented and relatively autonomous. While with chronic administration of relatively
large amounts of amphetamine, dysjunctive postures and dyskinesias
are developed more prominently (Ellinwood et al., 1972). In humans,
the chronicity factor is especially important. We have noted that
skin sensations associated with initial amphetamine use, e.g., tingling, etc., invoke with chronic use behavior patterns similar to
"grooming behavior," with the person repetitively examining and picking his skin. These behaviors often evolve into delusions of parasitosis (Ellinwood, 1972a). Similarly, inquiring and questioning
thinking patterns can evolve from suspiciousness and prying to more
paranoid manifestations.

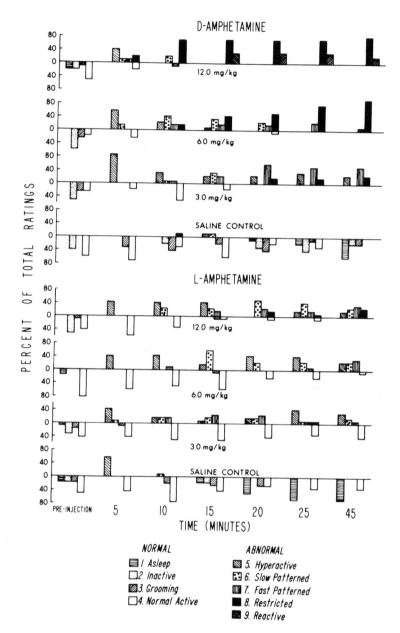

Fig. 3. Number of ratings in each behavioral category expressed as % of the total ratings for three doses of d- and l-amphetamine with saline control. Each determination represents two ratings and six rats, (from Ellinwood and Balster, 1974; reprinted by permission from European Journal of Pharmacology).

Because of the cognitive-perceptual nature of the evolving psychosis in humans, it is difficult to correlate directly its manifestations with the behavior of animals chronically administered amphetamine in the model of amphetamine psychosis. However, various remarkable similarities do exists, and, in general, we have observed that the evolution of behavior in animal studies is partially analogous to that noted in human studies. Figure 4 presents a triple-layer model with amphetamine psychosis serving as a model of functional paranoid psychosis, and chronic intoxication studies of animals serving as a behavior model of amphetamine psychosis. We have found this model a useful tool in organizing data relevant to amphetamine psychosis (Ellinwood and Sudilovsky, 1973a).

It should be noted that while the early and middle stages of the amphetamine-induced stereotyped behavioral pattern may be analogous to manifestations of a paranoid psychosis, in humans, the animal end-stage behavioral pattern has characteristics more similar to paranoid panic or catatonic excitement. We (Ellinwood and Sudiolvsky, 1973b) have pointed out that, as the older psychiatric literature recognized, there are many points of communality between paranoid and catatonic psychosis, which resemble the end-stage behaviors of the animal model.

Etiology

We have hypothesized (Ellinwood and Escalante, 1970a, 1970b; Ellinwood and Kilbey, 1975) that the etiology of stereotypies represents a malfunctioning of species-specific motor patterns, innervated by dopaminergic mechanisms, which underlie behaviors that can be considered reinforcing. This position is derived from the ethologist's point of view that there is an action-specific motivating energy associated with specific motor sequences that are highly prepotent for a given species (Lorenz, 1950). More recently in a similar biological theory of reinforcement, Glickman and Schiff (1967) proposed that reinforcement evolved as a mechanism to insure species-typical responses to appropriate stimuli. This theory is based on reviews of electrical stimulation of species-specific behaviors and overlapping loci for reinforcement for intercranial electrical self-stimulation. It proposes that species-specific behaviors are organized along the reinforcement pathways such that high probability of occurrence of these behaviors is maintained for survival purposes. Many of these species-specific behaviors involve curiosity and investigatory behaviors. Other examples are preying behaviors in the cat, and gnawing behavior in the rodent.

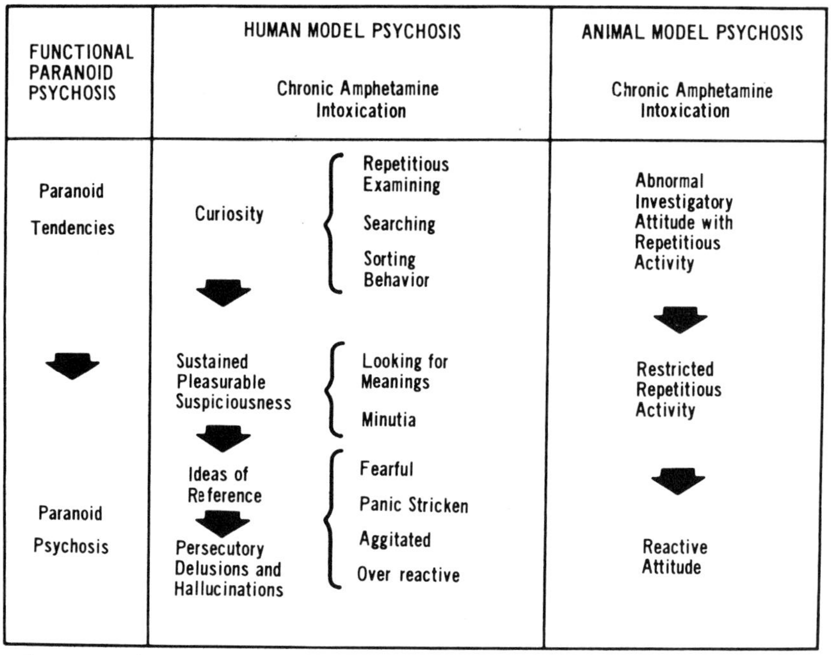

FUNCTIONAL PARANOID PSYCHOSIS	HUMAN MODEL PSYCHOSIS Chronic Amphetamine Intoxication		ANIMAL MODEL PSYCHOSIS Chronic Amphetamine Intoxication
Paranoid Tendencies	Curiosity	{ Repetitious Examining Searching Sorting Behavior	Abnormal Investigatory Attitude with Repetitious Activity
	Sustained Pleasurable Suspiciousness	{ Looking for Meanings Minutia	Restricted Repetitive Activity
Paranoid Psychosis	Ideas of Reference Persecutory Delusions and Hallucinations	{ Fearful Panic Stricken Aggitated Over reactive	Reactive Attitude

Fig. 4. Triple-layered representation of chronic amphetamine-
-induced behavior as a model of functional paranoid psychosis
(from Ellinwood and Sudilovsky, 1973b; reprinted by permission of
the Johns Hopkins University Press).

Similarly, O'Donahugh and Hagamen (1967) concluded that specific
attention mechanisms were associated with reinforcement properties
from various stimulated brain sites.

Wise and Stein (1970) have proposed that amphetamine acts by
releasing NE, and this release is correlated with preferential activation of operant behaviors which are at, or above, a critical
probability level for performance. Low probability behaviors are
not facilitated by amphetamine (Stein, 1964). Experimental results
supporting this concept have been obtained in studies using relatively low doses of amphetamine. In vivo work (Azzaro and Rutledge,
1973) has shown that NE is released by a much lower concentration
of amphetamine than that required to release DA, and that an even
higher concentration is necessary to release serotonin (5-HT).
Furthermore, in a comparison of brain areas, Azzaro and Rutledge
(1973) found the cerebral cortex to be maximally sensitive to
amphetamine's NE releasing action, and the corpus striatum to its
DA releasing action. These areas, plus the medulla, released 5-HT
at an approximately identical amphetamine concentration. Thus, it
seems feasible that at low levels, amphetamine has a primary effect
on NE, especially in higher brain centers, which may facilitate the
performance of recently acquired operant behaviors.

Recent evidence supports our hypothesis that activation of DA
receptors by amphetamine accounts for the expression of prepotent
behavioral patterns. Spatial preferences of rats in a T-maze were
found to reflect significantly higher contralateral striatal dopamine (Zimmerberg et al., 1974). This finding followed work by
Jerussi and Glick (1974) showing amphetamine-induced rotation in
non-lesion animals. Presumably, amphetamine acted to release DA
which enhanced the existing bilateral differences in DA content in
the rat brain. Similarly, we feel DA exists, differentially distributed in both amount and location, as a transmitter for various
fundamental behaviors which are expressed as stereotypies after
high doses and/or repeated administration of amphetamine. These
fundamental behaviors rest upon dopaminergically mediated reinforcement. This hypothesis is substantiated by recent work (Baxter et
al., 1974) showing that rats will self-administer apomorphine, a
DA receptor stimulator, an action which is blocked by pretreatment
by pimozide, a DA receptor blocker. Thus, the reinforcing effect
of apomorphine is seen as reflecting its action on central DA receptors.

Table 10

Results of Human Studies with Anesthesia cited by Porter (1972)

Score		Definition
1	Asleep	Lying down, eyes closed
2	Inactive	Lying down, eyes open
3	Inplace Activities (Grooming)	Normal grooming or chewing cage litter
4	Normal, Alert, Active	Moving about cage, sniffing, rearing
5	Hyperactive	Running movement characterized by rapid changes in position (jerky)
6	Slow Patterned	Repetitive exploration of the cage at normal level of activity
7	Fast Patterned	Repetitive exploration of the cage with hyperactivity
8	Restricted	Remaining in same place in cage with fast repetitive head and/or foreleg movement (includes licking, chewing and gnawing stereotypies)
9	Dyskinetic-Reactive	Backing up, jumping, seizures, abnormally maintained postures, dyskinetic movements

Dopamine

In their initial study, Randrup et al., (1963), attributed
stereotypies to the activation of DA receptors by amphetamine.
Various drugs, including apomorphine, cocaine, diethylpropion, fen-
camfamine, lysergic acid diethylamide, methamphetamine, methylphenidate, morphine, pemoline, phenmetrazine, pipradrol (Fog, 1969,
1970), l-dopa (Randrup and Munkvad, 1966a, 1966b), and ETA 495
(Costall and Naylor, 1972) induce stereotypies. Various strategies
have been employed to elucidate the mechanisms underlying this
action.

In order to test the central action of DA, investigators have
placed it directly in the various brain areas which histofluores-
ence microscopy has shown to be dopaminergically innervated (Anden
et al., 1966; Ungerstedt, 1971). Amphetamine, apomorphine, 3-meth-
oxytyramine, or DA, administered in the caudate nucleus elicited
stereotypies in cats (Cools and Van Rossum, 1970; Cools, 1971). In
rats, administration of DA, apomorphine, and hydroxyamphetamine, in
the striatum induced stereotyped gnawing (Ernst and Smelik, 1966;
Fog et al., 1967), and amphetamine placed in the globuspallidus or
caudate-putamen also resulted in stereotypies (Costall et al.,
1972a). This evidence comprises the most direct test of the idea
that activation of DA receptors underlies stereotyped behavior.
Supporting evidence has been provided also by investigations in
which DA receptor blocking agents have been used. Antagonism of
stimulant-induced stereotypies had been reported for haloperidol
(Willner et al., 1970) and perphenazine (Del Rio and Fuentes, 1969).
Using our rating scale, Table I, stereotyped behavior of rats was
rated after administration of pimozide (Ellinwood and Balster,
1974). A dose-dependent inhibitory effect, illustrated in Fig. 5,
was seen.

Recently, evidence describing the sites and relative amounts
of the various catecholamines (CA) has been presented. Examination
of CA distribution patterns across species by the histochemical
technique reveals considerable variation, not only in the brain
stem, but also in the forebrain (Ellinwood and Escalante, 1970a,
1970b; Sladek, 1971). In nonhuman primates, distribution of CA
fluorescence was noted to be different than that found in lower
species, and, in fact, there were reasonably widespread CA terminals
in the cortex, especially over the temporal and parietal regions.
In general, the CA pathways in lower animals such as the rat demonstrate a much more circumscribed outflow to the caudate and olfac-

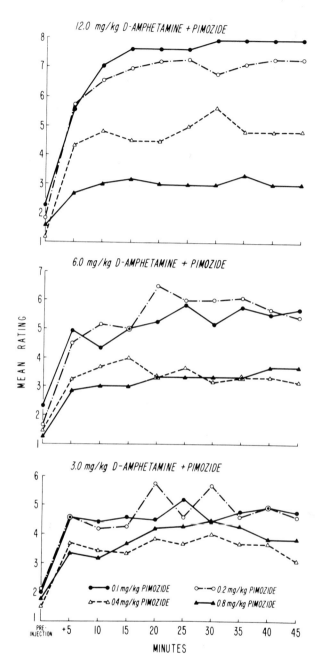

Fig. 5. The effects of pimozide pretreatment on the behavioral effects of d-amphetamine administration. Each value represents the mean of six rats (from Ellinwood and Balster, 1974; reprinted by permission from European Journal of Pharmacology).

tory forebrain, whereas in higher species, the distribution is
much more widespread. It is not documented, but certainly feasible
that this is reflected in the more constricted stereotyped behaviors noted in lower species following amphetamine intoxication.
The amphetamine-induced stereotyped sequences also appear at shorter
latencies in the rat, in comparison with the cat or dog. This may
be correlated with the relatively larger forebrain limbic and striatal systems of the rodent, and the increased concentrations of DA
[mg/gram brain mass], (Bertler and Rosengren, 1959; McGeer et al.,
1963; Wada and McGeer, 1966). There is evidence to support these
suggested relationships within species during the maturation process
which is discussed in the Ontogeny section of this chapter.

Norepinephrine

Since amphetamine also acts upon NE, much work has been done
to elucidate the relationship between this action and AISB. We have
quantified AISB using a nine-point rating scale (Ellinwood and
Balster, 1974), which is illustrated in Table I, and have found
d-amphetamine four times as effective in inducing mid-range stereotyped behaviors as is l amphetamine. These data, illustrated in
Fig. 6, are consistent with most of the observations in the literature regarding the effects of these stereoisomers on locomotion or
low intensity stereotypy (Rech and Stolk, 1970; Thornburg and Moore,
1973). They are inconsistent with Snyder et al., (1974) and Taylor
and Snyder's (1971) finding of a 10:1 d- to l-amphetamine effect on
locomotor activity. In addition, Taylor and Snyder (1971) also
found d-amphetamine to be twice as effective as l-amphetamine in
inducing stereotyped gnawing, a ratio which was found to hold in
humans for d- and l-amphetamine-induced psychoses (Angrist et al.,
1971). The contention that the potent d-amphetamine action on locomotion is mediated through a stereospecific action on the NE receptor, while the similar d-and l-stereotypy-inducing actions are mediated through DA receptors is controversial (Carlsson, 1970; Ferris
et al., 1972; Thornburg and Moore, 1973; Harris and Baldessarini,
1973). Our data suggest a uniform 4:1 ratio of activity for the
two isomers throughout the range of behaviors from hyperactivity
through medium intensity stereotypies. Because of the intriguing
and heuristic nature of the Snyder hypothesis (Snyder et al.,1974;
Snyder, 1972) the controversy should be resolved with further
studies in which the behavioral effects are specified more exactly.

We have attempted to determine the relative contribution of
NE to the amphetamine stereotypy. In an initial study, we reported

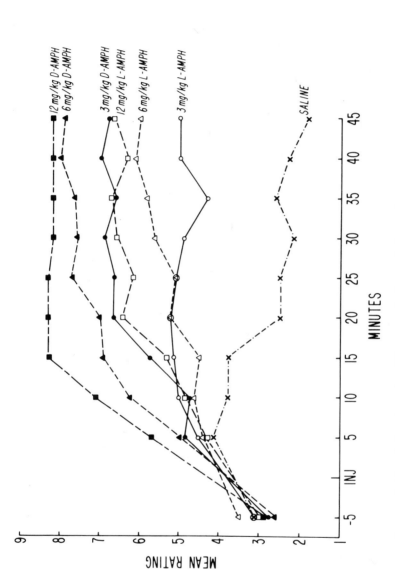

Fig. 6. A comparison of the behavioral effects of d- and l-amphetamine administration. Each volume represents the mean of six animals except saline where n = 12 (from Ellinwood and Balster, 1974; reprinted by permission from European Journal of Pharmacology).

that disulfiram, which decreased NE while increasing DA, significantly intensified and prolonged AISB in rats and cats (Ellinwood
et al., 1972). This effect in rats is illustrated in Fig. 7. We
hypothesized that the intensification of AISB by disulfiram was due
to the absence of an inhibition of dopaminergic activity usually
provided by NE. This finding was congruent with an earlier report
(Randrup and Scheel-Kruger, 1966) of prolonged amphetamine stereotypies in mice following disulfiram treatment, but incongruent with
another study which reported disulfiram to be ineffective in altering stereotypies (Maj and Przegalinski, 1967). We were interested
especially in continuing the investigation of NE mechanisms in the
model psychosis. In this respect, pretreatment with disulfiram had
not only potentiated AISB, but had been reported to produce psychosis in non-schizophrenic humans (Lidden and Satran, 1967), and
hallucinations and delusions in schizophrenic persons (Heath et al.,
1965). In a recent study (Kilbey and Ellinwood, unpublished data),
FLA-63 was administered in combination with amphetamine. While FLA
(10 and 25 mg kg) significantly blocked the hyperthermic effect of
amphetamine, it did not significantly enhance stereotyped behavior.
This raises two questions: first, since disulfiram has the dual
effect of lowering NE and raising DA levels (Goldstein and Nakajima,
1967), while FLA-63 has only the former action (Corrodi et al.,
1970), the intensification and prolongation of amphetamine stereotypies in the animal model (Ellinwood et al., 1972; Randrup and
Scheel-Kruger, 1966) as well as the induction of psychosis in humans
following disulfiram may result from its effect on DA. However, in
the FLA study, we did see a nonsignificant trend in our data toward
intensification and prolongation which might be significant using
other drug parameters. This possibility is being investigated currently in our laboratory.

                              Serotonin

    While the relationship of DA to stereotyped behavior following
amphetamine administration is beginning to be understood, the function, if any, of 5-HT in the process is far from clear. Gelder and
Vane (1962) originally proposed that amphetamine stimulated not only
catecholamine receptors, but also tryptamine receptors in the CNS.
It was postulated that species differences existed insofar as the
serotonergic system of the avian brain was held to be especially responsive to amphetamine (Vane, 1960; Dewhurst and Marley, 1965).
The stereotypic postural effects of amphetamine produced in chicks
and pigeons are blocked by anti-serotonergic agents (Braestrup,
cited in Randrup and Munkvad, 1972). In contrast, apomorphine

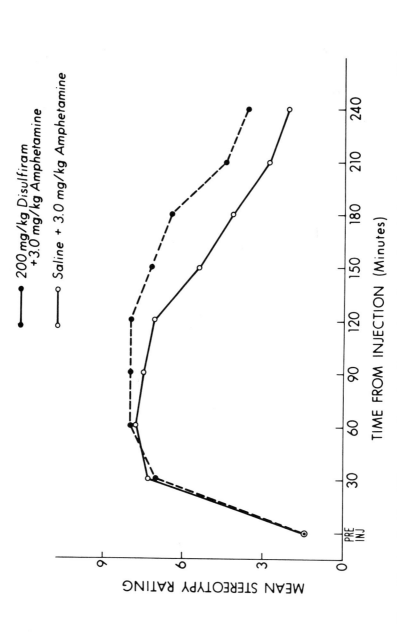

Fig. 7. The effect of disulfiram pretreatment on d-amphetamine-induced stereotypy. Eight rats comprise each treatment group.

elicited stereotyped pecking in the pigeon, but without the stereotyped postural effects noted after amphetamine. Thus, Randrup and
Munkvad (1972) suggest that amphetamine stimulates both catechol-
aminergic and serotonergic mechanisms, whereas apomorphine has only
the former effect. In rats, Randrup and Munkvad (1964) noted that
5-HT antagonists prolonged nonpostural components of AISB, and
Weiner et al., (1973) have demonstrated a facilitation of AISB with
simultaneous administration of methylsergide, a 5-HT antagonist, in
the guinea pig.

    In chronic amphetamine-intoxicated cats, one notes head twitch-
es and dyskinesias along with stereotypies (Ellinwood and Kilbey,
1975; Ellinwood and Sudilovsky, 1973a, 1973b) which indicates that,
although the serotonergic postural effect may be much weaker in
mammals than in avians, with chronic intoxication, it may be manifested. During chronic administration of amphetamine, especially
in those paradigms which periodically escalate the drug dosage, increasing concentrations of drug accumulate, and while low concentrations of amphetamine are associated with release of NE, higher
concentrations are associated with release of DA and 5-HT, as well.
Thus, it may follow that the dyskinetic effects noted in chronic
amphetamine intoxication result from higher concentrations of
amphetamine releasing 5-HT, which elicits postural components of
the stereotypy. This mechanism may also be involved in the production of hallucinations. Thus, Corne and Pickering (1967) have
found that substances which produced hallucinations in man induce
head-twitching in mice, which they attribute to 5-HT activity
(Corne et al., 1963). We have reported increased fluorescence of
5-HT in animals chronically administered methamphetamine (Escalante
and Ellinwood, 1972) which may reflect this process.

    The ontogeny of stereotypy following amphetamine selfadminis-
tration (Ellinwood and Kilbey, 1975) has been observed to proceed
from intense sniffing and examining through a constriction of these
behavioral patterns, and the initial appearance of a variety of abnormal behaviors including abortive grooming and disjunctive postures to an end-stage represented by dyskinesia, ataxia, and, sometimes, catatonia. The disjunctive behavior we have described
(Ellinwood and Escalante, 1970a, 1970b; Ellinwood et al., 1972) as
an abortive grooming response emerges after several days of amphetamine administration. It resembles the abnormal grooming behavior
described by Randall and Trulson (1974) which resulted from pontine
lesions and the abortive grooming response found by Cools (1973)
following application of 5-HT to the anteroventral caudate nucleus.

Randall and Trulson presented evidence indicating that the abnormal grooming response resulted from a transection of serotonergic input to the superior colliculus, while Cools' and our findings suggest an increase in striatal 5-HT underlies this behavior.

Several investigators have examined the level of 5-HT or 5-hydroxyindolacetic acid (5-HIAA) following administration of stereotypy producing doses of amphetamine. Lewander (1973) found that the levels of brain 5-HT were unaffected by an acute single dose or the last injection of amphetamine in the chronically treated rat, while the steady state level (between injections) of 5-HT in the chronic amphetamine treatment was reduced to approximately 75% normal levels. Levels of 5-HIAA in rat brain have been demonstrated to increase after amphetamine (Reid, 1970; Tagliamonte et al., 1971), which has been ascribed to increased brain tryptophan concentrations (Tagliamonte et al., 1971) which may result in an increased 5-HT turnover. Lewander (1973) reported a biphasic response; that is, brain 5-HIAA was reduced to 80% of the control level at one hour, and increased to 130% at four hours after a single injection of amphetamine. However, 5-HIAA was reduced in the chronic amphetamine-treated animal. Using other biochemical techniques to achieve a more direct assessment, the turnover of 5-HT has been reported not to change, or to decrease, after single injections of amphetamine (Schubert et al., 1972; Gorlitz and Frey, 1972), or to increase after chronic amphetamine treatment (Sparber and Tilson, 1972; Diaz and Huttonen, 1972). Clearly, further investigation is needed to clarify the action of amphetamine on 5-HT, and the role of 5-HT in AISB.

Ontogeny

Lal and Sourkes (1973) measured the ontogeny of stereotyped behavior after amphetamine or apomorphine injections in rats from Day 1 through Week 9. They found clearly identifiable stereotyped behavior after both drugs as early as two days of age. However, adult patterns of stereotypy were not present until Day 21 for apomorphine, and Day 35 for amphetamine. As the rat matured, onset of stereotyped behavior following drug administration became faster, and its duration shorter. As the authors did not measure brain levels of drug, monoamines, or their catabilites, it is not possible to interpret these data in any exact sense, but it does appear reasonable to ssume that adult stereotyped behavior patterns are dependent upon maturation of the CA system. Since NE neurons develop earlier than DA neurons (Kellogg and Lundborg, 1973), the

shift noted from a response to amphetamine characterized by locomotion effects (prior to Day 18) to one characterized by stereotypy
(completed by Day 35) might be thought to reflect development of
receptor processes. However, since apomorphine elicits mature
stereotyped behaviors by Day 21, it would appear that the receptor
processes underlying stereotypy and the motor processes by which it
is expressed are fully functioning by that time. Maturation of DA
receptor enzyme mechanisms or enzymatic metabolic processes regulating DA release or reuptake processes through Day 35, when fully
developed AISB is seen, may account for the observed data.

Anatomy

While the necessity of an intact striatum for the development
of stereotypies was an early observation (Randrup and Munkvad,
1968), recent investigations have suggested that specific brain
areas control expression of various components of the AISB (Naylor
and Olley, 1972, 1972b; Costall and Naylor, 1974a, 1974b;
Ungerstedt and Ljungberg, 1973). Ungerstedt (1971) has described:
(1) a nigro-striatal system with DA neurons in the zona compacta
and its rostro-medial extension in the area ventralis tegmenti
(cell group A9) which ascends through the lateral hypothalamus,
the mid-hypothalamus, the capsula interna, and the globus pallidus
to terminate in the caudate-putamen. Extensions of the system, in
turn, terminate in the nucleus amygdaloideus centralis. Axons from
A8, DA cell bodies which are caudal to the substantial nigra and
dorsal to the medial lemniscus, are thought to be part of this
system, also, as lesions in the corpus striatum cause degeneration
of both A8 and A9 neurons; and (2) a mesolimbic DA system with
nuclei dorsal and lateral to the interpeduncular nucleus (cell
group A10) which ascends with the axons of the nigrostriatal system
following a medial route to terminate in the nucleus accumbens,
olfactory tubercule and nucleus interstitialis stria terminalis.

The possibility of a response topology and a mesolimbic DA
system contribution to AISB was raised by work which showed that
lesions in the zona compacta of the substantia nigra did not modify, significantly, AISB (Iversen, 1971; Simpson and Iversen, 1971,
Costall et al., 1972b), while lesions which may have involved both
nigro-striatal and mesolimbic structures were shown to abolish
stereotypies (Creese and Iversen, 1973; Fibiger et al., 1973).
The implication of these studies was that the mesolimbic system
might be essential for AISB. To our knowledge a direct test of
this hypothesis by lesioning the A10 cell group has not been

reported.

Lesions of the terminal of the nigro-striatal system, i.e.,
the caudate nucleus, as well as the globus pallidus reduced or
abolished AISB depending on the amphetamine dose (Naylor and Olley,
1972a). Ungerstedt and Ljungberg (1973) showed that lateral hypothalamic lesions which effected stereotyped behavior did so via
their effect on striatal structures. They found a denervation of
the striatum to follow these lesions and an absence of AISB when
there were no demonstrable dopaminergic terminals in the striatum.
Likewise, reduction by 99% of striatal tyrosine hydroxylase activity prevented AISB (Creese and Iversen, 1975). Recently, Costall
and Naylor (1974a) were able to lesion selectively the neostriatum
(caudate and putamen) and the paleostriatum (globus pallidus), and
found the latter to be critical for the expression of AISB. They
also reported that lesions of the tuberculum olfactorium abolished
the sniffing components of AISB. These latter data appear to be
the clearest implication of a role for the mesolimbic DA system in
AISB. They have not been replicated, however, since Asher and
Aghajanian (1974) reported that 6-hydroxydopamine lesions of the
olfactory tubercule inhibited stereotypy only when the animal also
showed a significant loss of striatal DA. These investigators also
found an absence of AISB following caudate lesions. In addition,
reduction of nucleus accumbens DA following tubercule lesions did
not lead to inhibition of AISB. Thus, these data assert the importance of the nigro-striatal system of AISB. These conflicting findings are diagrammed in Fig. 8.

While Asher and Aghajanian (1974) have inspected visually the
fluorescence of the tubercule and caudate in their investigation,
it appears that a spectrofluorophotometric analysis to quantify the
DA loss in various nigro-striatal and mesolimbic system structures
as a function of lesions in A8, 9 and 10 areas, as well as a sophisticated behavioral study of the intensity, time of onset, and duration of the AISB is needed to answer finally whether or not a response topography exists for this behavior.

Cross-Species/Cross-Strain Investigations

In investigating AISB, Randrup and Munkvad (1968) interpreted
their inability to obtain AISB in the lamprey, a primitive vertebrate species, as due to an absence of DA in this species. However,
more recent evidence indicates that lampreys do possess dopamine
(Fange and Hanson, 1973), although their receptors may not show

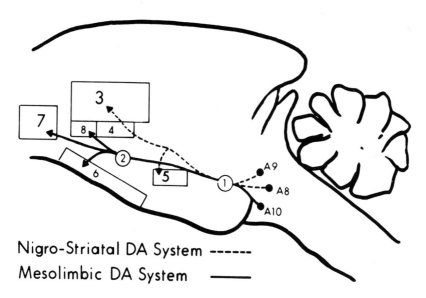

Nigro-Striatal DA System ------
Mesolimbic DA System ——

Fig. 8. (A9) Zona Compacta of the Substantia Nigra: Lesions have
no effect on AISB.[1,2,3] Lesions abolished AISB.[4] a) Ascending
mesolimbic (MLB) and nigrostriatal (NS) dopaminergic pathways at
the levels of the mid-hypothalamus: lesions have no effect on
AISB.[5] b) Mesolimbic dopaminergic pathways at the rostral level
of the nucleus paraventricularis: lesions blocked sniffing or repetitive head movements.[5] c) Neostriatum (caudate-putamen): lesions have no effects on AISB.[5] f) Olfactory tubercule: lesions
blocked - sniffing component.[5] Lesions had no effect on AISB.[6]
g) Accumbens septi nucleus: lesions had no effect on AISB.[5]
h) Interstitial stria terminalis nucleus: lesions had no effect on
AISB.[5] 1.(Iverson, 1971; 2. Simpson and Iversen, 1971; 3. Costall et
al., 1972b; 4. Creese and Iversen, 1975; 5. Costall and Naylor,
1974; 6. Asher and Aghajanian 1974).

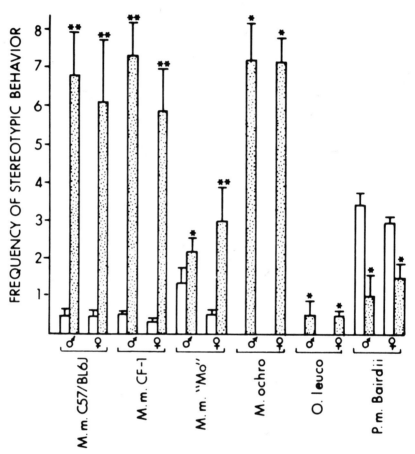

Fig. 9. The effects of acute methamphetamine treatment on stereotypic behavior of several mice species and strains. □ , Control;
▓ , methamphetamine (7 mg/kg). The frequencies are expressed as
averages of 20 "City" runs with the drugged and 20 "City" runs with
the control mice (from Richardson et al., 1972; reprinted by permission from Psychopharmacologia).

pharmacological specificity. Additionally, the absence of AISB in the Onychomys leucogastic (Ony) strain of mouse has been reported (Richardson et al., 1972). Moreover, these authors report that amphetamine reduced stereotypies in the Peromyscus maniculatus bairdii (Per) strain of mouse (Fig. 9). These findings are not easily related to DA levels. Richardson et al. (1972) present data which show cortical DA, 5-HT, and ACH levels to be higher in Ony and Per strains than they are in those strains showing AISB. Thus, cross-species and cross-strain investigations of AISB indicate that three patterns of response exist which can be thought of as the typical (AISB), paradoxical (amphetamine reduction of endogenous stereotypies), and intermediate (no change or biphasic) response patterns. In addition, the cross-species and/or cross-strain data indicate that the presence of DA, while it appears essential, is not sufficient for the development of stereotypies. The functioning of critical presynaptic nerve terminals also appears to be essential. This has been shown most clearly in the rat by Creese and Iversen (1973), who found that administration of 6-hydroxydopamine to neonatal rats blocked the appearance of AISB when amphetamine was administered to the rats at maturity. That this effect was due to an alteration of effect by amphetamine on presynaptic nerve terminals or reuptake mechanisms, but not the complete destruction of dopamine receptors, was shown by the fact that apomorphine administration resulted in stereotypies of normal intensity. The author attributed this to supersensitivity of the remaining post-synaptic receptors. In this respect, it would be interesting to determine whether or not apomorphine induces stereotypies in the Ony and Per strains of mouse. This would establish the presence or absence of functional DA receptors. If these were present, it would indicate that the differential amphetamine response in these species reflects a difference in presynaptic release or reuptake mechanisms.

Richardson et al. (1972) speculated that whatever mechanism may account for the typical, apradoxical, and intermediate response to methamphetamine they saw in mice might also account for other differential behavior patterns. These authors showed that two strains which have atypical responses to methamphetamine (Ony and Per) also exhibit less exploratory behavior, sleep more, have more carrying behavior, and groom other mice less than strains having typical responses. Both strains are nocturnal and have high monoamine levels. Based on this, the authors posited that amphetamine stereotypy responses reflect a convergence of three factors related to amine, exploration, and stereotypy levels. Animals which have

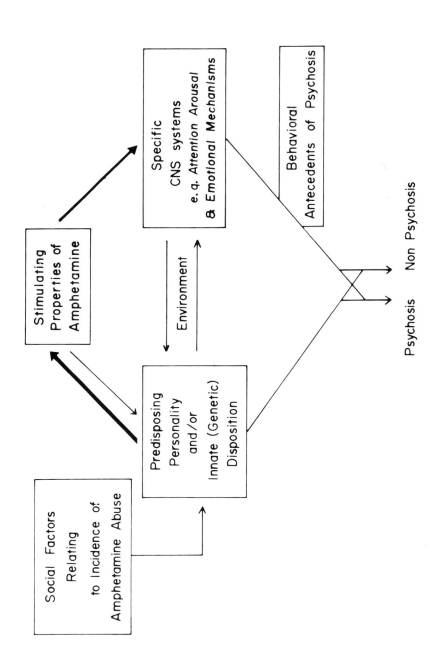

Fig. 10. Illustration of factors which contribute to the development of amphetamine psychosis (from Ellinwood, 1969; reprinted by permission from Seminars in Psychiatry).

a low level of monoamines, high exploration, and few stereotypies comprise those species showing increased stereotypies with amphetamine administration. In those animals or strains having the opposite characteristics, amphetamine would be expected to reduce stereotypies or to have no effect.

Differential drug responses related to activity levels have been reported by other investigators, also. Recent work (Oliverio et al., 1973; Oliverio et al., 1974) has shown that BALB/cJ mice which have low exploratory behavior show high levels of exploration when treated with scopolamine, while C57B1/6J mice show high levels of exploratory behavior respond to scopolamine with lowered exploration. Likewise, Richardson et al.(1972) report that their non-exploratory strain (Per) showed increased exploration with prolonged methamphetamine treatment, while other high--exploratory strains showed decreases. Oliverio et al. (1973, 1974) were able to identify a single gene, Exa, controlling exploratory activity, and one controlling the scopolamine response (Sco). Amphetamine responses, however, appeared to be polygenetically determined. Thus, the cross-strain investigations indicate that amphetamine-induced stereotypies are best viewed as a multi-determined process, if we are to describe eventually and evaluate the mechanisms contributing to this response.

AMPHETAMINE-INDUCED THERMAL RESPONSES

Recent investigations have targeted thermal responses associated with amphetamine administration for extensive examination. While the number of studies completed is large and individual differences among subjects is often noted (although rarely described), systematic studies employing different strains as an independent variable in assessing these responses are few. This type of analysis offers a potentially powerful means of identifying biological bases of behavioral variation, which should encourage investigators to broaden their research designs to include species and/or strain factors.

Peripheral and Central Factors

Systematic administration of amphetamine results in a dose-dependent hyperthermia in mice, rats, rabbits, and cats (Horita and Hill, 1972). Most of the studies in this area have suffered, however, from confounding of drug effects and effects of restraint or handling on temperature. According to Brown and Julian (1968), the

restraint factor may account for more than 50% of the observed hyperthermia. In spite of extensive study, the neural basis of
amphetamine-induced thermal responses has not been specified, and
the relative contributions of peripheral and central nervous system
mechanisms have not been delineated. Since amphetamine has an
effect on central and peripheral indices of NE, 5-HT and DA activity,
these amines have been implicated in mechanisms hypothesized to
explain experimentally observed amphetamine-temperature relationships. Exploration of these proposed mechanisms in the four species
mentioned has not yielded a generalized mechanism underlying what
had been presumed to be a uniform hyperthermic response. Rather,
inter/intra species comparisons have documented three basic response
patterns on this parameter similar to those seen for stereotyped
behavior.

Gessa et al (1969) attributed amphetamine-induced hyperthermia
to peripheral mechanisms as it is seen following administration of
hydroxyamphetamine, which has little central nervous system activity.
Caldwell et al. (1974) manipulated central and peripheral levels of
NE, DA and 5-HT independently in male and female rats. Reduction
of central and peripheral CA synthesis through administration of
d-methyl-p-tyrosine ester (Buethin et al., 1972), or peripheral CA,
through use of 6-hydroxydopamine hydrobromide abolished the hyperthermic response. When only peripheral dopamine was depleted,
using a treatment of dismethylimipramine followed by 6-hydroxydop-
amine (Breese et al., 1973), amphetamine-induced hyperthermia was
found. Thus, Caldwell et al. (1974) concluded, in the rat, amphetamine-induced hyperthermia appears dependent upon an intace peripheral NE system. The findings of Mantegazza et al. (1968) and of
Gessa et al (1969) that β-adrenergic blockers prevented amphetamine
hyperthermia and lipolysis in adipose tissue also suggested a peripheral site for amphetamine action. However, other investigators
have reported a dissociation of the metabolic and thermic actions
of amphetamine (Bizzi et al., 1968; Matsumoto and Shaw, 1971) and
in the rabbit amphetamine does not effect lipolysis nor is the
hyperthermia blocked by β-adrenergic blocking agents (Hill and
Horita, 1970). Thus, the comparative data argues against a general
peripheral mechanism underlying amphetamine-induced hyperthermia
in the various species in which this response is seen.

In contrast to those data suggesting peripheral mechanisms in
amphetamine-induced hyperthermia, in our laboratory, we have found
that FLA-63, which depletes central NE without altering peripheral
levels (Corrodi et al., 1970), blocked amphetamine-induced hyper-

thermia in rats (Kilbey and Ellinwood, unpublished data). Our finding is congruent with other work which suggests that central mechanisms regulate amphetamine-induced hyperthermia in the mouse as it
is unaffected by depletion of peripheral CA (Wolf and Bunce, 1973).
In the rabbit (Hill and Horita, 1971) and the rat (Matsumoto and
Shaw, 1971), central DA activity seems to be important for amphetamine-induced hyperthermia, as this response is blocked by pretreatment with pimozide.

Hyperthermia

Inter-strain comparisons of amphetamine-temperature relationships in mice, carried out by Caccia et al. (1973), suggest that
DA turnover is critical for hyperthermic amphetamine effect in mice.
These authors observed an amphetamine dose-dependent hyperthermia
in NMRI mice and HVA increases. A correlation between increasing
HVA concentrations and increasing hyperthermic effects of amphetamine was reported by Jori and Bernardi (1968, 1972) which suggests
dopaminergic participation in hyperthermia. Other evidence, however, has implicated central and peripheral NE mechanisms, as
stated (Kilbey and Ellinwood, unpublished data; Caldwell et al.,
1974). Thus, both NE and DA mechanisms must be considered to contribute to the amphetamine hyperthermia effect. Serotonin does not
appear to contribute to amphetamine-induced hyperthermia as pretreatment with p-chlorophenylalanine is without effect (Caldwell
et al., 1974).

Systematic information on thermal responses to amphetamine in
humans appears not to exist. However, hyperthermia or fever occurs
in persons hospitalized for amphetamine poisoning (Jordan and
Hampson, 1969; Harvey et al., 1949; Ellinwood, 1972b), and an
increase in temperature to about 100 degrees has been noted with
doses of amphetamine large enough to induce paranoid symptoms. The
hyperthermic response to amphetamine is blocked by 7 to 14 days pretreatment with α-methyl-p-tyrosine (Griffith, personal communication).

Hypothermia

A hypothermic response to peripherally administered amphetamine also has been reported in C57BL/6J mice (Scott et al., 1971),
CF-1 mice, at low doses only, (McCullough et al., 1970) and rats
(Jellinek, 1971). Caccia et al. (1973) reported that low doses of
amphetamine in C3H mice resulted in hypothermia while doses as high
as 15 mg/kg did not produce hyperthermia. These investigators
suggested that the absence of a hyperthermia response to amphetamine in C3H mice (Dolfini et al., 1970; Brown and Julian, 1968)
may be related to slower DA turnover, although faster 5-HT turnover is a possible mechanism also. While striatal DA turnover for
C57BL/6J mice following amphetamine is not known, DA turnover under

normal conditions is intermediate between that of other species
showing amphetsmine-induced hyperthermia. However, of three common
strains, 5-HT turnover is fastest in C57BL/6J mice (Kempf et al.,
1974). This suggests that faster 5-HT turnover may exist prior to
amphetamine administration in strains which show a hypothermic response to amphetamine.

In summary, while the mechanisms of amphetamine-induced thermal responses are still to be delineated, studies employing strain
differences in rodents as in independent variable have documented
some interesting correlations of differential responses, some of
which have been found also in investigations employing other species
as well. Three basic patterns of response are found: (1) an
increasing temperature with increasing amphetamine; (2) a decreasing temperature with increasing dosage; and (3) a decrease with
administration of low doses, and either [a] increases with high
doses, or [b] normal temperatures with high doses. The positive
response appears to be correlated with increases in striatal levels
of HVA, which implies increased striatal DA activity. Strains of
animals which show paradoxical response patterns appear to be characterized by a lack of increased striatal HVA activity and high
5-HIAA activity following amphetamine administration.

DIFFERENTIAL METABOLISM OF AMPHETAMINE

Although species and sex differences often result in a confus-
ing picture of the amphetamine-induced thermal responses, specific
differences in metabolism of amphetamine have been used to eliminate one mechanism proposed to explain the development of amphetamine tolerance. Administration of d- or d-l-amphetamine, in contrast to l-amphetamine, produces a prolonged depletion of NE in
rats and an incorporation of p-hydroxy-norephedrine into NE storage
vesicles (Groppetti and Costa, 1969; Brodie et al., 1970; Lewander,
1970, 1971a, 1971b). The accumulation of p-hydroxy-norephedrine
has been used to explain development of tolerance to amphetamine.
The p-hydroxy-norephedrine metabolite is thought to be stored, released, and taken up by the neuronal processes in the same way as
NE. Thus, it can function as a false transmitter. With chronic
amphetamine administration there is relatively more p-hydroxy-norephedrine and less NE at the nerve terminal. This hypothesis assumed that one of the major actions of amphetamine, the release of NE,
underlies the drug's effect on numerous responses; e.g. temperature,
food intake, activity.

P-hydroxy-norephedrine is not formed from l-amphetamine, and
neither guinea pigs nor rabbits parahydroxylate amphetamine (Doring
et al., 1970). This provides a method of testing the proposed role
of p-hydroxy-norephedrine. One set of investigations which manipulated species and drug conditions demonstrated that in guinea pigs
and rabbits, in which no central nervous system p-hydroxy-norephe-

drine can be detected after amphetamine, NE was depleted after
single and/or repeated injections (Lewander, 1971b, 1973). Thus,
NE depletion after amphetamine does not depend upon the formation
of p-hydroxy-norephedrine. Furthermore, decreased NE was observed
following: (1) l-amphetamine which is not converted to p-hydroxy-
-norephedrine in the rat (Lewander, 1971a); (2) either d-l or
d-amphetamine given to rats pretreated with desmethylimipramine
(Lewander, 1971a) or inprindole, drugs which block parahydroxylation of amphetamine (Freeman and Sulser, 1972). Tolerance to
anorexigenic effects developed to chronic administration of d- and
l-isomers of amphetamine (Lewander, 1973).

These studies suggest that the para-hydroxy-norephedrine mechanism is not a necessary component of tolerance seen in NE-mediated
amphetamine effects. Further evidence that it is not of major importance, however, was provided by Sever et al. (1974) who demonstrated that pretreatment of Wistar male and female rats with
p-hydroxy-amphetamine, a precursor of p-hydroxy-norephedrine, protected only the males from the hyperthermic effects of amphetamine
even though males and females develop a tolerance to the hyperthermic response. In addition, they reported a strain difference,
since male Wistar rats demonstrate a small temperature rise following amphetamine after p-hydroxy-amphetamine pretreatment, whereas
in the male Sprague-Dawley rat, the hyperthermic response is abolished totally. Thus, the hyperthermic response appears to be
related differentially to p-hydroxy-norephedrine in males and females, and thus would not appear to provide a general explanation
of tolerance. Even though Sever et al. (1974) suggest that more
extensive metabolism of p-hydroxy-amphetamine by the male may
account for their observation, the fact that tolerance is seen in
species without a parahydroxylation mechanism would seem to negate
this mechanism as being uniformly critical.

DIFFERENTIAL RESPONSES IN MAN

Euphoria - Dysphoria

In man, differential responses to amphetamine have often been
noted, but seldom have been the focus of systematic investigation.
As early as 1938, Bahnsen and co-workers (Bahnsen et al., 1938)
reported that while 28 of 46 volunteer normal subjects reported the
subjective effects of amphetamine to be pleasant, 18 reported the
opposite. Flory and Gilbert (1943) also evaluated first-person
accounts and reported that the incidence of dysphoric reactions
was greater in female than male college students. Recently, Tecci
and Cole (1974a, 1974b) have reported a biphasic response to amphetamine in women. Thirteen of 20 subjects tested by them exhibited
a one-half hour period of drowsiness associated with a lower contingent negative variation (CNV) index on the EEG, followed by behavioral alertness and increased CNV. Another seven subjects dem-

onstrated increased CNV throughout the session, and also reported
spontaneously euphoria. Recalling that Flory and Gilbert (1943)
reported that the incidence of dysphoric responses is greater in
females, one wonders if the biphasic CNV response to amphetamine
would be found less frequently among males.

The aminergic correlates of amphetamine-induced euphoria have
been investigated. The euphorigenic effects of amphetamine
(200 mg i.v.) remained constant throughout multiple administrations,
but were blocked by pretreatments with α-methyl-p-tyrosine (Jönsson
et al., 1971), an effect the authors attributed to α-methyl-p-tyrosine's blocking action (Weissman et al., 1965). Peripheral actions
of amphetamine were blocked also by α-methyl-p-tyrosine pretreatment.
Treatment over a seven-day period did not result in recovery of the
peripheral amphetamine responses, while euphoric responses returned
to 70% normal within a week. This effect was not found, however,
after a 14-day pretreatment with α-methyl-p-tyrosine, when amphetamine-induced euphoria was produced (Griffith, J. D., personal
communication), while peripheral responses were still blocked. If
the euphoric reaction is dependent on normal levels of CA, -methyl-
-p-tyrosine could be expected to attenuate it because the drug
blocks CA synthesis. With chronic treatment, unless there is tolerance to the blocking action, the antiamphetamine effect should
remain constant. This question has been investigated in animals.
Beuthin et al. (1972) report that chronic treatment with -methyl-
-p-tyrosine resulted in tolerance of the blocking effect seen for
amphetamine-induced activity. Tolerance development appeared to be
independent of DA and NE levels as they remained depressed at the
time (13 days) tolerance developed. Other investigators reported
that chronic (18 days) α-methyl-p-tyrosine administration did not
prevent recovery of NE to approximately 80% normal and DA to normal
levels, while it continued to block amphetamine-induced motor activity (Khalsa and Davis, 1974). In a recent experiment, conducted in
our laboratory, chronic treatment with α-methyl-p-tyrosine for 21
days did not result in recovery of amphetamine-induced stereotypy,
and whole brain levels of NE and DA remained depressed (Kilbey and
Ellinwood, unpublished data).

Amphetamine Psychosis

With humans, it is quite difficult to demonstrate genetic contributions to the drug intoxication outcome, especially in such a
complex array of phenomena as is manifested in the amphetamine psychosis syndrome. As was mentioned earlier, even the physiological
reactions which are much more amenable to familial and genetic analysis have yet to be evaluated systematically in humans. With such
complex results as the amphetamine psychosis, typically we ask the
question as to the contribution of the personality to the drug
interaction outcome. Personality itself is an interaction product
(although enduring) of the individual's traits with the environment

Table II. Personality Diagnosis Abstracted from Amphetamine Psychosis Literature

Diagnosis	Herman and Nagler (1954)	Hampton (1961)	Bartholomew and Marley (1959)	Beamish and Kiloh (1960)	Bell and Trethowan (1961)	Ellinwood (1967)	Total % (N=82)
Antisocial Personality	7	9	11	7	2		45%
Passive Aggressive Personality					3	2	6%
Schizoid Personality					2	2	5%
Inadequate Personality					4		5%
Hysterical Personality					3	1	5%
Psychoneurosis	1		1				4%
Schizophrenia		16				4	25%
Manic-depressive		5		7		1	8%

over his life history. The amphetamine psychosis syndrome is a
reasonably circumscribed entity characterized by primary delusions
(often delusions of persecution), idease of reference, visual and
auditory hallucinations, changes in body image, hyperactivity,
excitation and stereotyped, repetitious behavior. The severity of
symptomatology is dependent on the duration of the chronic intoxication process in that symptoms successively evolve over time, and
are dependent on the dose and as we will discuss, personality
factors interacting with the environment. The content of this syndrome is quite dependent on the underlying personality in that individuals with a relatively more stable personality tend to have delusions of persecution about events that have a greater probability
of occurrence, e.g., government spying, police surveillance, etc.
Individuals with more psychotic or borderline personalities, more
often have delusions involving persecution by Martians, evil spirits,
and various abstract forces. The relationship between amphetamine
psychosis and the underlying psychotic traits has been debated
widely since the initial observation of amphetamine psychosis reported by Young and Scoville (1938) who ascribed the syndrome to
the release of latent paranoid traits. While it is reasonable to
assume that any individual given a sufficient dose of amphetamine
over a long enough period of time may be expected to develop a
psychosis, there is evidence that the psychotic threshold is lower
in individuals with pre-psychotic or borderline disorders. An
interesting complication when assessing this relationship is that
borderline, psychotic and psychopathic individuals have a greater
tendency to experiment with and to respond positively to the effects
of amphetamines (Ellinwood, 1967), and any tabulation of personality
structure of individuals developing psychosis needs to take this
into account. Table II demonstrates such a tabulation abstracted
from amphetamine psychosis literature (Ellinwood, 1969). One can
note that sociophathic personality and schizophrenia represent a
disproportionate 70% of the total. The preponderance of these two
diagnostic categories may reflect the communality of some biological mechanism, perhaps deficit arousal mechanisms as we have previously postulated (Ellinwood, 1968). Other work has also suggested that these two groups share a common genetic basis as significant increases in schizophrenia and psychopathic disorders are
noted in children of schizophrenic parents raised by non-schizophrenic, non-psychopathic adoptive parents (Mednick, et al., 1974).
That borderline individuals and schizophrenics are more susceptible
to the acute and chronic effects of amphetamine is readily apparent
from the well known use of amphetamine in moderate doses (10-30 mg)
to induce the exacerbation of a latent psychotic symptomatology in
borderline individuals as a diagnostic test (Sargant and Slater,
1963). Also, Davis and Janowsky (1973) have reported an exacerbation of a variety of preexisting schizophrenic symptoms when small
(29 mg) doses of methylphenidate or amphetamine (d-20; l-28 mg)
were administered to psychotic patients. We have attempted to diagram the interaction of variables of importance in the ontogeny of

amphetamine psychosis (Ellinwood, 1969). This conceptualization is presented in Fig. 10.

As a rule, amphetamine psychosis develops gradually over a period of chronic intoxication (Kalant, 1966, Ellinwood, 1967). The more rare reports of psychosis from a single large dose (Connell, 1958; Rickman et al., 1961) are difficult to differentiate from the induction of psychosis in borderline individuals just discussed. Occasionally, one also notes a toxic delirium with very high acute doses, but these can certainly be differentiated from psychosis. The induction of amphetamine psychosis in the experimental situation also suffers problems of interpretation. Griffith et al. (1970) induced psychotic reactions in experienced amphetamine users with administration of i.v. amphetamine in doses from 120 mg total given over one day to 700 mg total infused over five days. Angrist et al. (1971) had similar results indicating that amphetamine psychosis in experienced users could be induced in a relatively short period of time. The difficulty is that all experiments utilized experienced amphetamine abusers for ethical reasons, and these individuals may have previously experienced amphetamine psychotic symptoms. Certainly, when an experienced amphetamine abuser develops a psychosis on 80 to 150 mg it is reasonable to expect that he will have in the past used such an amount; therefore, it is reasonable to expect that he has experienced an amphetamine psychosis previously. In our opinion, once the individual has developed the amphetamine psychosis, it is triggered more readily by smaller doses following a period of abstinence. Similar observations have been made by Kramer (1969). Utena (1974) has emphasized the increased potential for psychotic reaction to physical and psychological stress as well as subsequent exposure to amphetamine. Also, our observations in the amphetamine animal models (previously discussed in this chapter) have demonstrated that chronic treatment involving high doses of amphetamine leads to the development of end-stage behaviors which can be reinstated, thereafter, by administration of low doses of drug. In emphasizing the predisposing personality factors and the previous chronic experience with amphetamine, we most certainly do not wish to relegate the dose level to a minor role in the contribution to psychosis. We have reported previously (Ellinwood, 1967) that the dose level was maintained at a significantly higher level in individuals who developed psychosis than in those who did not.

Biological Bases

Although data from experimental models of amphetamine intoxication is abundant, there is little direct evidence bearing on the biological bases of amphetamine-induced psychotic reactions in humans, and only a few studies have manipulated the biochemical processes believed to be related to them. The evidence supporting a theory of a biochemical etiology of schizophrenia has been reviewed

recently (Snyder et al., 1974) as has that supporting the utility
of conceptualizing amphetamine-induced psychosis as a model of
paranoid schizophrenia (Snyder, 1972), or as a model for a paranoia-
-catatonia continuum of schizophrenia (Ellinwood and Sudilovsky,
1973b). Other recent experimental evidence bearing on these questions also has been organized (Usdin, 1974; Usdin and Snyder, 1973).
A ratio of 2:1 (Angrist et al., 1971) or 3:2 (Davis and Janowsky,
1973) was reported for the d-isomer of amphetamine in comparison
with the l-form in inducing psychotic symptoms, which is consistent
with the relative effect of these two isomers on dopaminergically
innervated behaviors in animals in studies reviewed in this chapter.
Gunne and Anggard (1973) administered 150 mg amphetamine for two
days to abusers experiencing a paranoid psychosis. Urinary elimination of amphetamine was enhanced or retarded by administration of
ammonium chloride or sodium bicarbonate, respectively. Psychotic
symptoms showed no correlation with plasma amphetamine levels, but
they were correlated with urinary output of hydroxylated metabolites.

Griffith et al (1970) found that chronic (14 days) treatment
with α-methyl-p-tyrosine reduced the amount of amphetamine necessary
to induce paranoid symptomatology by half. This result would not
have been predicted on the basis of animal experiments showing
chronic administration of α-methyl-p-tyrosine to block amphetamine-
-induced stereotypies (Kilbey and Ellinwood, unpublished data).

SUMMARY

The differential responses to amphetamine for several response
parameters (behavioral stereotypies, thermal responses, and, in
humans, affective and pathological responses) have been described.
To identify which possible segments of these response patterns are
under genetic control is not an easy task. The work of one group
of investigators (Richardson et al., 1973; Karczmar et al., 1973)
has shown clearly strain-specific patterns in the stereotyped behavioral responses to amphetamine. Unfortunately, the examination
of whole brain amine levels did not produce clear predictors of
differential responses. Recent work (Barchas et al., 1974) has
established genetically determined differences between strains in
the ability to synthesize catecholamines. The relation of these
genetic factors to behavior and pharmacological actions have not
been investigated, but should provide data relevant to current
theories of the biological bases of behavior as well as differential
response patterns. However, the best present information (Oliverio
et al., 1973, 1974) indicates that amphetamine-induced activity responses are polyginecally determined. Unfortunately, our technology
has not yet caught up with our curiosity in this area, and we know
practically nothing about polygenetically determined behaviors, and,
at present, to the best of our knowledge, there does not exist a
useful theoretical orientation upon which to base investigations.

In terms of other responses to amphetamine, the investigations necessary to indicate whether or not genetic variation exists and, if so, whether it is mono- or polygenetically determined have not been done. The differential patterns seen in every response parameter examined in this chapter certainly indicate that this approach would be a useful and a powerful way of expanding our knowledge of the relationship among genetic, psychological, and pharmacological factors as they are expressed in behavior.

REFERENCES

ANDEN, N. E., DAHLSTROM. A., FUXE, K., LARSSON, K., OLSON, L., & UNGERSTEDT, U. 1966. Ascending monoamine neurones to the telecephalon and diencephalon. Acta. physiol. Scand. 67:313.

ANGRIST, B., SHOPSIN, B., & GERSHON, S. 1971. Comparative psychotomimetic effects of stereoisomers of amphetamine. Nature 234:152.

ASHER, I. M., & AGHAJANIAN, G. K. 1974. 6-hydroxydopamine lesions of olfactory tubercules and caudate nuclei: Effect on amphetamine-induced stereotyped behavior in rats. Brain Res. 82:1.

AZZARO, A. J., & RUTLEDGE, C. O. 1973. Selectivity of release of norepinephrine, dopamine and 5-hydroxytryptamine by amphetamine in various regions of rat brain. Biochem. Pharmacol. 22:2801.

BAHNSEN, P., JACOBSEN, E., & THESLIFF, H. 1938. The subjective effect of beta-phenyliso-propylaminsulfate on normal adults. Acta med. Scand. 97(1-3):89.

BARCHAS, J. D., CIARANELLO, R. D., DOMINIC, J. A., DEGUCHI, T., ORENBERG, E., RENSON, J., & KESSLER, S. 1974. Genetic aspects of monoamine mechanisms. In E. Usdin (Ed.) Neuropsychopharmacology of Monoamines and Their Regular Enzymes. New York: Raven Press. Pp. 195.

BARTHOLOMEW, A. A., & MARLEY, E. 1959. Toxic responses to 2--phenyl-3-methyl tetrahydr-1, 4 oxazine hydrochloride (Preludin) in humans. Psychopharmacologia 1:124.

BAXTER, B. L., GLUCKMAN, M. I., STEIN, L., & SCERNI, R. A. 1974. Self-injection of apomorphine in the rat: Positive reinforcement by a dopamine receptor stimulant. Pharmacol. Biochem. Behav. 2:387.

BEAMISH, P., & KILOH, L. G. 1960. Psychoses due to amphetamine consumption. J. Ment. Sci. 106:337.

BELL, D. S., & TRETHOWAN, W. H. 1961. Amphetamine addiction. J. Nerv. Ment. Dis. 133:489.

BERTLER, A., & ROSENGREN, E. 1959. Occurrence and distribution
    of catecholamines in brain. Acta physiol. Scand. 47:350.

BIZZI, A., CODEGONI, A. M., LIETTI, A., & GARATTINI, S. 1968.
    Different responses of white and brown adipose tissues affect-
    ing lipolysis. Biochem. Pharmacol. 4:573.

BRAESTRUP, C. 1972. Dopaminergic and tryptominergic effects of
    amphetamine in pigeons, cited by Randrup and Munkvad. In
    Correlation between specific effects of amphetamine on the
    brain and on behavior, In Current Concepts on Amphetamine
    Abuse. Government Printing Office. Pp. 17.

BREESE, G. R., COOPER, B. R., & SMITH, R. D. 1973. Biochemical
    and behavioral alterations following 6-hydroxydopamine admin-
    istration into brain. In E. Usdin & S. H. Snyder (Eds.)
    Frontiers in Catecholamine Research. New York: Pergamon Press.
    Pp. 701.

BRODIE, B. B., CHO, A. K., & GESSA, G. L. 1970. Possible role of
    p-hydroxynorephedrine in the depletion of norepinephrine in-
    duced by d-amphetamine and in tolerance to this drug. In E.
    Costa & S. Garattini (Eds.) International Symposium on Amphet-
    amines and Related Compounds. New York: Raven Press. Pp. 217.

BROWN, A. M., & JULIAN, T. 1968. The body temperature response
    of two inbred strains of mice to handling, saline, and amphet-
    amine. Internat. J. Neuropharmacol. 7:531.

BUETHIN, F. C., MIYA, T. S., BLAKE, D. W., & BOUSQUET, W. F. 1972.
    Enhanced sensitivity to noradrenergic agonists and tolerance
    development to alpha-methyltyrosine in the rat. J. Pharmacol.
    exp. Ther. 181:446.

CACCIA, S., CECCHETTI, G., GARATTINI, S., & JORI, A. 1973. Inter-
    action of (+)-amphetamine with cerebral dopaminergic neurons
    in two strains of mice, that show different temperature re-
    sponses to this drug. Brit. J. Pharmacol. 49:400.

CALDWELL, J., SEVER, P. S., & TRELINSKI, M. 1974. On the mecha-
    nism of hyperthermia induced by amphetamine in the rat. J.
    Pharm. Pharmacol. 26:821.

CARLSSON, A. 1970. Amphetamine and brain catecholamines. In E. Costa & S. Garattini (Eds.) International Symposium of Amphetamines and Related Compounds. New York: Raven Press. Pp. 289.

CONNELL, P. H. 1958. Amphetamine psychosis. Maudsley Monographs No. 5. New York: Oxford University Press.

COOLS, A. 1971. The function of dopamine and its antagonism in the caudate nucleus of cats in relation to the stereotyped behaviour. Arch. int. Pharmacodyn. 194:259.

COOLS, A. R. 1973. Serotonin: a behaviourally active compound in the caudate nucleus of cats. Israel J. Med. Sci. 9:5.

COOLS, A., & VAN ROSSUM, J. M. 1970. Caudate dopamine and stereotypes behavior of cats. Arch. int. Pharmacodyn. 197:163.

COOPER, J. R., BLOOM, F. E., & ROTH, R. H. 1974. The Biochemical Basis of Neuropharmacology. New York: Oxford University Press.

CORNE, S. J., & PICKERING, R. W. 1967. A possible correlation between drug-induced hallucinations in man and behavioural responses in mice. Psychopharmacologia (Berl.) 11:65.

CORNE, S. J., PICKERING, R. W., & WARNER, B. T. 1963. A method for assessing the effects of drugs on the central actions of 5-hydroxytryptamine. Brit. J. Pharmacol. 20:106.

CORRODI, H., FUXE, K., HAMBERGER, B., & LJUNGDAHL, A. 1970. Studies on central and peripheral noradrenaline neurons using a new dopamine-β-hydroxylase inhibitor. Eur. J. Pharmacol. 12:145.

COSTALL, B., & NAYLOR, R. J. 1972. Possible involvement of noradrenergic area of the amygdala with stereotyped behavior. Life Sci. 11:1135.

COSTALL, B., & NAYLOR, R. J. 1974a. Extrapyramidal and mesolimbic involvement with the stereotypic activity of d- and l-amphetamine. Eur. J. Pharmacol. 25:121.

COSTALL, B., & NAYLOR, R. J. 1974b. The nucleus amygdaloideus centralis and neuroleptic activity in the rat. Eur. J. Pharmacol. 25:138.

COSTALL, B., NAYLOR, R. J., & OLLEY, J. E. 1972a. Stereotypic and anticatalyptic activities of amphetamine after intracerebral injections. Eur. J. Pharmacol. 18:83.

COSTALL, B., NAYLOR, R. J., & OLLEY, J. E. 1972b. The substantia nigra and streotyped behavior. Eur. J. Pharmacol. 18:95.

CREESE, I., & IVERSEN, S. D. 1973. Blockage of amphetamine-induced motor stimulation and stereotypy in the adult rat following neonatal treatment with 6-hydroxydopamine. Brain Res. 55:369.

CREESE, I., & IVERSEN, S. D. 1975. The pharmacological and anatomical substrates of the amphetamine response in the rat. Brain Res. 83:419.

DAVIS, J. M. & JANOWSKY, D. S. 1973. Amphetamine and methylphenidate psychosis. In E. Usdin & S. Snyder (Eds.) Frontiers in Catecholamine Research. New York: Pergamon Press. Pp. 977.

DEL RIO, J., & FUENTES, J. A. 1969. Further studies on the antagonism of stereotyped behaviour induced by amphetamine. Eur. J. Pharmacol. 8:73.

DEWHURST, W. G., & MARLEY, E. 1965. The effects of alphamethyl derivatives of noradrenaline phenylethylamine and tryptamine on the central nervous system of the chicken. Brit. J. Pharmacol. 25:682.

DIAZ, J. L. & HUTTONEN, M. O. 1972. Altered metabolism of serotonin in the brain of the rat after chronic ingestion of d-amphetamine. Psychopharmacologis (Berl.) 23:365.

DOLFINI, E., RAMIREZ DEL ANGEL, A., GARATTINI, S., & VALZELLI, L. 1970. Brain catecholamines released by dexamphetamine in three strains of mice. Eur. J. Pharmacol. 9:333.

DORING, L. G., SMITH, R. L., & WILLIAMS, R. T. 1970. The metabolic fate of amphetamine in man and other species. Biochem. J. 116:425.

ELLINWOOD, E. H. JR. 1967. Amphetamine psychosis: I. Description of the individuals and the process. J. nerv. ment. Dis. 144:273.

ELLINWOOD, E. H. JR. 1968. Amphetamine psychosis: II. Theoretical implications. J. Neuropsychiat. 4:45.

ELLINWOOD, E. H. JR. 1969. Amphetamine psychosis: A multi-dimensional process. Seminars in Psychiatry. 1:208.

ELLINWOOD, E. H. JR. 1971. Effect of chronic methamphetamine intoxication in rhesus monkeys. Biol. Psychiat. 3:25.

ELLINWOOD, E. H. JR. 1972a. Amphetamine psychoses: Individuals, settings, and sequences. In E. H. Ellinwood & S. Cohen (Eds.) Current Concepts on Amphetamine Abuse. Dept. Health, Education and Welfare Publication No. (HSM) 72-9085. Washington, D.C. Pp. 143.

ELLINWOOD, E. H. JR. 1972b. Emergency treatment of acute reactions to CNS stimulants. J. Psychedelic Drugs. 5(2):147.

ELLINWOOD, E. H. JR., & BALSTER, R. L. 1974. Rating the behavioral effects of amphetamine. Eur. J. Pharmac. 28:35.

ELLINWOOD, E. H. JR., & ESCALANTE, O. 1970a. Behavior and histopathological findings during chronic methedrine intoxication. Biol. Psychiat. 2:27.

ELLINWOOD, E. H. JR., & ESCALANTE, O. 1970b. Chronic amphetamine effect on the olfactory forebrin. Biol. Psychiat. 2:189.

ELLINWOOD, E. H. JR., & KILBEY, M. MARLYNE. 1975. Amphetamine stereotypy: the influence of environmental factors and prepotent behavioral patterns on its topography and development. Biol. Psychiat. 10:3.

ELLINWOOD, E. H. JR., & SUDILOVSKY, A. 1973a. Chronic amphetamine intoxication: behavioral model of psychoses. In Jonathan O. Cole, Alfred M. Freedman, & Arnold J. Friedhoff (Eds.) Psychopathology and Psychopharmacology. Baltomore: Johns Hopkins University Press. Pp. 51.

ELLINWOOD, E. H. JR., & SUDILOVSKY, A. 1973b. The relationship of the amphetamine model psychosis to schizophrenia. In I. A. Ban et al., (Eds.) Psychopharmacology, Sexual Disorders, and Drug Abuse. Amsterdam: North=Holland Publishing Co. Pp. 189.

ELLINWOOD, E. H. JR., SUDILOVSKY, A., & NELSON, L. 1972. Behavioral analysis of chronic amphetamine intoxication. Biol. Psychiat. 4:215.

EMELE, J., SHANAMAN, J., & WARREN, M. 1961. Chlorphentermine hydrochloride, p-chlor-α-α-dimethylphen-ethylamine hydrochloride, a new anorexigenic agent. II. Central nervous system activity. Fed. Proc. 20(Part I):328.

ERNST, A. M., & SMELIK, P. G. 1966. Site of action of dopamine and apomorphine on compulsive gnawing behavior in rats. Experientia 22:837.

ESCALANTE, O., & ELLINWOOD, E. H. JR. 1972. Effects of chronic amphetamine intoxication on adrenergic and cholinergic structures in the central nervous system: histochemical observations in cats and monkeys. In E. H. Ellinwood, Jr., (Ed.) Current Concepts on Amphetamine Abuse. Department of Health, Education and Welfare Publication No. 72-9085, U.S. Pp. 97.

FANGE, R., & HANSON, A. 1973. Comparative pharmacology of catecholamines. In G. Petrie & M. J. Michelson (Eds.) International Encyclopedia of Pharmacology and Therapeutics. New York: Pergamon Press. Pp. 391.

FERRIS, R. M., TANG, F. L. M., & MAXWELL, R. A. 1972. Comparison of the capacities of isomers of amphetamine, deoxypipradrol and methylphenidate to inhibit the uptake of tritiated catecholamines into rat cerebral cortex slices, synaptosomal preparations of rat cerebral cortex, hypothalamus and striatum and into adrenergic nerves of rabbit aorta. J. Pharmacol. exp. Ther. 181(3):407.

FIBIGER, H. C., FIBIGER, H. P., & ZES, A. P. 1973. Attenuation of amphetamine induced motor stimulation and stereotypy by 6-hydroxydopamine in the rat. Brit. J. Pharmacol. 4:683.

FITZ-GERALD, F. L. 1967. The effects of d-amphetamine upon behavior of young chimpanzees reared under different conditions. Excerpta Medica. International Congress Series. 129:1226.

FLORY, C. D., & GILBERT, J. 1943. The effects of benzedrine sulphate and caffeine citrate on the efficiency of college students. J. Appl. Psychol. 27(2):121.

FOG, R. 1969. Stereotyped and non-stereotyped behavior in rats induced by various stimulant drugs. Psychopharmacologia 14: 299.

FOG, R. 1970. Behavioural effects in rats of morphine and amphetamine and of a combination of the two drugs. Psychopharmacologia (Berl.) 16:305.

FOG, R. L., RANDRUP, A., & PAKKENBERG, H. 1967. Aminergic mechanisms in the corpus striatum and amphetamine induced stereotyped behaviour. Psychopharmacologia (Berl.) 11:179.

FREEMAN, J. J. & SULSER, F. 1972. Iprindole-amphetamine interactions in the rat: the role of aromatic hydroxylation of amphetamine in its mode of action. J. Pharmacol. exp. Ther. 183:307.

GELDER, M. G. & VANE, J. R. 1962. Interaction of the effects of tyramine, amphetamine and reserpine in man. Psychopharmacologia (Berl.) 3:231.

GESSA, G. L., CLAY, G. A., & BRODIE, B. B. 1969. Evidence that hyperthermia produced by d-amphetamine is caused by a peripheral action of the drug. Life Sci. 8:135.

GLICKMAN, S. E., & SCHIFF, B. V. 1967. A biological theory of reinforcement. Psych. Rev. 74:81.

GOLDSTEIN, M., & NAKAJIMA, K. 1967. The effect of disulfiram on catecholamine levels in the brain. J. Pharmacol. exp. Ther. 157:96.

GORLITZ, B. D., & FREY, H. H. 1972. Central monoamines and antinociceptive drug action. Eur. J. Pharmacol. 20:171.

GRIFFITH, J. D., CAVANAUGH, J. H., HELD, J., & OATES, J. A. 1970. Experimental psychoses induced by the administration of d-amphetamine. In E. Costa & S. Garattini (Eds.) Amphetamines and Related Compounds. New York: Raven Press. Pp 897.

GROPPETTI, A., & COSTA, E. 1969. Tissue concentration of p-hyddroxynorephedrine in rats injected with d-amphetamine: effect of pretreatment with desipramine. Life Sci. 8:653.

GUNNE, L. M., & ANGGARD, M. D. 1973. Amphetamine metabolism in amphetamine-induced psychoses. In E. Usdin & S. H. Snyder (Eds.) Frontiers in Catecholamine Research. New York: Pergamon Press. Pp. 983.

HAMPTON, W. H. 1961. Observed psychiatric reactions following use of amphetamine and amphetamine-like substances. Bull. N. Y. Acad. Med. 37:167.

HARRIS, J. E., & BALDESSARINI, R. J. 1973. Uptake of [^{3}H]-catecholamines by homogenates of rat corpus striatum and cerebral cortex: effects of amphetamine analogues. Neuropharm. 12: 669.

HARVEY, J. K., TODD, C. W., & HOWARD, J. W. 1949. Fatality associated with benzedrine ingestion: a case report. Delaware Med. J. 21:111.

HEATH, R. G., NESSELHOF, W., BISHOP, M. P., & BYERS, L. W. 1965. Behavioral and metabolic changes associated with administration of tetraethylthiuram disulfide (antabuse). Dis. Nerv. Syst. 26:99.

HERMAN, M., & NAGLER, S. H. 1954. Psychoses due to amphetamine. J. Nerv. Ment. Dis. 120:268.

HILL, H. F., & HORITA, A. 1970. Amphetamine-induced hyperthermia in rabbits. Pharmacologist 12:197.

HILL, H. F., & HORITA, A. 1971. Inhibition of (+)-amphetamine hyperthermia by blockade of dopamine receptors in rabbits. J. Pharm. Pharmacol. 23:715.

HORITA, A., & HILL, H. F. 1972. Hallucinogens, amphetamines and temperature regulation. In E. Schonbaum & P. Lomax (Eds.) The Pharmacology of Thermoregulation. New York: S. Karger. Pp. 417.

IVERSEN, S. D. 1971. The effect of surgical lesions to frontal cortex and substantia nigra on amphetamine responses in rats. Brain Res. 31:195.

JANSSEN, P., NIEMEGEERS, C., & SCHELLENKENS, K. 1965. Is it possible to predict the clinical effects of neuroleptic drugs (major tranquilizers) from animal data. Arzneim. Forsch. 15:104.

JELLINEK, P. 1971. Dual effect of dexamphetamine on body temperature in the rat. Eur. J. Pharmac. 15:389.

JERUSSI, T. P., & GLICK, S. D. 1974. Amphetamine-induced rotation in rats without lesions. Neuropharmacology 13:283.

JÖNSSON, L. E., ANGGARD, E., & GUNNE, L. M. 1971. Blockade of intravenous amphetamine euphoria in man. Clin. Pharmacol. Therapy. 12:889.

JORDAN, S. C., & HAMPSON, F. 1960. Amphetamine poisoning associated with hyperpyrexia. Brit. Med. J. 2(Part I):844.

JORI, A., & BERNARDI, D. 1969. Effect of amphetamine and amphetamine-like drugs on homovanillic acid concentration in the brain. J. Pharm. Pharmacol. 21:694.

JORI, A., & BERNARDI, D. 1972. Further studies on the increase of striatal homovanillic acid induced by amphetamine and fenfluramine. Eur. J. Pharmacol. 19:276.

KALANT, O. J. 1966. "The Amphetamines: Toxicity and Addiction," Springfield, Illinois: Thomas.

KARCZMAR, A. G., & SCUDDER, C. L. 1967. Behavioral responses to drugs and brain catecholamine levels of mice of different strains and genera. Fed. Proc. 26:1186.

KARCZMAR, A. G., SCUDDER, D. L., & RICHARDSON, D. L. 1973. Interdisciplinary approach to the study of behavior in related mice types. In S. Ehrenpreis & I. G. Kopen (Eds.) Chemical Approaches to Brain Function. New York: Academic Press. Pp. 159.

KELLOGG, C., & LUNDBORG, P. 1973. Inhibition of catecholamine synthesis during ontogenic development. Brain Res. 61:321.

KEMPF, E., GREILSAMER, J., MACK, G., & MANDEL, P. 1974. Correlation of behavioral differences in three strains of mice with differences in brain amines. Nature 247:483.

KHALSA, J. H., & DAVIS, W. M. 1974. Neurochemical effect of chronic pretreatment with -methyltryosine or U-14,624 in rat, Society for Neuroscience, 4th Annual Meeting, Abstract #345. Pp. 281.

KILBEY, M. M., FRITCHIE, G. E., MCLENDON, D. M., & JOHNSON, K. 1972. Delta-9-tetrahydrocannabinol induced inhibition of attack behavior in the mouse. Nature 238:643.

KRAMER, J. C. 1969. Introduction to amphetamine abuse. J. Psyched. Drugs 2:1.

LAL, S., & SOURKES, T. L. 1973. Ontogeny of stereotyped behavior induced by apomorphine and amphetamine in the rat. Arch. int. Pharmacodyn. 202:171.

LEWANDER, T. 1970. Catecholamine turnover studies in chronic amphetamine intoxication. In E. Costa & S. Garattini (Eds.) International Symposium on Amphetamines and Related Compounds. New York: Raven Press. Pp. 317.

LEWANDER, T. 1971a. On the presence of p-hydroxynorephedrine in the rat brain and heart in relation to changes in catecholamine levels after administration of amphetamine. Acta. pharmac. et tox. 29:33.

LEWANDER, T. 1971b. Effects of acute and chronic amphetamine intoxication on brain catecholamines in the guinea pig. Acta. pharmac. et tox. 29:209.

LEWANDER, T. 1973. Effect of chronic treatment with central stimulants on brain monoamines and some behavioral and physiological functions in rats, guinea pigs, and rabbits. In E. Usdin (Ed.) Neuropsychology of Monoamines and their Regulatory Enzymes. New York: Raven Press. Pp. 221.

LIDDEN, S., & SATRAN, R. 1967. Disulfiram (antabuse) psychoses. Amer. J. Psychiat. 123:1284.

LORENZ, KONRAD Z. 1950. The comparative method of studying innate behaviour patterns. In Physiological Mechanisms in animal behaviour. Symposia of the Society for Experimental Biology 4:221.

LYON, M., & RANDRUP, A. 1971. The dose-response effect of amphetamine upon avoidance behavior in the rat seen as a function of increasing stereotypy. Pharmacologia 23:334.

MAAS, J. W. 1962. Neurochemical differences between two strains of mice. Science 137:621.

MAAS, J. W. 1963. Neurochemical differences between two strains of mice. Nature 197:255.

MAJ, J., & PRZEGALINSKI, E. 1967. Disulfiram and some effects of amphetamine in mice and rats. J. Pharm. Pharmacol. 19:341.

MANTEGAZZA, P., NAIMZADA, K. M., & REVA, M. 1968. Effects of prop-
    ranolol on some activities of amphetamine. Eur. J. Pharmacol.
    4:25.

MATSUMOTO, C., & SHAW, W. N. 1971. The involvement of plasma free
    fatty acids in (+)-amphetamine-induced hyperthermia in rats.
    J. Pharm. Pharmacol. 23:387.

MCCULLOUGH, D. O., MILBERG, J. N., & ROBINSON, S. M. 1970. A
    central site for the hypothermic effect of (+)-amphetamine
    sulfate and p-hydroxyamphetamine hydrobromide in mice. Brit.
    J. Pharmacol. 40:219.

MCGEER, P. L., MCGEER, E. G., & WADA, J. A. 1963. Central aromat-
    ic amine levels and Behavior II., serotonin and catecholamine
    levels in various cat brain areas following administration of
    psychoactive drugs or amine precursors. Arch. Neurol. 9:81.

MEDNICK, S. A., SCHULSINGER, F., HIGGINS, J., & BELL, B. 1974.
    Genetics, Environment, and Psychopathology. Amsterdam: North-
    -Holland Publishing Co.

MILLER, F. P., COX, R. H., JR., & MAICKEL, R. P. 1968. Intra-
    strain differences in serotonin and norepinephrine in discrete
    areas of rat brain. Science 162:463.

NAYLOR, R. J., & OLLEY, J. E. 1972a. Modification of the behav-
    ioral changes induced by amphetamine in the rat by lesions in
    the caudate nucleus, the caudate-putamen and globus pallidus.
    Neuropharmacology 11:91.

NAYLOR, R. J., & OLLEY, J. E. 1972b. Modification of the behav-
    ioral changes induced by Haloperidol in the rat by lesions in
    the caudate nucleus, the caudate-putamen and globus pallidus.
    Neuropharmacology 11:81.

O'DONAHUGH, N. F., & HAGAMEN, W. D. 1967. A map of the cat brain
    for regions producing self-stimulation and unilateral atten-
    tion. Brain Res. 5:289.

OLIVERIO, A., ELEFTHERIOU, B. E., & BAILEY, D. W. 1973. Explora-
    tory activity: genetic analysis of its modification by scopol-
    amine and amphetamine. Physiol. Behav. 10:893.

OLIVERIO, A., CASTELLANO, C., EBEL, A., & MANDEL, P. 1974. A gen-
    etic analysis of behavior: a neurochemical approach. Ad.
    biochem. Psychopharmacol. 11:411.

RANDALL, W., & TRULSON, M. 1974. A serotonergic system involved in the grooming behavior of cats with pontile lesions. Pharm. Biochem. & Behav. 2:355.

RANDRUP, A., & MUNKVAD, I. 1964. On the relation of tryptaminic and serotonergic mechanisms to amphetamine-induced abnormal behavior. Acta Pharmac. et tox. 21:272.

RANDRUP, A., & MUNKVAD, I. 1966a. Role of catecholamines in the amphetamine excitatory response. Nature 211:540.

RANDRUP, A., & MUNKVAD, I. 1966b. DOPA and other naturally occurring substances as causes of stereotypy and rage in rats. Acta psychiat. Scand. Suppl. 42:193.

RANDRUP, A., & MUNKVAD, I. 1967. Stereotyped activities produced by amphetamine in several animal species and man. Psychopharmacologia 11:300.

RANDRUP, A., & MUNKVAD, I. 1968. Behavioural stereotypies induced by pharmacological agents. Pharmakopsychiatr./Neuro-psychapharmakol. 1:19.

RANDRUP, A., & MUNKVAD, I. 1972. Correlation between specific effects of amphetamine on the brain and on behavior. In E. H. Ellinwood, Jr. & Sidney Cohen (Eds.) Current Concepts on Amphetamine Abuse. Rockville, Maryland:National Institutes of Mental Health. Pp. 17.

RANDRUP, A., & SCHEEL-KRUGER, J. 1966. Diethyldithiocarbamate and amphetamine stereotype behavior. J. Pharm. Pharmacol. 18:752.

RANDRUP, A., MUNKVAD, I., & USDIN, E. 1963. Adrenergic mechanisms and amphetamine induced abnormal behaviour. Acta Pharmac. et tox. 20:145.

RECH, R. H., & STOLK, J. M. 1970. Amphetamine-drug interactions that relate brain catecholamines to behavior. In E. Costa & S. Garattini (Eds.) Amphetamines and Related Compounds. New York: Raven Press. Pp. 385.

REID, W. D. 1970. Turnover rates of brain 5-hydroxytryptamine increased by d-amphetamine. Brit. J. Pharmacol. 40:483.

RICHARDSON, D., KARCZMAR, A. G., & SCUDDER, C. L. 1972. Intergeneric behavioral differences among methamphetamine treated mice. Psychopharmacologia 25:347.

RICKMAN, E. E., WILLIAMS, E. Y., & BROWN, R. K. 1961. Acute toxic psychiatric reaction related to amphetamine medication. Med. Ann. D. C. 30:209.

ROSENBLATT, J. S. 1972. Learning in newborn kittens. Sci. Amer. 227:18.

SARGANT, W., & SLATER, E. 1963. Introduction to Physical Treatment in Psychiatry. Edinburgh: Livingstone.

SCHLESINGER, K., BOGGAN, W. D., & FRIEDMAN. D. 1965. Genetics of audiogenic seizures: I. Relation to brain serotonin and norepinephrine in mice. Life Sci. 4:2345.

SCHUBERT, J., FYRO, B., BYBACK, H., & SEDVALL, G. 1972. Effects of cocaine and amphetamine on the metabolism of tryptophan and 5-hydroxytryptamine in mouse brain in vivo. J. Pharm. Pharmacol. 22:860.

SCHUSTER, C. R., & BALSTER, R. L. The discriminative stimulus properties of drugs. In T. Thompson & P. B. Dews (Eds.) Advances in Behavioral Pharmacology. New York: Academic Press, in press.

SCOTT, J. P., LEE, CHING-TSE., & HO, JOHN, E. 1971. Effects of fighting, genotype, and amphetamine sulfate on body temperature of mice. J. Comp. Physiol. Psychol. 76:349.

SEGAL, D. S., & MANDELL, A. J. 1974. Long-term administration of d-amphetamine: Progressive augmentation of motor activity and stereotypy. Pharm. Biochem. Behav. 2:249.

SEVER, P. S., CALDWELL, J., & WILLIAMS, R. T. 1974. Evidence against the involvement of false neurotransmitters in tolerance to amphetamine-induced hyperthermia in the rat. J. Pharm. Pharmacol. 26:823.

SIMPSON, B., & IVERSEN, S. D. 1971. Effects of substantia nigra lesions on the locomotor and stereotypy responses to amphetamine. Nature 230:30.

SLADEK, J. R. 1971. Differences in the distribution of catecholamine varicosities in the cat and rat reticular formation. Science 174:410.

SNYDER, S. H. 1972. Catecholamines in the brain as mediators of amphetamine psychoses. Arch. gen. Psychiat. 27:169.

SNYDER, S. H., BANERJE, S. P., YAMAMURA, H. I., & GREENBERG, D. 1974. Drugs, neurotransmitters and schizophrenia. Science 184:1243.

SPARBER, S. B., & TILSON, HUGH A. 1972. The releasability of central norepinephrine and serotonin by peripherally administered d-amphetamine before and after tolerance. Life Sci. 11(I): 1059.

STEIN, L. 1964. Self-stimulation of the brain and the central stimulant action of amphetamine. Fed. Proc. 23:836.

SUDAK, H. S., & MAAS, J. W. 1964a. Central nervous system serotonin and norepinephrine localization in emotional and non-emotional strains in mice. Nature 203:1254.

SUDAK, H. S., & MAAS, J. W. 1964b. Behavioral neurochemical correlation in reactive and nonreactive strains of rats. Science 146:418.

TAGLIAMONTE, A., TAGLIAMONTE, P., PEREZ-CRUET, J., STERN, S., & GESSA, G. L. 1971. Effect of psychotropic drugs on tryptophan concentration in the rat brain. J. Pharmacol. exp. Ther. 177(3):475.

TAYLOR, K. M., & SNYDER, S. H. 1971. Differential effects of d- and l-amphetamine on behavior and on catecholamine disposition in dopamine and norepinephrine containing neurons of rat brain. Brain Res. 28:295.

TECCE, J. J., & COLE, J. O. 1974a. Effect of amphetamine on CNV and behavior in man. In W. C. McCallum & J. R. Knott (Eds.) Event Related Slow Potentials of the Brain. England: John Wright & Sons, in press.

TECCE, J. J., & COLE, J. O. 1974b. Amphetamine effects in man: paradoxical drowsiness and lowered electrical brain activity (CNV). Science 185:451.

TEITELBAUM, P., & DERKS, P. 1958. The effect of amphetamine on forced frinking in the rat. J. Comp. Physiol. Psychol. 51: 801.

THORNBURG, J. E., & MOORE, K. E. 1973. Dopamine and norepinephrine uptake by rat brain synaptosomes: relative inhibitory potencies of l- and d-amphetamine and amantadine. Res. Commun. Chem. Pathol. Pharmacol. 5(1):81.

UNGERSTEDT, U., 1971. Stereotaxic mapping of the monamine pathways in the rat brain. Acta physiol. Scand. Suppl. 367:1.

UNGERSTEDT, U., & LJUNGBERG, T. 1973. Behavioral-anatomical corr-
elates of central catecholamine neurones. In E. Usdin & S.
Snyder (Eds.) Frontiers in Catecholamine Research. New York:
Pergamon Press. Pp. 689.

USDIN, E. 1974. (Ed.) Neuropsychopharmacology of Monoamines and
Their Regulatory Enzymes. New York: Raven Press.

USDIN, E., & SNYDER, S. 1974. (Eds.) Frontiers in Catecholamine
Research. New York: Pergamon Press.

UTENA, H. 1974. On relapse-liability; Schizophrenia, amphetamine
psychoses and animal model. In H. Mitsuda & I. Fukuda (Eds.)
Biological Mechanisms of Schizophrenia and Schizophrenia-like
Psychosis. Tokyo: Igaku Shorn Ltd. Pp. 285.

VANE, J. R. 1960. The actions of sympathomimetic amines on trypt-
amine receptors. In J. Vane & G. W. M. O'Connor (Eds.)
Adrenergic Mechanisms. London: CIBA Foundation Symposium,
Churchill Ltd. Pp. 356.

WADA, J. A., & MCGEER, E. G. 1966. Central aromatic amines and
behavior III. Correlative analysis of conditioned approach behavior and brain levels of serotonin and catecholamines in
monkeys. Arch. Neurol. 14:129.

WALLACH, M. B. 1974. Drug-induced stereotyped behavior: similarities and differences. In E. Usdin (Ed.) Neuropsychopharmacology of Monoamines and the Regulatory Enzymes. New York:
Raven Press. Pp. 241.

WEINER, W. J., GOETZ, C., WESTHEIMER, R., & KLAWANS, H. J., JR.
1973. Serotonergic and antiserotonergic influences on amphetamine-induced stereotyped behavior. J. Neurol. Sci. 20:373.

WEISSMAN, A., KOE, B. K., & TENEN, S. S. 1965. Antiamphetamine
effects following inhibition of tyrosine hydroxylase. J.
Pharmacol. exp. Ther. 151:339.

WILLNER, J. H., SAMACH, M., ANGRIST, B. M., WALLACH, M. B., &
GERSHON, S. 1970. Drug-induced stereotyped behavior and its
antagonism in dogs. Comm. Behav. Biol. 5:135.

WISE, C. DAVID., & STEIN, LARRY. 1970. Amphetamine: facilitation
of behavior by augmented release of norepinephrine from the
medical forebrain bundle. In E. Costa & S. Garattini (Eds.)
Amphetamine and Related Compounds. New York: Raven Press. Pp.
463.

WOLF, H. H., & BUNCE, M. E. 1973. Hyperthermia and the amphetamine aggregation phenomana: absence of a causal relation. J. Pharm. Pharmacol. 25:425.

YOUNG, D., & SCOVILLE, W. B. 1938. Paranoid psychosis in narcolepsy and the possible dangers of benzedrine treatment. Med. Clin. N. A. (Boston) 22:637.

ZIMMERBERG, BETTY., GLICK, S. D., & JERUSSI, T. P. 1974. Neurochemical correlates of a spatial preference in rats. Science 185:623.

SOME DRUG-DRUG INTERACTIONS INVOLVING PSYCHOTROPIC AGENTS[1]

William E. Fann, M.D. and Bruce W. Richman, M.A.

Departments of Psychiatry and Pharmacology, Baylor
College of Medicine, and the Psychiatry Service,
Veterans Administration Hospital, Houston, Texas

CONTENTS

INTRODUCTION

The idiosyncracies of drug response and drug-drug interaction
are often secondary to the idiosyncracies of individual organ systems because they are affected by such factors as age, youth,
disease, or genetically transmitted characteristics. With the
multiplicity of psychopharmacologic agents now available, and with
the tendencies of many psychiatrists toward prescription of polypharmacy, the frequency and variety of psychotropic drug interactions are increasing faster than our ability to discover and adequately analyze the causative components. Our knowledge of the
genetic factors influencing these activities is particularly

---

[1]This work was supported in part by a grant from the Veterans
Administration.

deficient, and the necessary body of animal data upon which to base
careful human studies has not yet been suitably developed. Reports
of unanticipated psychotropic drug-drug interactions in which genetic factors appear to figure significantly are few and tentative.
Some cases of genetically influenced responses involving singly
administered agents interacting with organ systems have been reported (Kalow, 1971). Well documented instances of one drug altering
the activity of another as a result of genetic factors, such as
the inhibition of diphenylhydantoin metabolism by iproniazid in
slow acetylators (Kutt & McDowell, 1968) are particularly scarce.
Rather than attempt a compendium of annecdotal reports of such
cases here, we will devote this brief chapter to an outline of some
of the broader mechanisms which we can state with some assurance
are fairly consistent components in the interactivity of multiple
drugs within living organisms. As further information concerning
the role of genetics in these processes is developed in the future,
it will probably have to be done with reference to the patterns
with which we have thus far seen drug-drug interactions occur when
they are influenced by advanced age, disease or trauma to effected
organs and tissues, or matters of biochemical compatibility. The
following information is presented, therefore, as a construct of
both established and theoretically possible occurrences.

ALTERATION OF TISSUE AND PLASMA BINDINGS

Binding of drugs to plasma proteins or inactive tissue sites
provide important variables in the overall function of therapeutic
compounds. Such binding may create depots for the compound; being
bound to body proteins thus protects the drug from immediate metabolic degredation or other changes that may inactivate it; where
the drug possesses high lipid solubility it may become localized
in body fat and when released from these stores may cause prolongation of drug action. Drugs that are bound to plasma proteins are
inactive while so bound, the free drug concentration being available for therapeutic activity, metabolism and excretion. For drugs
that are highly protein bound (and thus have a small free drug com-
partment), even small changes in the ratio of bound to free drug
may markedly affect its therapeutic effects and, in addition, its
ability to bring about side effects. Most neuroleptic compounds
and tricyclic antidepressants are highly bound, and would thus be
expected to show susceptibility to interactions with other drugs
that compete with them for binding sites on plasma protein and at
tissue sites. A basic drug, such as diphenylhydantoin, which is
highly bound to human albumin might interfere non-competitively
with the basic tricyclic imipramine (Koch-Seser & Sellers, 1971).

In subjects in whom percentage of body weight contributed by
adipose tissue is particularly large, drugs that are highly lipid-
-soluble would tend to show longer duration of action because the
additional adipose tissue would represent a larger storage area

for the compounds. The stored compounds would continue to be released and act for some time after actual administration of the compound has been discontinued.

In patients who have marked alteration in content of body fat, there may be either an increase or a diminution in therapeutic response to the compound, consistent with the body type. In chronic diseases involving secondary changes in type and composition of plasma protein, alteration of binding of circulating therapeutic compounds is possible. Any condition which would alter these drug--protein affinities may result in changes in activity of the therapeutic agent; an inhibition of the affinity might result in more free drug being available; an increase in the binding capacity would, conversely, diminish the availability of the circulating drug. Although available data evaluating the precise influence of these states on drug activity is meager, when multiple system decompensation and chronic disease are present in patients experiencing unusual responses to psychotropic agents, the clinician should give due consideration to these mechanisms in tracing the etiology of the problem.

ONE DRUG BLOCKING TRANSPORT OF ANOTHER TO THE SITE OF ACTION

Some major tranquilizers of the phenothiazine class and the tricyclic antidepressant drugs inhibit the activity of the norepinephrine pump, the adrenergic membrane transport system which takes up and transports norepinephrine and a variety of ring-substituted bases such as guanethidine and similar adrenergic neuron blocking drugs. The antihypertensive guanethidine, secondary to transport by this pump, is concentrated in the adrenergic neuron, where it exerts a selective blocking action on the sympathetic postganglionic neurons. Blockade of the pump by the psychotropic compound prevents the accumulation of guanethidine and ultimately antagonizes its therapeutic hypotensive effect. The patient who has a tricyclic antidepressant or chlorpromazine added to a stable and effective guanethidine regimen will return to hypertensive levels, with associated consequences (Fann, Janowsky & Davis, 1971). Tyramine, a potent pressor amine, acts through similar uptake and delivery to the neuron by the norepinephrine pump. We can, therefore, posit an antagonism of guanethidine-related hypotension by demonstrating the antagonism of the pressor response to tyramine. We have been able to demonstrate the tricyclics desipramine and doxepin affect blood pressure response to infused tyramine by blocking the re--uptake pump, thereby antagonizing the effects of the tyramine and sustaining the blood pressure response to the indirectly acting pressor norepinephrine, which is inactivated by transport to the neuron. Blockade of the transport mechanism would, therefore, leave more of the active substance available to the postsynaptic receptor sites.

CHANGES IN EXCRETION OF ONE DRUG BY ANOTHER

Amphetamine is often taken in overdosage. Treatment of amphetamine overdosage can be assisted by rendering the patient's urine acidic (Davis et al., 1971). It has been shown that the rate of renal excretion of amphetamine is more than doubled in the presence of acid urine conditions when compared to conditions of basic urine pH. Altering the patient's urine to an acid pH would therefore hasten the clearance of the drug from the blood. A drug such as ammonium chloride, which produces acidosis and thereby urinary acidification, would function effectively in this pharmacological procedure.

Lithium is a safe and effective antimanic agent if properly administered and properly monitored. When serum levels rise beyond the generally accepted safe concentration of 2.0 mEq/liter, however, serious side effects can occur, ranging from mild sedation and confusion to coma and death. To avoid these responses during therapy with lithium, an adequate sodium intake must be maintained and a physiologically normal serum sodium level assured. When serum sodium drops below physiologic levels, lithium is selectively reabsorbed by the renal tubules and the ion can thereby rapidly accumulate to toxic levels. For this reason, sodium depleting drugs, such as chlorothiazide, are contraindicated when patients are receiving lithium. Studies of sodium and lithium metabolism show that the increased excretion of chlorothiazide is not associated with an increase in urinary lithium excretion, and when rapid salt depletion occurs lithium toxicity can develop (Davis & Fann, 1970). Many individuals with cyclic affective disorders who are candidates for lithium therapy may also have concurrent conditions militating for diuretic therapy.

ALTERATION OF METABOLISM OF ONE DRUG BY ANOTHER

Phenobarbital, a sedative prescribed variously for anxiety, as an anticonvulsant, to increase sedative effect of phenothiazines, and as a hypotensive agent in mild essential hypertension, accelerates liver microsomal metabolism of certain other drugs, such as some phenothiazines, warfarin (Coumadin) and diphenylhydantoin. Concomitant use of phenobarbital and a phenothiazine may actually lower the serum level of the phenothiazine thereby reducing the clinical effect, including sedation, of the phenothiazine.

Conversely, methylphenidate (Ritalin) a mild stimulant to the central nervous system (CNS) is prescribed to increase alertness and overcome drug-induced sedation. In addition to its CNS stimulant properties, methylphenidate also retards liver microsomal metabolism of certain other compounds including the anticonvulsant diphenylhydantoin, tricyclic antidepressants, phenothiazines, and anticoagulants, such as warfarin. In some instances, methylphenidate, given to counteract drug-induced sedation, blocks liver metabolism of the offending drug and thereby actually increases the blood level of the sedative agent (effectively increasing the dose) so that the net result is to increase the drug-induced sedation (Fann, 1973).

The phenomenon of a stimulant drug enhancing sedation and a sedative compound reducing soporific effects presents on the surface, at least, an unexpected therapeutic paradox.

ALTERATION OF DRUG MEDIATOR ACTIVITY BY ANOTHER DRUG

Monoamine oxidase inhibitors actively prevent deamination of catecholamines within the adrenergic neuron. In this manner, tranylcypromine, an antidepressant agent, reduces intraneuronal breakdown of norepinephrine, thereby causing more of this transmittor substance to be available after release by indirectly acting pressor amines such as tyramine, amphetamine and its congeners (e.g., sympathomimetics found in decongestants and other over-the counter cold preparations). By this inhibition of monoamine oxidase such compounds as tranylcypromine and pargyline (an antihypertensive drug) potentiate the pharmacologic action of these pressor agents. Because of this interaction, depressed persons taking tranylcypromine and hypertensive patients taking pargyline have suffered hypertensive crises after eating foods (e.g., cheese, chicken livers, certain wines) that contain high amounts of tyramine or from the concomitant ingestion of sympathomimetic amines such as amphetamine and its congeners. Since many of these sympathomimetic compounds are readily available as proprietary medications, this is an interaction that is common.

INTERFERENCE WITH DRUG ABSORPTION FROM THE GASTROINTESTINAL TRACT

Gel antacids containing magnesium and aluminum interfere with the absorption of a variety of drugs including the major tranquilizer, chlorpromazine, from the gastro-intestinal tract. Concomitant administration of one of the antacids with a tranquilizer may reduce the effectiveness of the tranquilizer by impairing absorption of this psychotropic agent. Though there may be no direct threat to the physical well-being of the patient from such combinations, other unwanted effects such as recurrence of the psychosis or severe affective disorder, etc., may occur if such an interaction is not anticipated. It is also possible that cholestyramine, an ion exchange resin used for the treatment of hypercholesterolemia, might interfere with absorption of psychotropic agents since it will bind any drug with an appropriate charge at the pH at which the two coexist in the gut (Fann et al., 1973).

DISCUSSION

The factors involved in the prescription of polypharmacy are

complex, often so complex that we do not have the information necessary to control and anticipate them. We are just now beginning
to learn of significant age-related changes in drug absorption,
distribution, binding, metabolism, and excretion. The biological
conditions under which one drug can alter the activity of another
can conceivably be replicated by idiopathic changes in organ or
enzyme systems. Genetically transmitted mutations or systemic mal-
functions can impose additional variables on an already tenuous
relationship between toxic substances within the organism.

Studies of mechanisms and pathways of drug metabolism lend
themselves easily to research in animal models, but investigation
involving the role of genetic factors in human drug response is
particularly difficult to conduct and the researcher must await
rather than create his opportunities. Until such data is available
any practicing physician must, when planning multiple psychopharma-
cotherapeutic intervention, maintain a high index of suspicion for
adverse drug interactions when observing clinical phenomena.

REFERENCES

KALOW, W. 1971. Genetic factors in adverse drug reactions. J.
    Clin. Pharmacol. 5:38.

KUTT, H., & McDOWELL, F. 1968. Inhibition of diaphenylhydantoin
    metabolism in rats and in rat liver microsomes by antituber-
    cular drugs. Neurology 18:706.

KOCH-WESER, J., & SELLERS, E. M. 1971. Drug interactions with
    cumarin anticoagulants. New Eng. J. Med. 285:487.

FANN, W. E., JANOWSKY, D. S., & DAVIS, J. M. 1971. Antagonism of
    antihypertensive effect of guanethidine by chlorpromazine.
    Lancet 2:436.

DAVIS, J. M., FANN, W. E., GRIFFITH, J. E., & OATES, J. A. 1971.
    Pharmacological aspects of the treatment of amphetamine abuse:
    The effects of urinary pH. Adv. Neuropsychpharmacol. 279.

DAVIS, J. M., & FANN, W. E. 1970. Lithium. Ann. Rev. Pharmacol.
    2:285.

FANN, W. E. 1973. Some clinically important interactions of
    psychotropic drugs. S. Med. J. 66:661.

FANN, W. E., DAVIS, J. M., JANOWSKY, D. S., SEKERKE, J. J., &
    SCHMIDT, D. M. 1973. Chlorpromazine: The effects of antac-
    ids on its gastrointestinal absorption. J. Clin. Pharm. 388.

AUDIOGENIC SEIZURES AND ACOUSTIC PRIMING

Kurt Schlesinger, Ph.D.

and

Seth K. Sharpless, Ph.D.

Department of Psychology and Institute for Behavioral
    Genetics
University of Colorado
Boulder, Colorado   80302

CONTENTS

The Laterality of Acoustic Priming 394

Generality of Audiogenic Seizures and Acoustic
    Priming 396

    Relations between sound-, drug- and electrically-
        induced seizures 396

    Dilute mice and experimental phenylketonuria 398

    Relationship of acoustic priming to general
        seizure susceptibility 398

    Relationship of acoustic priming to "kindling" . . . 400

Morphological Correlates of Audiogenic Seizures 402

    Cortex 402

    Thalamus 402

    Inferior colliculi 403

    Ear 403

Neurophysiological Correlates of Audiogenic Seizures . . 404

    Cochlear microphonic 404

    Auditory thresholds 405

Neurophysiological Correlates of Acoustic Priming . . . 405

Biochemical Correlates of Audiogenic Seizures and
    Acoustic Priming 406

    5-HT, NE and GABA in audiogenic seizures and
        acoustic priming 407

        Strain differences in levels of 5-HT and NE . . . 408

        Pharmacological manipulations of levels of
            5-HT and NE 409

            Reserpine and tetrabenazine 409

            α-methyl tyrosine and parachlorophenylalanine . 410

INTRODUCTION

Susceptibility audiogenic seizures, judging from the number
of research papers published on this topic, is a phenomenon of considerable interest. The research literature on audiogenic seizures
has been reviewed previously by Finger (1947), by Bevan (1955), and
by Henry (1966). Busnel (1963) has edited an international symposium on this topic, and Welch & Welch (1970) have edited a monograph
in which several chapters are devoted to the subject. Lehman (1970)
and Schlesinger & Uphouse (1972) have published reviews on the pharmacological correlates of audigenic seizures. From these reviews,
as suggested by Schlesinger & Griek (1970), several trends are dis-
cernable. These are: (1) that work on this topic has become interdisciplinary involving, in many instances, the collaborative efforts
of geneticists, pharmacologists, psychologists, etc.; (2) that work
on audiogenic seizures has become cosmopolitan; e.g., in 1947 Finger
found 100% of the work done on this phenomenon to be North American,
in 1955, only 83% of the research was by North Americans, and in
Henry's 1966 review, 51% of the research on audiogenic seizures was
by American authors; (3) that work on audiogenic seizures has come,
more and more, to rely on the mouse as the biological material of

choice and, consequently, a heavier and heavier emphasis has been placed on discovering genetic determinants of susceptibility to audiogenic seizures. More recently, a fourth trend has emerged, as more and more research is reported on "acoustic priming", i.e., rendering animals which are resistant to sound-induced seizures susceptible to these convulsions by prior exposure to loud noise.

Why is so much effort devoted to research on audiogenic seizures and acoustic priming? There are at least 3 answers to this question. First, mice which are susceptible to audiogenic seizures also tend to be more susceptible to other seizure-inducing agents than are animals which are resistant to audiogenic seizures. Since audiogenic seizures have now been described in animals of a variety of species including the mouse, Peromyscus, rat, guinea pig, rabbit and man, it is hoped that investigations of this phenomenon will lead to some insight regarding the heritable mechanisms which underlie individual differences in central nervous system excitability. Second, acoustic priming can be thought of as a simple example of the plasticity of the central nervous system and, as such, can be studied to reveal some of the mechanisms which underlie this most important aspect of nervous tissue. Third, strains of mice susceptible to audiogenic seizures appear to share some common features with humans suffering from phenylketonuria and these animals are studied as models of this disease. Much the same case has been made with respect to certain epilepsies. We will discuss these 3 important aspects of the work on audiogenic seizures and acoustic priming in more detail in the body of this review.

The purpose of this paper is to review the more recent research on audiogenic seizures and acoustic priming. Emphasis will be placed on papers which deal with the biological aspects of this topic. Special attention will be given to the theory suggested by Sharpless (see Schlesinger & Uphouse, 1972) and by Saunders et al. (1972) that the effects of acoustic priming might be mediated through damage induced supersensitivity of disuse.

THE PHENOMENA

Audiogenic seizures

Sound-induced convulsions are a series of psychomotor reactions to an intense acoustic stimulus. Many different techniques have been employed to test for susceptibility to audiogenic seizures. These techniques differ with respect to two classes of variables: (1) The intensity, frequency and duration of the seizure-inducing stimulus differ from experiment to experiment. (2) The scoring system employed to evaluate the seizure response also differs across reports. Experiments have been performed which have studied the intensity and frequency specificity of the stimulus necessary to elicit a convulsion (Frings & Frings, 1953; Fuller & Wimer, 1966); in general, intensities in excess of 100 db's have been used, and mixed frequencies, e.g., noise generated by electric bells, have been used to elicit audiogenic seizures. In terms of scoring the response, and in view of acoustic priming, one of the more important variables in evaluating the susceptibility of any given animal is whether or not the animal is tested more than once. Several workers have characterized animals as susceptible or resistant on the basis of their response on four or five test trials (Witt & Hall, 1949; Ginsburg, 1954), whereas other investigators use a single test as an index of susceptibility (Fuller et al., 1950; Schlesinger et al., 1966).

In many laboratories, as a standard procedure, each animal is tested only once by being exposed to the sound of an electric bell for 60 to 90 seconds. The bells used in these experiments generate between 100 to 117 db's of noise at the level of the mouse. In response to this stimulus animals from seizure susceptible strains have audiogenic convulsions. The complete syndrome of audiogenic seizures typically consists of (1) a latency of variable duration during which the mouse may huddle, or wash and groom excessively; (2) a wild-running phase characterized by frenzied and stiff-legged running around the boundary of the container; (3) a myoclonic convulsion during which the animals fall on their sides while drawing up their hind legs towards their chin; (4) a myotonic seizure during which all four legs are extended caudally; and, (5) death due to respiratory failure. It should be noted that a large proportion of the mice can be revived by artificial resuscitation.

Extensive variations of this pattern have been described (Schlesinger & Griek, 1970). Nevertheless, the characteristic and distinct phases of this syndrome have made scoring of the response relatively easy.

Acoustic priming

Exposure to acoustic stimulation before testing for susceptibility to audiogenic seizures is known to affect susceptibility to sound induced convulsions (Fuller & Williams, 1951; Fuller & Smith, 1953; Henry, 1967). In the earlier literature these phenomena were termed "prestimulation effects;" more recently, they have been called "acoustic priming." Demonstrations of acoustic priming involve two procedures: a priming procedure and a subsequent retest. Typically, animals from a seizure resistant genotype are used as experimental subjects. These animals are exposed to an intense acoustic stimulus during a critical period of neural development, i.e., the animals are primed. Subsequently, the animals are retested, i.e., they are

again exposed to an intense acoustic stimulus. At this time, audiogenic seizures are observed in the primed animals which are indis-
tinguishable, in all respects, from those observed in mice from
normally seizure susceptible genotypes. In other words, priming
produces a phenocopy of a "seizure susceptible" animal in a mouse
from a normally seizure resistant genotype.

Several parameters of acoustic priming have been investigated.
These include studies on (1) the critical age at which priming is
most effective, (2) the optimal priming-retest interval, and (3)
the optimal duration for which the priminal stimulus is applied to
produce the maximal effect. With respect to these variables, the
following observations have been made: First, for most genotypes
investigated, a critical period has been found during which priming
is most effective. This critical period differs for mice of different genotypes, both in terms of the best age for effecting priming and the duration of the critical period. Second, optimal priming-retest intervals have been found to vary from genotype to genotype. For example, the optimal priming-retest interval for C57Bl/6J
mice is on the order of 192 hours; in HS mice, i.e., in a heterogeneous population of mice derived from crossing eight inbred strains,
the optimal priming-retest interval is approximately 96 hours. It
is of interest to note that significant residual effects of priming
can be demonstrated for periods up to 3 weeks after the application
of the priming stimulus. Third, priming for periods as short as 1
second have been demonstrated to produce significant priming effects.
Thirty to 60 seconds of priming appears to be the best duration for
effecting priming. Periods of priming which are longer, or repeated
applications of the priming stimulus, reduce the effectiveness of
priming. These parameters of acoustic priming have been reported
by Henry & Bowman (1970), Collins (1970) and Boggan et al. (1971).

A phenomenon which is, in a sense, the opposite of acoustic
priming has been described. In animals of certain genotypes, prestimulation significantly reduces susceptibility to audiogenic
seizures; such observations have typically been reported for mice
of seizure susceptible genotypes (Fuller & Williams, 1951; Fuller
& Smith, 1953).

GENETIC AND ONTOGENETIC ASPECTS OF AUDIOGENIC
SEIZURES AND ACOUSTIC PRIMING

The genetics of audiogenic seizures

The importance of genetic factors in determining susceptibility
to audiogenic seizures has been demonstrated in a number of laboratories and in animals of several species. In the main, three types
of experiments have been employed in attempts to determine the nature

of the genetic mechanisms underlying susceptibility to audiogenic
seizures; these three approaches have been selective breeding experiments, strain comparison studies and single gene experiments.

Selective breeding experiments: Maier & Glaser (1940) and
Maier (1942) have reported the results of selective breeding experiments in several lines of rats where the phenotype selected for was
susceptibility to audiogenic seizures. Although selection was carried out for only a few generations, some success in selecting for
this phenotype was observed. Griffiths (1942) was also successful
in selecting for this trait in rats. Frings & Frings (1953) carried out a far more extensive selection program for susceptibility
to audiogenic seizures in the mouse. These investigators were successful in selecting for seizure susceptibility and seizure resistance in these mice; the major response to selection was observed
within the first two generations of selective breeding. Nellhaus
(1963) has reported the results of a selective breeding experiment
in rabbits, in which he was successful in selecting for high and low
susceptible lines.

The results of all of these selective breeding experiments are
prima facie evidence for the involvement of genetic factors in determining the expression of this trait in animals of these species.

Strain comparison studies: Strain comparison studies of susceptibility to audiogenic seizures have also been carried out in
animals of a number of species. For example, Antonitis et al.
(1954) have studied sound-induced seizures in several breeds of
rabbits and found that susceptibility to these seizures was a function of the breed tested. Watson (1939) has studied audiogenic
seizures in several lines of Peromyscus maniculatus and also observed
that the lines differed with respect to seizure susceptibility. By
far the largest number of strain comparison studies have been carried out with inbred strains of mice which have been found to differ widely with respect to seizure susceptibility (Fuller & Sjursen,
1967; Schlesinger et al., 1966; Coleman & Schlesinger, 1965).

Phenotypic differences between inbred lines, in this case differences with respect to susceptibility to audiogenic seizures,
are also prima facie evidence for the involvement of genetic factors in determining the expression of the trait measured.

The animals most often used in research on audiogenic seizures
are inbred DBA/2J and C57Bl/6J mice: DBA/2J mice are susceptible
to audiogenic seizures whereas C57Bl/6J mice are resistant to these
seizures. DBA/2J mice are an example of a dilute strain, i.e., an
example of mice of dilute coat color homozygous for the autosomal
recessive allele d in linkage group II. It is an interesting fact
that mice of all dilute strains ever tested, i.e., DBA/2J, DBA/1J,

BDP/J, P/J, I/FnLn and DBA/Crgl mice, are susceptible to audiogenic
seizures. It is of additional interest to note that dilute lethal
mice (d^l/d^l) suffer from spontaneous seizures. Finally, the rabbits
susceptible to audiogenic seizures in Nellhaus' selective breeding
experiment were blue-eyed. In other words, dilute animals seem
to be peculiarly susceptible to sound-induced convulsions, although
this is not meant to imply that only dilute animals are seizure
prone. Indeed, some mice of non-dilute genotypes are susceptible
to sound-induced seizures (Fuller et al., 1967). The evidence is
also compelling that the dilute locus itself is unrelated to the
expression of this trait (Schlesinger et al., 1966), despite some
earlier reports to the contrarcy (Huff & Huff, 1962; Huff & Fuller,
1964). Nevertheless, it remains an interesting observation that
mice of dilute genotypes are so uniformly susceptible to audiogenic seizures, and this raises the interesting possibility that
some gene on linkage group II mediates some components of the convulsive response. Indeed, Ginsburg et al. (1967) have reported on
such a gene.

Single gene studies. The inbred strains studies referred to
above have been utilized in a number of breeding experiments aimed
at determining the number and chromosomal location of the genes
underlying susceptibility to audiogenic seizures. For example,
Dice (1935) and Watson (1939) concluded that seizure susceptibility
in Peromyscus maniculates is inherited as a single recessive gene
in some lines. Antonitis et al. (1954) proposed a similar genetic
mechanism as underlying susceptibility to audiogenic seizures in
the rabbit. Witt & Hall (1949), on the basis of breeding experiments with DBA and C57Bl/6J mice, came to a similar conclusion regarding the inheritance of seizure susceptibility in the mouse.

More recent, and perhaps more careful experiments with mice
have failed to confirm such a mechanism for audiogenic seizures.
Fuller & Thompson (1960) have suggested a polygenic mode of inheritance of susceptibility to audiogenic seizures and Ginsburg
& Miller (1963) have suggested a two-gene model. Schlesinger et
al. (1966) have suggested that the exact age of the mouse at the
time of testing and the phenotype used as an index of seizure susceptibility are important variables which must be controlled in
such studies; with such controls, most measures of seizure susceptibility did not fit a one-locus, two-allele hypothesis.

Nevertheless, several genes have been identified which contribute significantly to the expression of this trait. These are:
(1) The Asp locus, on linkage group VIII, identified by Collins &
Fuller (1968) and Collins (1971). It should be noted that the
mechanism of action of this locus with respect to seizure susceptibility is unknown. (2) Two loci identified by Ginsburg et al.
(1967); these loci are of considerable interest since one gene is
linked to the dilute locus on linkage group II and affects the

granular cell layer of the dentate gyrus of the hippocampus. The
second gene, not as yet mapped, appears to affect the metabolism
of glutamic acid in nerve cells.

The Ontogenetics of Audiogenic Seizures

Mice of genotypes susceptible to audiogenic seizures are not
uniformly susceptible through their development. In animals of
most genotypes peak susceptibility occurs during some "critical
period" of neural development. This developmental aspect of susceptibility to audiogenic seizures was first recognized by Vicari
(1951) in DBA/2J mice. Subsequently, other investigators indenti-
fied other critical periods of susceptibility in mice of other
genotypes: For example, Swinyard et al. (1963) have reported
on this phenomenon in O'Grady susceptible mice. Depending on genotype and the index of susceptibility employed, these differences
can be quite dramatic. Schlesinger et al.(1965) have reported
the results of such an experiment in which susceptibility to audiogenic seizures was assessed in DBA/2J, C57Bl/6J and F_1 hybrid mice,
14-, 21-, 28-, 35- and 42-days of age on the day of testing. Using
the index of lethal convulsions as a criterion of susceptibility,
87% of the DBA/2J mice were susceptible at 21-days of age, but only
14% were susceptible at 14- and 28-days of age. C57Bl/6J animals
showed no lethal convulsions at any age, and F_1 hybrid mice were
closer to the non-susceptible parent line, but showed a developmental pattern of susceptibility similar to that observed in DBA/
2J mice.

No evidence is available which explains these developmental
patterns. An experiment by Ralls (1967) bears on the developmental
aspect of susceptibility to audiogenic seizures in DBA/2J mice.
Using auditory evoked responses recorded from the inferior colliculi
as a measure of auditory threshold, this investigator found that
auditory sensitivity declines sharply in these mice as a function of
age. The most dramatic change in auditory sensitivity was observed
as frequencies optimal for eliciting audiogenic convulsions, i.e.,
between 10 and 15 kHz.

The Genetics of Acoustic Priming

Very few experiments have reported on genetic mechanisms in
acoustic priming. As a consequence, very little is known about
the nature of such mechanisms. However, there seems to be very
little doubt that genetic factors are important in acoustic priming, or at least in determining the extent to which priming is
effective. As we have already indicated, Henry (1967) first reported on acoustic priming in C57Bl/6J mice. Iturrian & Fink (1967)

next reported the phenomenon in CF # 1 mice. Fuller and Collins
have described acoustic priming in SJL/J mice. Boggan et al.,
(1971) have reported on acoustic priming in C57Bl/6J and HS mice.
The extent, or effectiveness, of acoustic priming depends on the
genotype of the organism being tested.

Two of the more systematic analyses of genetic mechanisms in
acoustic priming have been reported by Henry & Bowman (1969) and
by Henry and Bowman (1970). In the first experiment DBA/2J, C57Bl/
6J, BALB/cJ, DBA/2J x C57Bl/6J, BALB/cJ x C57Bl/6J and DBA/2J x
BALB/cJ mice were tested for the effectivenss of acoustic priming.
DBA/2J mice which are normally susceptible to audiogenic seizures
were not affected by priming. C57Bl/6J mice, normally seizure resistant, were made seizure susceptible by priming. BALB/cJ mice,
also normally seizure resistant, were made more seizure prone by
priming, although the effect produced in this inbred strain was
quantitatively smaller than that produced in C57Bl/6J mice. In
BALB/cJ mice, for example, priming enhanced the incidence of wild-
running fits and of clonic seizures, but myotonic and lethal seizure incidences remained unaffected by this treatment. Some effects of acoustic priming on subsequent seizure susceptibility
was noted in each of the three F_1 hybrid groups tested. The effect was largest in DBA/2J x C57Bl/6J mice, and smaller in the
other two groups. In the second experiment referred to above,
DBA/2J, C57Bl/6J and F_1 hybrid mice were used as experimental subjects. These mice were primed at various ages starting from birth
to 28-days of age; all mice were then retested for susceptibility to
audiogenic seizures at 28-days of age. Acoustic priming induced susceptibility to audiogenic seizures in C57Bl/6J and F_1 hybrid mice;
in DBA/2J mice, acoustic priming was observed to "further enhance"
seizure susceptibility.

These experiments indicate that the effectiveness of acoustic
priming varies as a function of the genotype of the animal being
tested. Therefore, it seems quite likely that genetic mechanisms,
in part, determine the degree of priming effectiveness.

In the experiment just discussed, the effects of acoustic
priming in F_1 hybrid mice were of two types, i.e., in some instances the effect resembled that observed in C57Bl/6J mice and sometimes
the effect resembled that observed in the other parent strains. Re-
semblance of the hybrid to one or the other of the parent strains
was a function of the age at which the F_1 hybrid was primed. Thus,
developmental factors appear to be of considerable importance in
producing acoustic priming.

The Ontogenetics of Acoustic Priming

Two factors are most important with respect to the developmental aspects underlying the effectiveness of acoustic priming. These are the following: (1) Critical periods exist during which acoustic priming is effective; these critical periods very for mice of different genotypes. (2) Acoustic priming, if applied during the critical period, shows residual effects days and sometimes weeks after the presentation of the priming stimulus. These two factors are important because of the following considerations: First, experiments appear possible which would reveal the developmental genetic aspects of priming effectiveness. Such experiments might answer certain important questions regarding the genetic control of neural development. Second, because animals respond to acoustic priming only during certain critical periods - and because these critical periods vary from strain to strain - certain control procedures are made relatively simple. For example, if acoustic priming during the critical period is observed to have a certain physiological or biochemical effect, then the same stimulus given at another time might be expected to produce a different effect if the observed change is causally related to priming effectiveness. Third, since the effects of acoustic priming persist for relatively long periods of time one can think of the changes produced by the stimulus as instances of the plasticity of the central nervous system. It is this aspect of acoustic priming, i.e., the implied plasticity of the nervous system, which is most intriguing. In other words, it is possible to think of this phenomenon as an interesting model system in which to study the plasticity of the nervous system.

A number of experiments have investigated the developmental parameters of acoustic priming. We will discuss two of these experiments, both of which have been mentioned in slightly different contexts before.

Henry & Bowman (1970) found a "sensitivity" period in C57Bl/6J mice; this period of sensitivity to acoustic priming extended from approximately 14 to 21-days of age, peak sensitivity occurring at approximately 16-days of age. In C57Bl/6J x DBA/2J F_1 hybrid mice a bimodal sensitivity period is observed; peak sensitivity was observed when the priming stimulus was applied between 14 and 16-days of age, and, again, between 22 and 24-days of age.

Boggan et al. (1971) primed HS mice in two day intervals between 12 and 34 days of age; all animals were retested 48 hours later. The effects of priming were significant in animals exposed to the auditory stimulus between 12 and 26 days of age; peak sensitivity was noted in animals primed between 16 and 20 days of age. The degree of sensitization was also found to depend on the test-

retest interval. In HS mice an increase in seizure susceptibility
was first noted 16 hours after priming; the sensitivity reached a
peak 48 hours after priming and remained relatively high for at
least 384 hours (16 days). In C57Bl/6J mice increased seizure
susceptibility was noted 1 hour after the presentation of the priming stimulus, reached a peak 192 hours afterwards and then declined.
Increased susceptiblity to audiogenic seizures after sensitization
was noted to be reflected first by an increase in the incidence of
wild-running fits, then clonus, then tonus and, finally, lethal
seizures. Generally, as the optimal age for priming effectiveness
is passed, the incidence of lethal seizures, tonic seizures and
clonic seizures declines first and finally those of wild-running
fits decline. Seizure susceptibility also varied as a function
of the duration of priming. As little as 1 second exposure to
the acoustic stimulus will cause priming in C57Bl/6J mice. The
optimal duration appears to be 30 seconds, 60 seconds being less
effective in terms of inducing sensitization. Fuller & Collins
(1968), working with SJL/J mice, noted that 5 seconds of priming
was effective in producing sensitization. Increased seizure susceptibility was noticed 30 to 36 hours after priming; this onset
of sensitivity could be delayed if the animals were repeatedly
stimulated at 6 to 12 hour intervals.

    Although there is abundant evidence that mice become especial-
ly susceptible to priming during a certain period of development,
a period which is quite reasonably referred to as "critical" for
priming, it is nevertheless true that priming can be induced at
other ages provided the stimulus is sufficiently intense. Chen
et al (1973) observed that BALB/c mice, which had previously been
reported to be insensitive to priming at 14 days, could be primed
by increasing the intensity of the stimulus to 128-130 db (re:
10002 dyne/cm2). Gates & Chen (1973) have reported that older mice
(BALB/c at 150 days of age) can also be primed by very high intensity stimuli. Thus, the critical period for priming, like many other
"critical periods" is a matter of quantitative rather than qualitative differences in susceptibility (Denenberg & Kline, 1964).

                    THE LATERALITY OF ACOUSTIC PRIMING

    A very interesting observation with respect to acoustic prim-
ing was first reported by Fuller & Collins (1968). These investigators studied the effects of acoustic priming in one ear only on
subsequent susceptibility to audiogenic seizures. The experiments
were conducted in SJL/J mice; all animals were exposed to the priming stimulus when 21-days of age and retested for susceptibility to
audiogenic seizures 2 days later. Blockage of one auditory canal
was achieved by insertion of a glycerine plug. These authors observed that animals primed in one ear only were susceptible to aud-

iogenic seizures if subsequently retested through the ear open at the time of priming. However, if the retest stimulus was administered through the ear plugged at the time of priming no increased susceptibility to audiogenic seizures was observed.

The results of this experiment suggest that some mechanism mediating this phenomenon has a unilateral representation. As Fuller & Collins point out, either the ear itself or parts of the auditory system which are innervated only ipsilaterally are strongly implicated as the sites of sensitization.

Henry & Bowman (1970) also studied binaural interactions of priming effectiveness. Seizure severity was related to the number of ears open at the time of priming; for example, animals primed through both ears had seizures more severe than animals primed through one ear. Latency of onset of the seizure elicited at retest was shorter in animals primed through both ears.

Collins (1970) has reported on unilateral inhibition of sound-induced convulsions in SJL/J mice. At 21 days of age mice were primed; subsequently, at 12 hour intervals, the animals were re-exposed to the priming stimulus with one or the other ear plugged. Forty-eight hours after priming, all animals were tested for susceptibility to audiogenic seizures, through one or the other of the two ears. Significantly fewer seizures were observed in animals retested through the ear which had been repeatedly stimulated. A small degree of inhibition of seizure susceptibility was observed in animals retested through both ears, but repeatedly stimulated through one ear only.

Finally, Collins & Ward (1970) have reported an interesting experiment in which asymmetries in seizure susceptibility were observed. Mice of seizure susceptible strains DBA/1J, DBA/2J and SJL/J mice acoustically primed through both ears were used. The results were that (1) seizures induced with one ear blocked were symmetrical, i.e., there was no association between the direction of the wild-running fit and the side of the ear blocked; (2) seizure risk, here taken as the incidence of myoclonic seizures, is not affected by plugging one ear; (3) for SJL/J mice mean latency to seizure increases with either ear plugged; (4) for DBA/2J mice mean latency to seizure also increases with either ear plugged, but curiously, genetically susceptible DBA mice were found to be differentially sensitive to stimulation through the right and left ear. Mean latency to seizure was 6.2 seconds shorter in mice stimulated through the left ear; this difference is highly significant.

These data are of considerable importance since they immediately suggest appropriate control procedures. Since the effects of acoustic priming have a laterality component, left versus right ear,

or left versus right parts of the brain, can serve as experimental
and control tissues. The availability of such appropriate controls
within the same animal could be of immense value in discovering
causal relationships which determine sensitivity to seizures following acoustic priming.

GENERALITY OF AUDIOGENIC SEIZURES AND ACOUSTIC PRIMING

The question has been asked as to whether audiogenic seizures
and acoustic priming are merely biological curiosities or whether
these pheonomena are of more general interest. In this section, we
will address ourselves to 4 questions: (1) Are animals genetically
susceptible to audiogenic seizures also more susceptible to seizures
induced by other means, especially drug- and electrically-induced
seizures? (2) Are dilute mice, which are seizure susceptible, a
good experimental model of experimental phenylketonuria, and can
they be used to study the "seizure aspects" of human phenylketonuria (PKU)? (3) Are acoustically primed animals which are made
more susceptible to audiogenic seizures also more susceptible to
seizures induced either chemically or electrically? (4) Is the
phenomenon of acoustically induced sensitivity to seizures analogous
to sensitivities induced in nervous tissue by other means? Specifically, is there a relationship between acoustic priming and
"kindling" as that phenomenon has been described by Goddard et al.
(1969)?

Relations between sound-, drug- and electrically-induced seizures

We will next review some evidence which suggests a relation
between drug-, electrically- and sound-induced seizures. Some of
this evidence has been reviewed by Fuller & Wimer (1966) who have
concluded that in general some relationship exists between chemical-
ly- and electrically-induced seizures on the one hand, and susceptibility to audiogenic seizures on the other hand. Busnel & Lehman (1961), for example, have reported that mice susceptible to
audiogenic seizures have lower pentylenetetrazol seizure thresholds
than mice resistant to audiogenic seizures. Swinyard et al. (1963)
on the other hand, failed to observe a relationship between sound-
and pentylenetetrazol-induced seizures. Schlesinger et al. (1968)
have also studied susceptibility to sound- and pentylenetetrazol-
induced seizures in DBA/2J, C57B1/6J and F_1 hybrid mice. With respect to pentylenetetrazol-induced seizures DBA/2J mice, which are
susceptible to audiogenic seizures, were found to have lower seizure thresholds than C57B1/6J mice. F_1 hybrid mice were found to
be intermediate in susceptibility to pentylenetetrazol seizures as,
indeed, they are with respect to audiogenic seizures. These dif-

ferences in pentylenetetrazol seizure thresholds were quantitatively quite small, but statistically significant. The discrepancies in the results of these experiments could be due to a number
of variables, although it seems most likely that they are due to
the fact that mice of different genotypes were used in the various
experiments.

Busnel & Lehman (1961) have also reported that caffeine, produced more seizures in mice susceptible to audiogenic seizures than
in mice of resistant genotypes. These same investigators have reported that the ED_{50} for strychnine-induced seizures in mice of a
genotype susceptible to audiogenic seizures was 1.35 mg/kg, whereas this same threshold was 1.75 mg/kg for mice from a genotype resistant to audiogenic seizures. Similar differences have been reported for nicotine-induced seizures (Frings & Kivert, 1953). Results from our laboratory (Schlesinger & Uphouse, 1972) indicate
that DBA/2J mice are more susceptible to physostigmine-induced seizures than are C57Bl/6J animals; DBA/2J mice were also found to be
more susceptible to thiosemicarbazide-induced seizures than were
C57Bl/6J animals. Davis & Webb (1964), however, have failed to observe a correlation between hexafluorodiethyl ether and sound-induced seizures.

A number of investigators have reported that electroconvulsive seisure thresholds are lower in mice susceptible to audiogenic
seizures than in mice of resistant genotypes (Goodsell, 1955; Hamburgh & Vicari, 1960; Swinyard et al., 1963). Schlesinger et al.
(1968) have reported that DBA/2J mice have significantly lower elec-
troconsulsive seizure thresholds than either C57Bl/6J or F_1 hybrid
mice.

These data can be interpreted as evidence to suggest that mice
of strains susceptible to audiogenic seizures, e.g., DBA/2J mice,
are more susceptible to seizures induced by other means than are
mice of strains resistant to audiogenic seizures, e.g., C57Bl/6J
mice. However, the kind of generality implicit in the above statement is very difficult to establish unequivocally, since not all convulsants can be tested. Also, even if this kind of generality could
be established for a given strain susceptible to audiogenic seizures
it would remain an empirical questions as to whether or not other
genotypes susceptible to audiogenic seizures are also more susceptible to seizures induced by other means than another strain resistant
to audiogenic seizures. Nevertheless, it seems a reasonable first
assumption that DBA/2J mice are an excellent choice of biological
material for studying genetic and biochemical variables which determine seizure susceptibility.

Dilute Mice and Experimental Phenylketonuria

Several behavioral symptoms are associated with PKU, an inborn error or metabolism caused by a deficiency in the liver enzyme phenylalanine hydroxylase. These symptoms include mental retardation, the most interesting and certainly the best known symptom of this disease. Other symptoms commonly found in PKU are an accentuation of superficial and deep reflexes (Harris, 1962), irritability and a high incidence of epileptic seizures (Partington, 1961). It is this last symptom of PKU, namely the high incidence of epileptic seizures, which is of particular interest here. In this context, it is of considerable importance to note that the un ffected heterozygote carrier of the disease has a lower pentylenetetrazol seizure threshold than do normal individuals (Nakai et al., 1966).

There are several intriguing similarities between dilute seizure susceptible mice and human phenylketonurics; these will be discussed in a later section of this paper. Here we will only review some data which shows that phenylketogenic treatments render mice susceptible to audiogenic seizures. Karrer & Cahilly (1963) have pointed out that attempts to produce PKU experimentally have been of 3 types: (1) Administration of excess phenylalanine in diets or by other means; (2) pharmacological manipulations of phenylalanine hydroxylase activity as with parachlorophenylalanine (pChPhe); and (3) use of genetic stocks deficient in phenylalanine hydroxylase activity, such as dilute strains of mice. Schlesinger et al. (1969) have reported the results of experiments in which all of these techniques were employed and the effects of these treatments noted with respect to susceptibility to audiogenic seizures. The effects of injections of pChPhe and phenylalanine and the injection of diets varying in phenylalanine and tyrosine content were studied in mice of several genotypes. All of these treatments were observed to enhance susceptibility to audiogenic seizures. When these phenylketogenic treatments were combined with injections of α-methyl tyrosine, further increases in the incidence of audiogenic seizures was observed.

These data suggest that a neglected symptom of phenylketonuria, i.e., high incidence of epileptic seizures, can be studied experimentally in dilute seizure susceptible strains of mice.

Relationship of Acoustic Priming to General Seizure Susceptibility

An important question with respect to acoustic priming is whether or not animals rendered more susceptible to audiogenic seizures by acoustic priming are also more susceptible to seizures induced by other means. Two experiments, Henry & Bowman (1969) and Iturrian & Fink (1969), have been reported in the literature

which bear on this point. Since on the basis of these two experiments one comes to precisely the opposite conclusions the studies
will be reported in some detail. Henry & Bowman (1969) worked with
mice of six different genotypes; at 16-days of age all mice were
anesthetized and acoustically primed in this condition. When 21-
days of age all animals were retested, some for susceptibility to
audiogenic seizures, other for electroconvulsive seizures and a
third group for pentylenetetrazol seizures. Unprimed mice were
used as control subjects. Electroconvulsive seizure tests were
conducted through corneal electrodes, 7.65 ma current was applied
for 300 msec. Pentylenetetrazol seizure tests were conducted by
injecting 100 mg/kg of the drug intraperitoneally and observing
the animals for 5 minutes. No increased incidence of chemo-con-
sulsive or electroconvulsive seizures were noted in the primed,
as compared to the control, animals

Iturrian & Fink (1969) have reported the results of a similar
experiment in which CAW-CF-1(SW) mice were used as experimental
subjects. Primed and control animals were used, and the effects
of priming on electroconvulsive and pentylenetetrazol seizures
was studied. Maximal electroshock seizures were determined by
the intensity of the current necessary to evoke hind-leg tonic extension in 50% of the animals tested. Low frequency or minimal
electroshock seizures were measured by the intensity of the current necessary to evoke "some response" followed by at least 3
seconds of persistent clonic activity in 50% of the mice. Pentylenetetrazol seizure thresholds were determined by a timed and continuous intravenous infusion method. Infusions were contined until two
time points were reached; these were (1) the occurance of 3 seconds
of persistent clonus and (2) tonic extension. Seizure thresholds
were expressed as averaged infusion times. The results were that
priming did affect low frequency electroconvulsive seizures and
chemoconvulsive thresholds, but maximal seizure thresholds were unaffected by acoustic priming.

The results of these two experiments, of course, lead to opposite and contradictory conclusions. On the basis of the Henry
& Bowman experiment one would conclude that acoustic priming specifically enhances sensitivity to audiogenic seizures; on the other
hand, on the basis of the Iturrian & Fink experiment one would conclude that acoustic priming enhances susceptibility to seizures in
a more general sense. This difference in results must be due to
the difference in the procedures used. Henry & Bowman did not obtain seizure thresholds; their data are incidences of seizures in
primed versus non-primed mice. For both the electroconvulsive seizure tests and the pentylenetetrazol seizure tests stimulus parameters far in excess of the seizure thresholds for mice were used.
Iturrian & Fink did obtain seizure thresholds for individual animals

and in this sense their data give a clearer picture of the effects
of acoustic priming on seizure susceptibility in general. However,
the effects of acoustic priming on drug- and electrically-induced
seizures need to be further investigated. The results of these experiments should be important because if acoustic priming is specific
to auditory sensitivities then one would look for causal mechanisms
in the auditory system; on the other hand, if acoustic priming enhances seizure susceptibility in general then the effects may not be
limited to the auditory system.

Relationship of Acoustic Priming to "Kindling"

Delgado & Sevillano (1961), working in cats, have reported
the results of an experiment which showed that in certain structures of the central nervous system, namely the hippocampus, afterdischarges to electrical stimulation become more widespread after
the stimulus is repeatedly presented. In a more recent paper,
Goddard and associates (1969) have reported that repeated low-intensity stimulation of subcortical areas can trigger behavioral
convulsions if these sites are stimulated for long periods of time.
Goddard (1969) has also reported the results of an experiment in
which chemical stimulation was used; daily injections of carbachol,
at very low doses, were observed to increase the probability of
seizure development after repeated application of the compound.
These observations suggest that contunied low intensity stimulation,
either electrical or chemical, or certain areas of the brain can
cause functional alterations in these tissues which lower their
thresholds to seizure.

Goddard et al. has recently described a series of experiments
in which brief bursts of electrical stimulation were presented one/
day to certain areas of the brain. Initially, these stimuli did
not affect behavior nor were electrographic afterdischarges observed.
After repeated presentations of this stimulation, once per day, the
stimulus which was previously ineffectual was observed to elicit
localized afterdischarges, stereotyped behaviors and, eventually,
bilateral clonic convulsions. These changes in the response to the
stimulus after an appropriate "incubation" period were termed "kindling." Further experiments were performed which revealed the following characteristics of kindling: (1) Many areas of the brain
did not respond to repeated stimulation in the manner just described.
Positive, i.e., kindling-type responses were observed in a so-called
olfactory-limbic system set of structures. This area included structures from the olfactory bulb to the entorhinal cortex; the septum,
hippocampus and particularly the amygdala were positive. Certain
extra-pyramidal motor system structrures such as the globus pallidus
were also positive. (2) Certain loci were uniform in their response;
for example, the amygdaloid nuclei were all positive. Other loci,

for example the caudate and the putamen, were variable in their response, i.e., certain electrode placements gave positive results and
other placements gave negative results. (3) Transfer of kindling
effects were observed between different structures and between right
and left sides of the brain. For example, if kindling was produced
in the septum fewer trials were required to produce kindling in the
amygdala. (4) The stimulation parameters which lead to kindling
were examined in detail. The findings were that stimulation frequencies between 25 and 150 Hz were equally effective in eliciting
kindling. A frequency of 60 Hz was found to be most effective as
the triggering frequency regardless of the kindling frequency. The
number of stimulations (trials) required to elicit the first behavioral convulsion was observed to vary as a function of the locus
being stimulated and as a function of the time interval between
trials. A 24-hour time interval between trials was found to be
optimal; longer and even shorter intervals were less effective in
eliciting kindling. (5) The effects of kindling, i.e., the functional changes in the nervous system, were found to persist for
relatively long periods of time. A 12-week rest after kindling did
not eliminate the response. (6) It was claimed that the phenomenon
of kindling was not due to tissue damage. Electrolytic lesions de-
liverately produced at the tips of the stimulating electrodes did
not affect the results in the direction of producing more seizures;
if anything, such lesions had the opposite effect. (7) Significant
strain and individual differences in the effectiveness of producing
kindling were observed. For example, experiments were performed on
three breeds of rats: Holtzman albino rats, Wistar albino rats
and Royal Victoria hooded rats were used. In Holtzman rats the convulsions observed after kindling were mush more pronounced than
those observed in the other two lines. Other differences between
these lines were that in Holtzman rats additional convulsions were
observed following the electrically triggered seizures; these convulsions were observed in 50% of the Holtzman rats studied and these
seizures followed by 2 to 3 minutes the electrical stimulation. The
number of trials to produce kindling was also observed to vary as a
function of genotype; it was significantly lower in Holtzman rats
than in animals of the other two lines.

All of these experiments suggest that the exercise of neural
tissue results in functional changes in that tissue which renders
it more susceptible to epilepti-form-like seizure discharge. The
experiments also suggest that the nature of the exercise is not an
important variable; electrical, chemical or sensory stimulation may
all lead to similar results. Whatever the nature of these changes,
they do not appear to be transitory; in the case of kindling and of
acoustic priming the changes persist for periods of weeks. Finally,
both kindling and priming effectiveness seems to vary in animals of
different genotypes. It is, of course, hazardous to speculate that
both phenomena are mediated by similar processes; however, the simi-

larities between these two phenomena are sufficiently impressive to
make it a tempting speculation that a common mechanism exists which
mediates both kindling and acoustic priming.

MORPHOLOGICAL CORRELATES OF AUDIOGENIC SEIZURES

A good deal of research has been reported on the anatomical
loci involved in susceptibility to audiogenic seizures. Most of
this research has been performed through the use of the classical
lesion techniques. Interestingly, no anatomical research has ever
been reported on the anatomical structures involved in acoustic
priming. This is probably due to the fact that the pehnomenon was
only recently described and because it is most readily elicited in
mice, which because of their small size are not the favorite biological material for neuroanatomical work.

Cortex

A number of investigators have explored the function of the
neocortex in audiogenic seizures. Beach & Weaver (1943), working
in rats, have tested the effects of decortication on susceptibility
to sound-induced seizures. These investigators report that virtual
decortication enhances susceptibility to audiogenic seizures, both
in terms of overt seizure incidence and severity. However, the
lesions produced in this early study also invaded subcortical areas.
Winer & Morgan (1945) have studied the effects of auditory, motor and
frontal cortical lesions on susceptibility to audiogenic seizures.
In this study a reduction in seizure frequency was noted in all operated groups, particularly in the group with damage to the auditory
cortex. Kesner et al. (1965) have reported that KCl-induced spreading depression does not eliminate susceptibility to audiogenic seizures. Although there are some discrepanceis in these studies, it
appears evident that the cortex is not the principal locus at which
audiogenic seizures are precipitated; although these lesions do affect seizure incidence, they do not eliminate the response.

Ward & Sinnett (1971) have repoted that biolateral spreading
cortical depression in mice susceptible to audiogenic seizures does
not lower seizure incidence, but does increase the latency to seizure. Cortical depression does not appear to alter priming effectiveness. If only one side of the cortex is depressed asymetrical
convulsions are observed, mice falling to the side on which the depression produces ataxia.

Thalamus

Koenig (1957) has studied the effects of lesions of the medial geniculate bodies on susceptibility to audiogenic seizures in rats. Bilateral lesions of these thalamic nuclei did not reduce seizure incidence, although the severity of the seizures was somewhat reduced.

Inferior Colliculi

Kesner (1966), working in rats, has reported that lesions of the inferior colliculi completely abolished susceptibility to audiogenic seizures. Kesner, in this same experiment, reports on the effects of other subcortical lesions: (1) Animals with lesions of the midbrain reticular formation failed to exhibit clonic-tonic seizures, but still had wild-running fits in response to the sound. (2) Lesions of the caudate nuclei substantially increased the frequency and severity of audiogenic seizures. (3) Lesions of the intralaminar nuclei, hippocampus, amygdala and septum had only minor effects on seizure susceptibility; septal lesions tended to reduce the incidence of audiogenic seizures. Wada et al. (1970) have reported the results of an interesting experiment in which inferior collicular lesions were made and the effects of these lesions on susceptibility to audiogenic seizures was studied. Both genetically sensitive and genetically insensitive animals were used; in genetically insensitive animals (both rats and cats) a transient sensitivity to sound-induced convulsions was produced by administration of thiosemicarbazide, methionine sulfoximine and pentylenetetrazol. Both genetically determined and drug-induced susceptibility to audiogenic seizures were eliminated in animals with bilateral lesions of the inferior colliculi.

Ear

Geller et al. (1966) have reported that the administration of 6-aminonicotinamide, a powerful inhibitor of nicotinamide, completely abolishes susceptibility to audiogenic seizures. Ten to twenty mg/kg doses of 6-aminonicotinamide completely eliminated susceptibility to sound-induced seizures within 4 days after drug administration. Some pathologic l effects of the drug were noted in nuclei of the medulla, pons and midbrain; these lesions consisted of small foci, 0.2 to 0.5 mm in diameter, of nerve cell loss. In a subsequent paper, Kornfeld et al. (1970) noted very severe damage in the inner ear of 6-aminonicotinamide treated animals. Twenty-four hours after the administration of a single 20 mg/kg dose of the inhibitor, the first signs of pathological degeneration were noted in the inner ear; acute degeneration was maximal 3 to 4 days following treatment. The lower basal and upper second turn of the origin of Corti were most severely damaged. These authors noted that the damage was severe enough to impair responses to sound, and judged that these lesions were incompatible with the elaboration of sound-induced seizures.

NEUROPHYSIOLOGICAL CORRELATES OF AUDIOGENIC SEIZURES

Cochlear Microphonic

Niaussat & Legouix (1967) have reported the results of experiments in which both cochlear microphonics and auditory ction potentials were recorded in seizure susceptible and seizure resistant mice following click stimulation. The cochlear microphonic was recorded through electrodes in contact with the round window and the mice were stimulated with tones ranging in frequency between 2 and 12 kHz. In normal mice typical cochlear microphonis potentials were recorded for the frequenices mentioned above; amplitudes of these potentials were approximately 0.6 mV. for a 10 kHz tone. In addition, the two classical negative deflections corresponding to the action potential of the VIIIth nerve were recorded from this electrode; the amplitude of this potential reached 0.5 mV. Surprisingly, no cochlear microphonic potential could be recorded from mice of seizure susceptibile genotypes. With very high intensity sounds, 120 to 130 db's, and with electrodes in the perilymph of the scali tympani, microphonics of very low amplitudes (on the order of 50 uV) could be recorded from these animals. On the other hand, the action potential in seizure susceptible mice appeared normal in every respect.

In a later paper Niaussat (1968) has reported further studies on the relation between audiogenic seizure susceptibility and neurophysiological recordings from the inner ear of rodents. In mice, the same results as described above were obtained, i.e., seizure susceptibile mice had no, or very low amplitude, cochlear microphonics; however, normal auditory evoked responses to sound stimulation were obtained. Seizure resistant mice, on the other hand, had both normal cochlear microphonics and auditory evoked potentials. In rats different results were obtained; seizure susceptible rats had slightly lower amplitude cochlear microphonics than seizure resistant animals, but in both strains the amplitude of the evoked potential was proportional to the size of the cochlear microphonic. These results with rats must, however, be taken with a good deal of caution since most of the animals used in this experiment suffered from otitis. Darrouzet et al. (1968) have reported the results of a histological study of the organ of Corti from seizure resistant and seizure susceptible strains of mice. Two techniques were used, one a staining technique and the other a phase-contrast procedure, and degeneration of external hair cells was examined. In seizure resistant mice up to 70% degeneration of external hair cells in the apex of the membrane was noted with one method, and 25% degeneration was noted with the other method. In seizure susceptible mice both methods indicate

up to 50% degeneration of external hair cells in the basal region of
the membrane.

Auditory Thresholds

Ralls (1967), in an experiment which has been referred to previously, has reported on differences in auditory evoked responses in
several species of Peromyscus and several strains of Mus musculus.
The animals were stimulated with sounds varying in intensity and frequency, and auditory evoked potentials were recorded from the inferior colliculi. Auditory thresholds, defined as the lowest intensity of sound, for different frequencies, which produced measur
able evoked responsed, were calculated. Studies on DBA/2J and BALB/cJ
mice were reported;   mice of the former strain are susceptible to
audiogenic seizures whereas mice of the latter strain are resistant
to these seizures. Thresholds for 16 to 19-day old DBA/2J mice was
approximately 15 db's for frequencies at 12.5 kHz; this age corre
sponds approximately to the age of maximal seizure risk in these
animals. Unfortunately, BALB/cJ mice were not tested at this age;
nevertheless, this threshold for DBA/2J mice is considerably lower
than the lowest threshold reported for BALB/cJ animals; the lowest
threshold in BALB/cJ mice was approximately 30 db's, obtained in 48-
day old animals for frequencies at 15 kHx. Whether these differences
in auditory thresholds are causally related to seizure susceptibility
is, of course, unknown. In DBA/2J mice auditory sensitivity, especially to high frequency sounds, decreases rapidly with age; this
might account for the decre ise in susceptibility to audiogenic seizures with age noted in these animals. Such decreased sensitivity
to high frequency sounds were also observed in BALB/cJ mice, but the
effect was not nearly as great in mice of this genotype.

NEUROPHYSIOLOGICAL CORRELATES OF ACOUSTIC PRIMING

Recently, Saunders et al. (1972) have studied the cochlear microphonic response to tone and click stimulation in control and acoustically primed animals. BALB/c mice were used as subjects and animals were primed at 21-days of age and retested at 28-days of age.
Cochlear microphonic thresholds as a fuction of frequency were recorded in primed and in control animals. At every frequency tested,
except at 1 and 30 kHz, the primed animals had significantly higher
thresholds than the control mice; at 17 kHz, for example, the thresholds in primed amimals were 25 db's higher than in control mice.

Intensity functions recorded at 5, 17 and 25 kHz also indicate
a severe loss in sensitivity in primed animals. For example, at 17
kHz a tone of 60 db's elicited a 96 μV cochlear microphonic in control animals, whereas a similar stimulus presented to primed mice

produced only a 1.1 μV response.

Auditory responses to click stimulation were also significantly different in primed and control mice. In control animals a click of 75 db's produced a clear cochlear microphonic response with N_1-N_2 components of relatively large amplitude. Clicks of 110 db's were necessary to produce an auditory response in primed animals and even then the cochlear microphonic and the N_1-N_2 components of the response were of reduced amplitude.

These authors conclude that priming results in damage to the basilar membrane, specifically hair cell injury. They suggest that the effect of such damage might result in disuse of nervous tissue and a consequent supersensitivity of higher neural centers.

Saunders & associates (1972) have also investigated evoked potentials at the level of the cochlear nucleus in primed mice. The amplitude of the potentials evoked by low-intensity clicks (below 95 db) in the primed animals was less than that of the potentials evoked in the unprimed animals; the primed animals had a higher threshold as judged by the minimally detectable averaged evoked response. At higher intensities of stimulation, on the other hand, the amplitude of the evoked potentials was greater in the primed animals. Evoked potentials from the inferior colliculus (Saunders et al., 1972; Henry & Saleh, 1973; Willott & Henry, 1974) yield a similar picture, being smaller at low intensities and larger at high intensities in the primed animals. The similarity between these changes and the clinical phenomenon of "recruitment deafness" in humans, which is sometimes associated with chronic exposure to intense sound, has been emphasized by Henry & Saleh (1973). Recruitment deafness is often ascribed to damage to the outer hair cells, and Willott & Henry (1974) have described inflections in the curves relating evoked potential amplitude to stimulus intensity which may separate contributions of the outer and inner hair cells ("L" and "H" curves). The part of the curve presumably dependent on outer hair cell function was most diminished by priming. One might expect that the cochlear microphonic would also be affected most by damage to the outer hair cells.

BIOCHEMICAL CORRELATES OF AUDIOGENIC SEIZURES AND ACOUSTIC PRIMING

An enormous literature has been accumulated on possible biochemical and pharmacological differences between seizure susceptible and seizure resistant mice. Much of this literature can be summarized in terms of two hypotheses which have been advanced to account for audiogenic seizures: One of these hypotheses suggests that serotonin (5-HT), norepinephrine (NE) and gamma-aminobutyric acid (GABA) are importantly involved in seizure susceptibility. We

will discuss these experiments under the general rubric of this
hypothesis. The other hypothesis suggests that differences in
carbohydrate metabolism might account for susceptibility to audiogenic seizures in mice of various genotypes. Again, we will discuss these experiments from the point of view of this hypothesis.
Finally, some biological and biochemical experiments have been reported which do not fit either of these models; we will discuss
these results under the title of misscellaneous experiments.

5-HT, NE and GABA in Audiogenic Seizures and
Acoustic Priming

Many experiments aimed at understanding the mechanisms underlying susceptibility to audiogenic seizures are based on an observation
originally reported by Coleman (1960). Coleman found that dilute
mice were deficient in pheylalanine hydorxylase activity in liver.
The extent of this deficiency depended on the particular line of
dilute mice tested, varying between a 90% deficiency in dilute lethal mice to a 50% deficiency in DBA/2J animals. Coleman also reported that dilute mice, if challenged by excess pheylalanine, metabolize
this amino acid more slowly than do non-dilute animals similarly
challenged. Finally, dilute mice were also observed to excrete certain abnormal phenylalanine metabolites such as phenylacetic and
phenylactic acid. Rauch & Yost (1963) have reported the results of
similar experiments in which they found that the activity of the
enzyme phenylalanine hydroxylase increase in dilute and non-dilute
mice up to age 17. Thereafter, the activity of this enzyme continues
to increase in animals of non dilute genotypes but not in dilute
animals. The defect in phenylalaine hydroxylase activity does not
appear to be due to a failure to make the enzyme. If crude liver
homogenates are centrifuged at 17,000 x g enzyme activity in the
supernatant fraction becomes normal. It has therefore been suggested that in dilute mice an endogenous inhibitor of phenylalanine hydroxylase is associated with the mitochondrial fraction; this inhibitor is soluble in deoxycholate.

Some controversy exists with respect to these findings: Zannoni
et al. (1963), working with dilute lethal mice, failed to find a
deficiency in pheylalanine hydroxylase activity in these animals.
On the other hand, dilute lethal mice, if challenged with either
phenylalanine or phenylpyruvic acid, show a degree of inhibition of
phenylalanine hydroxylase inhibition far in excess of that exhibited
by non-dilute animals. Mauer & Sideman (1961), also working with
dilute lethal mice, have failed to find a deficiency in phenylalanine hydroxylase activity in these animals. Results in our laboratory (Schlesinger & Uphouse, 1971), in DBA/2J and C57Bl/6J mice, in-
diate that in crude liver homogenates animals of the former geno-

type have approximately 30% less phenylalanine hydroxylase activity;
levels of circulating phenylalanine, however, are the same in animals of these genotypes.

In terms of this model, Coleman made the suggestion that the
abnormal phenylalanine products produced by dilute mice, namely
phenylacetic acid, inhibit decarboxylating reactions. This has
indeed been described in a number of tissues (Hanson, 1958; Sandler
& Close, 1959). Results reported by Schlesinger & Uphouse (1972)
indicate that phenylacetic acid acts as a competitive inhibitor
for 5-hydroxytryptophan decarboxylase activity in brain tissue.
When thinking of decarboxylating reactions in brain tissue one naturally thinks of 5-HT, NE and GABA, and Coleman postulated that
animals of seizure susceptible genotypes are deficient in these
compounds and that these deficiencies, in turn, account for the
high proportion of audiogenic seizures typically observed in mice
of dilute genotypes. [One must make several assumptions, and there
are several complications, in this model: It is necessary to assume
that phenylacetic acid, in the amounts present in dilute mice, inhibits decarboxylation. Further, a serious complication arises
from the fact that hydroxylation rather than dec rboxylation is the
rate-limiting reaction in the synthesis of, for example, NE (Spector
et al., 1965). In the human PKU, however, abnormal phenylalanine
metabolites have been shown to be excreted conjugated with pyridoxine
(Yen & Ritman, 1964). Since supplemental pyridoxine administration
protects dilute mice against audiogenic seizures (Schlesinger, 1968)
and since diets deficient in this vitamin increase seizure susceptibility in dilute mice (Coleman & Schlesinger, 1965), it seems possible that dilute seizure susceptible mice are functionally deficient
in pyridoxine. If this is the case, and this is entirely speculative
then decarboxylation might become the rate-limiting reaction in these
animals.]

What is the evidence that dilute seizure susceptible mice are
deficient in levels of 5-HT, NE and GABA in brain, and what is the
evidence to suggest that these deficiencies are causally related
to audiogenic seizures?

Strain Differences in Levels of
5-HT and NE

Schlesinger et al. (1965) have measured levels of 5-HT and NE
in brain tissue of 14-, 21-, 28-, 35- and 42-day old DBA/2J, C57Bl/
6J and F_1 hybrid mice. Significant differences in levels of these
amines were observed in animals of these genotypes: DBA/2J mice
had 32% less 5-HT and 44% less NE in brain than C57Bl/6J animals.
These differences were only observed in 21-day old mice, which cor-
responds to the time of maximal seizure risk in DBA/2J mice. Schles-

inger et al. (1968) have also examined the subcellular distribution
of 5-HT in mice of these genotypes; DBA/2J mice had significantly
less 5-HT in both the particulate and supernatant fractions.

Scudder et al. (1966) have reported the results of experiments
in which levels of DOPA, dopamine, NE and 5-HT were measured in six
genera and three strains of mice. Threshold current intensities to
produce electroconvulsive seizures were also determined. Electroshock seizure latencies were negatively correlated with levels of
these biogenic amines; longer latencies occurred in those strains
which had higher amine levels. Karczmar et al. (1968) have also
reported an inverse correlation between brain levels of catecholamines and cholinesterase activity in brains of mice.

Nellhaus (1968) has found that rabbits of seizure prone lines
had lower levels of 5-HT in brain than rabbits from non-susceptible
genotypes.

McGeer et al. (1969) failed to find a correlation between levels of amines and susceptibility to audiogenic seizures in DBA/2J
and C57B1/6J mice. This experiment, however, was conducted in 6-
week old mice, when DBA/2J animals are no longer susceptible to
audiogenic seizures.

Most recently, Kellogg (1971) has reported an experiment in
which 5-HT metabolism was studied in C57B1/6J and DBA/2J mice. In
young and old mice, DBA/2J animals had significantly less 5-HT in
brain than C57B1/6J animals. Rates of synthesis of 5-HT were significantly greater in DBA/2J than in C57B1/6J animals, the rate
constant of disappearance of 5-HT and 5-hydroxyindoleacetic acid
were greater in DBA/2J than in C57B1/6J mice, and DBA/2J mice had
lower monoamino oxidase activity than C57B1/6J animals.

All of these studies suggest that differences in 5-HT and NE
mechanisms exist between seizure susceptible and seizure resistant
mice. It would be important to localize these differences anatomically and to study the turnover of NE in mice of these genotypes.

Pharmacological manipulations of levels of 5-HT and NE:

A number of experiments have been reported in which levels of
5-HT and NE were manipulated with drugs and the effects on audiogenic seizures were noted.

Reserpine and tetrabenazine: A number of studies have shown
that these two drugs, which lower levels of both 5-HT and NE, increase susceptibility to audiogenic seizures (Lehman & Busnel, 1963;
Foglia et al., 1963; Schlesinger et al., 1968; Schlesinger et al.,

1970; Bevan & Chinn, 1957). We have also reported experiments which
indicate that reserpine increases susceptibility to electroconvulsive and pentylenetetrazol induced seizures (Schlesinger et al.
1968).

α-Methyl tyrosine and parachlorophenylalanine: Several studies
have reported on the effects of α-MT and pChPhe, which lower levels
of NE and 5-HT respectively, on susceptibility to a variety of seizure inducing agents. These compounds increase susceptibility to
audiogenic seizures (Lehman, 1965; Lehman, 1968; Schlesinger et al.,
1968; Schlesinger et al., 1970). In our experience lowering levels
of 5-HT or NE singly causes a small increase in susceptibility to
audiogenic seizures; lowering levels of both 5-HT and NE, by injecting both compounds, causes a large increase in susceptibility
to audiogenic seizures. We have also observed that these drugs maximally increase seizure susceptibility in animals which are pyridoxine deficient (Schlesinger & Schreiber, 1969).

Monoamine oxidase inhibitors: A variety of monoamine oxidase
inhibitors have been studied for their effects on audiogenic seizures.
In our laboratory iproniazid also protects animals against electroconvulsive seizures (Schlesinger et al., 1968). Monoamine oxidase
inhibitors have also been shown to counteract the increased susceptibility to audiogenic seizures induced by reserpine (Lehman & Busnel,
1962).

Thymoleptics and inhibitors of catechol-0-methyl transferase:
These drugs increase NE release into receptor sites, either by inhibiting reuptake or by inhibiting COMT. These compounds do not
increase total levels of NE (Iversen, 1967). Examples of such drugs
are imipramine, amitryptyline, pyrogallol and propriophenase. All
of these drugs have been studied and all protect animals against
audiogenic seizures (Lehman, 1970).

Injections of substrates (5-HTP and Dopa): Injections of 5-
HTP, the metabolic precursor of 5-HT, increases levels of 5-HT in
brain and protects the mice against audiogenic seizures, as well as
protecting animals against electrically- and pentylenetetrazol-induced
seizures (Schlesinger et al., 1968; Schlesinger et al., 1970). Increased sensitivity to sound-induced seizures by reserpine is antagonized by dopa (Boggan & Seiden, 1971). This antagonism depended on
the conversion of dopa to dopamine, since blockage of the decarboxylase prevented this dopa effect. Decreased susceptibility to audiogenic seizures was observed when brain levels of dopamine were significantly elevated, suggesting a role of dopamine in protection a-
gainst audiogenic seizures.

Direct injections of 5-HT and NE: Direct intracranial injections of 5-HT and NE were found to protect mice against audiogenic
seizures; similar results were obtained with respect to pentylene-

tetrazol-induced seizures (Schlesinger et al., 1969).

GABA and Seizure Susceptibility

Ginsburg et al. (1967) have studied glutamic acid decarboxylase (GAD) activity in seizure prone and seizure resistant mutants. In one seizure prone mutant GAD activity was lower than in the seizure resistant strain. Levels of GABA, however, were not different in mice of any of these genotypes.

Lowering levels of GABA with hydrazines has been shown to increase susceptibility to audiogenic seizures (Lehman, 1963). On the other hand, drugs which increase levels of GABA, for example aminooxyacetic acid, protect mice against audiogenic, electroconvulsive and pentylenetetrazol induced seizures (Lehman, 1963; Schlesinger et al., 1970; Schlesinger et al., 1968; Kuriyama et al., 1966).

Direct intracranial application of GABA has also been reported to protect mice against sound-, electrically- and pentylenetetrazol-induced seizures (Ballantine, 1963; Schlesinger et al., 1969).

Pyridoxine and Audiogenic Seizures

Lyon et al. (1958) have reported on the effects of varying amounts of pyridoxine on measures of body weight, food intake and organ levels of pyridoxine. These experiments were carried out in I/FnLn and C57Bl/FnLn mice; the former strain is dilute, the latter strain is not. In I/FnLn mice, diets deficient in pyridoxine were observed to increase susceptibility to audiogenic seizures.

Coleman & Schlesinger (1965) have reported the results of a similar experiment; DBA/2J, BDP/J, P/J, C57Bl/6J and DBA/2J x C57Bl/6J F_1 hybrid mice were pl ced on diets varying in vitamin B_6 content. Mice of the former three genotypes are dilute, whereas mice of the latter two genotypes are not dilute. In mice of dilute strains, diets deficient in pyridoxine increased susceptibility to audiogenic seizures.

Schlesinger & Schreiber (1969) tested F_2 hybrid mice derived from DBA/2J and C57Bl/6J animals for susceptibility to sound- and electrically-induced seizures following treatment with pyridoxine deficient diets. In addition, these animals were maintained on terramycin in an attempt to make the pyridoxine deficiency more severe. Susceptibility to both sound- and electroconvulsive-seizures were increased in these animals. As we have previously indicated, treatment with α-MT and pChPhe leads to a further increase in seizure susceptibility in pyridoxine deficient animals. Levels of 5-HT and NE were unchanged by this dietary treatment. However, Tews & Lovell (1967), working in mice of the genotypes, have reported that such diets decrease levels of GABA, suggesting that the effects of pyridoxine deficient diets on audiogenic seizures are mediated through some GABA mechanism.

Finally, preliminary experiments in our laboratory have indicated that supplemental pyridoxine protects mice against audiogenic seizures (Schlesinger, 1968). These results are very reminiscent of similar data on human patients; Tower (1969) has summarized data on a "familial" pyridoxine dependent syndrome, one of the symptoms of which are convulsions, which can be controlled by supplemental vitamin B_6.

Circadian Rhythms and Audiogenic Seizures

A number of investigators have reported a circadian rhythm of susceptibility to audiogenic seizures; susceptibility to audiogenic seizures has been reported to be particularly high just after the onset of darkness (Halberg et al., 1955; Halberg et al., 1958; Halberg et al., 1955). Similar data have been reported for electro-convulsive seizure thresholds (Davis & Webb, 1963; Webb & Russell, 1966).

Since levels of the biogenic amines, i.e., levels of 5-HT, also show a circadian periodicity, peak concentrations occurring during the day and lower concentrations at night (Dixit & Buckley, 1967; Friedman & Walker, 1968; Quay, 1965); we have undertaken a series of experiments which attempt to correlate levels of 5-HT and NE and circadian susceptibility to audiogenic seizures.

Schreiber & Schlesinger (1971) have reported significant day-night differences in sound- and electrically-induced seizures in DBA/2J and F_1 hybrid mice; small circadian differences in seizure susceptibility were reported in C57B1/6J mice. Levels of 5-HT and NE were determined in three parts of the brain. No differences in levels of NE were observed in any part of the brain as a function of the time of day at which the samples were taken. Statistically significant differences in levels of 5-HT were observed in all parts of the brain as a function of the time of day during which the samples were obtained; levels of 5-HT were lower at night, a period during which seizure susceptibility was greatest. The results of this study suggest a correlation between circadian rhythms of seizure susceptibility and levels of 5-HT in the brain. In order to test this relation more directly, Schreiber & Schlesinger (1971) performed an experiment in which light cycles were manipulated directly and the effects of these treatments on levels of biogenic amines and on seizure susceptibility were studied. Animals were

maintained under four conditions of lighting: normal, reverse cycle,
all dark and all light conditions were used. The circadian rhythm of
seizure susceptibility could be completely reversed under reverse
light conditions. Most interestingly, conditions of all light and
all dark dramatically increased susceptibility to audiogenic seizures.
These conditions of lighting also significantly decrease levels of
both 5-HT and NE in all parts of the brain.

Since drug treatments which increase susceptibility to audiogenic seizures also lower thresholds for epileptic seizures in humans (Laufer et al., 1954; Pfeiffer et al., 1956) and since epileptic patients have been reported to fall into 1 of 3 categories with
respect to the onset of epileptic convulsions, i.e., nocturnal, diurnal and indifferent (Bercel, 1964; Furuchi, 1969), susceptibility
to audiogenic seizures might be a useful model system in the study
of epilepsy.

BIOCHEMICAL CORRELATES OF ACOUSTIC PRIMING

Several studies have been reported on the effects of various
drugs on susceptibility to audiogenic seizures induced by acoustic
priming.

Boggan et al. (1971) has reported the results of an experiment
in which drugs alter levels of 5-HT and/or NE were tested for their
effects on acoustic priming; specifically, the actions of reserpine,
catron, 5-HTP and Dopa were studied. These drugs were administered
at two times, either before priming or before the retest. None of
these compounds, administered before priming, changed the effectiveness of priming. On the other hand, these drugs did alter susceptibility to audiogenic seizures if given before the retest; compounds
which increased levels of the biogenic amines tended to protect a-
gainst seizures, whereas compounds which lowered levels of the amines
tended to enhance seizure risk. In these experiments the effects
of catron and reserpine, in protecting against or enhancing seizure
risk respectively, were quite small.

Sze (1970) has reported the results of an interesting series
of experiments in which the effects of acoustic priming were determined on levels of GABA in whole brain homogenates. Auditory stimulation was observed to cause an immediate decrease in levels of
GABA in brain, a decrease which reached its maximum 10 to 20 minutes
after stimulation and then returned to control values. Similar effects were not observed for levels of 5-HT and NE. Injections of
aminooxyacetic acid, a compound which increases levels of GABA in
brain, before the application of the priming stimulus completely
blocked the effectiveness of acoustic priming in eliciting subsequent seizure susceptibility. It is difficult to interpret the re-

sults of these experiments; however, they do tend to implicate some
GABA system in causing priming effectiveness.

SUMMARY

The data summarized in this report can be interpreted as indicating that 5-hydroxytryptamine, norepinephrine, gamma-aminobutyric
acid and possible dopamine are not without significance in determining susceptibility to sound-induced seizures. Similar evidence, although not nearly as extensive, exists with respect to seizure susceptibility induced through acoustic priming. In general, these
data are of two types: (1) Correlational data suggest such a relationship, inasmuch as seizure susceptibility has been correlated
with levels of the biogenic amines across genotype, age and experimental treatments. (2) Pharmacological and dietary manipulation
of levels of 5-HT, NE and GABA has been shown to alter seizure susceptibility in directions predicted from this model.

However, much more evidence is necessary to further support
the idea that amine and GABA metabolism are causally related to
audiogenic seizures. For example, we do not know the anatomical
locus of this relationship; are the differences in levels of amines
between seizure susceptible and seizure resistant mice found in
nearly all areas of the brain, or are they restricted to areas involved in auditory function, or are they found in regions of the
brain which are known to have low seizure thresholds such as the
hippocampus? Are the differences in levels of these amines in mice
of these various genotypes caused by the observed differences in
phenylalanine hydroxylase activity? This question is testable
since single gene revertents (mutants) on DBA/2J background exist;
these mutants are as susceptible to audiogenic seizures as are the
dilute mice, but phenylalanine hydroxylase activity and levels of
the biogenic amines have not yet been measured in these animals.
The neurophysiological effects of compounds which alter susceptibility to audiogenic seizures have yet to be explored. For example,
auditory evoked potentials need to be measured as a function of
drug treatments which are known to affect susceptibility to audiogenic seizures. Similar behavioral experiments, i.e., acoustic
startle reactions, should be performed as a function of these drug
treatments. Finally, a number of experiments have already indicated that steady state levels of the biogenic amines, although important, do not by themselves adequately account for susceptibility to audiogenic seizures as measured in dose-response experiments.
The dynamic state of the adrenergic, serotonergic and GABA systems
also appears to be an important variable in seizure susceptibility,
and enzyme measurements and turnover studies need to be performed.

Such experiments would contribute enormously to our understand-

ing of the relationship between audiogenic seizures and levels of
these compounds in the brain.

THE ATPase HYPOTHESIS

Ginsburg & Roberts (1951) originally reported that glycolytic
substrates protect mice of certain genotypes against audiogenic
seizures. This finding led to the formulation of a model which
postulated that variations in available ATP affects susceptibility to sound-induced convulsions. Subsequent research has added
some support to this model.

Abood & Gérard (1955) have reported on a phosphorylation defect in mice susceptible to audiogenic seizures. At 28 to 36 days
of age, i.e., when DBA/1 mice are susceptible to audiogenic seizures, Mg-activated ATPase activity was 20% lower in these mice as
compared to C57 animals. At 45-days of age these differences were
no longer observed. With pyruvate and glutamate as substrates,
DBA/1 had a 14 to 27% lower P/O ratio than C57 animals. DBA/1 mice
also had less ATP in brain tissue than did C57 animals. Results
in our laboratory, using DBA/2J and C57B1/6J mice, are contratic-
tory to those reported by Abood & Gerard in that our data indicate
that mice of the former genotype have significantly more ATP in
brain tissue than C57B1/6J animals; in crude and purified brain
mitochondrial preparations from DBA/2J and C57B1/6J mice, ADP to
ATP conversion was significantly greater in DBA/2J mice and these
differences could be attributed to differences in ATPase activity
(MacInnes et al., 1970).

Ginsburg (1963) has reported the results of extensive experiments
in which the effects of a variety of compounds related to the tri-
carboxylic acid cycle and/or to energy turnover were studied. Substances such as lactic acid, succinic acid, and glutamic acid reduced seizure susceptibility, whereas compounds such as glutamine,
pyruvic acid, and α-ketoglutaric acid increased seizure susceptibility. Schlesinger (1968) has reported that glutamic acid as well as
blutamine protects DBA/2J mice against audiogenic seizures.

Buday et al. (1961) have noted that intraventricular injections
of ATP cause severe convulsions in rats. MacInnes et al. have reported that intracranial injections of relatively small amounts of
ATP increase susceptibility to audiogenic seizures in both DBA/2J
and C57B1/2J mice.

Pasquini et al. (1968) have reported on the effects of audiogenic seizures on amino acid changes in brains of mice. Levels of
glutamine and glutamate decreased during the wild running fit of
the seizure and than continued to decrease during the clonic-tonic

phase of the response. Levels of aspartate and GABA remained unchanged during the wild running fit, but decreased during the seizure. Systemic injections of GABA increased brain levels of this
compound and protected mice against audiogenic seizures.

Ginsburg et al. (1967) have reported the results of genetic
experiments in which ATPase activity was studied in DBA/1J, DBA/
2J, C57B1/6J and C57B1/10J mice and in crosses derived from these
inbred mice. Significant differences in ATPase activity were observed in the granular cell layer of the fascia dentata of the
hippocampus. These differences in enzyme activity appeared to be
mediated by a single autosomal gene which was linked to the dilute
locus on the second linkage group. ATPase activity was also correlated with seizure susceptibility in the manner predicted by
Ginsburg & Miller (1963), i.e., the gene controlling ATPase activity behaved as one of the two genes underlying seizure susceptibility in this model.

All of these data suggest that variations in available ATP
affect nervous system functioning in general and seizure susceptibility in particular. The precise mechanisms of action of high-
energy phosphate metabolism on genetically determined differences
in seizure susceptibility remain to be determined.

MISCELLANEOUS EXPERIMENTS

Hamburgh et al. (1970) have reported the results of experiments in which seizure prone animals were joined parabiotically
to seizure resistant mice and the effects on audiogenic seizures
were studied. In seizure susceptible mice joined to seizure resistant animals the incidence of audiogenic seizures decreased
dramatically; joining of two seizure susceptible animals with each
other did not affect seizure risk. In some parabiotic pairs between seizure resistant and seizure susceptible mice audiogenic
seizures still occurred; in these animals the establishment of
joint circulation, as tested by the injection of vital dyes, proved
to be either defective or absent. Several interpretation of these
data seem plausible: Either a circulating anticonvulsant factor
passes from the seizure resistant to the seizure susceptible animal, or a neurotoxic compound is metabolized by an enzyme present
in the seizure resistant, but not the seizure susceptible, mouse.
Unfortunately, many of the animals joined parabiotically succumbed
to parabiosis intoxication; this complication could be resolved
through the use of inbred, histocompatible strains of mice.

Jameson et al. (1971) have studied the effects of acetoxycycloheximide induced protein synthesis inhibition on audiogenic
seizures. In DBA/2J mice sensitivity to audiogenic seizures de-

clines with age; however, in acetoxycycloheximide treated mice
this decline is greatly retarded and even 50-day old mice seize in
response to auditory stimulation. In other words, a transitory
inhibition of protein synthesis renders otherwise seizure resistant
DBA/2J mice susceptible to audiogenic seizures.

Henry (1967) has reported the results of experiments in which
the effectiveness of acoustic priming was studied in unanesthetized,
pentobarbital anesthetized and ether anesthetized C57B1/6J mice.
Acoustic priming was observed in all animals and no quantitative
differences in the effectiveness of acoustic priming were noted between awake and anesthetized preparations. Henry suggests that the
results of this experiment indicate that the reticular formation is
probably not involved in acoustic priming.

Finally, the effects of a variety of other drugs have been
studied for their effects on sound-induced seizures. Sedatives,
minor tranquilizers and phenothiazone derivatives, e.g., phenobarbital, benactyzine and chlorpromazine, have all been found to protect animals against audiogenic seizures; these data have been summarized by Lehman (1970).

THE DISUSE HYPOTHESIS

In the early work on acoustic priming, it was considered that
the phenomenon might represent a form of neuronal plasticity analagous to learning, or "imprinting", in which, however, the impress
of a brief intense experience had unusually dramatic consequences.
The fact that the phenomenon was lateralized led to some optimism
that it might be exploited to reveal the locus and mechanism of certain kinds of plastic changes brought about by experience. The
subsequent discovery by Goddard (1969, 1969) of the "kindling"
phenomenon, in which electrical or chemical stimulation of certain
brain structures led to increased susceptibility to epilepiform
discharges, suggested that the phenomenon might be general, not
confined to the auditory system of mice.

However, the sound pressure level required to produce acoustic
priming is near that which produces cochlear damage in larger animals, and the possibility that the effect is secondary to sound-induced cochlear damage must be considered. Cochlear damage might
result either in partial denervation or disuse of neurons in the
central auditory pathways. Many excitable structures which undergo a period of disuse become more excitable. We have elsewhere referred to this phenomenon as "disuse supersensitivity" (after Cannon's "denervation supersensitivity"; Sharpless. 1969).

Disuse supersensitivity has been most studied in peripheral

structures. Extrajunctional ACh receptors develop in skeletal muscle simple as a consequence of diuse (Lomo & Rosenthal, 1972; Drachman & Witzke, 1972; Cohen & Fischbach, 1973). A similar proliferation of extrajunctional ACh receptors occurs in denervated neurons
in the frog's heart (Kuffler et al., 1971). Autonomic effectors,
both smooth muscle and gland, also become supersensitive when disused, but in this case, the supersensitivity is unspecific (Hudgins
& Fleming, 1966), and cannot be attributed to the proliferation of
specific postjunctional receptors. It appears that disused autonomic effector organs and denervated skeletal muscles also undergo
changes in calcium binding and mobility, which may play an important
role in supersensitivity (Carrier & Jurevics, 1973; Isaacson &
Sandow, 1967).

In the central nervous system, there are numerous phenomena
which are superficially analagous to disuse supersensitivity in
peripheral organs (Stavraky, 1961; Sharpless, 1964; 1969; 1974).
Chronically undercut cerebral cortex, in which neurons are partially denervated and relatively inactive, gradually becomes more susceptible to epileptiform afterdischarges (Echlin & McDonald, 1954;
Sharpless & Halpern, 1962). This effect seems to be due to diuse
of cortical neurons; at least, it can be prevented by daily sub-
convulsive electrical stimulation (Rutledge et al., 1967). Sever-
ance of the optic nerve leads to the development of hyperexcita-
bility of visual cortex (Fentress & Doty, 1971). Visual (Spehlmann
et al., 1970), auditory (Desmedt & Franken, 1963), and somatosen-
sory cortex (Spiegel & Szekely, 1955) all appear to develop some
form of increased excitability following damage to sensory thalamus.

It would be possible to cite numerous other instances in which
some form of increased excitability gradually develops in central
nervous structures after partial deafferentation or prolonged suppression of activity by drugs. The mechanisms responsible for such
changes are generally unknown, but it appears that disuse of excitable cells engages very basic cellular processes involved in the
regulation of energy metabolism and transmitter release as well as
postjunctional sensitivity (Sharpless, 1974).

There are thus two diametrically opposed hypotheses with respect to the genesis of seizure susceptibility in coustically
primed animals. On the one hand, the effect may be due to excessive stimulation or exercise of auditory pathways during a labile
phase of their development; on the other hand, it may be due to
partial denervation or disuse following sound-induced damage of the
receptor organs. If the disuses hypothesis were correct, it ought
to be possible to reverse the effect or delay its development by
"exercising" the disused pathways, increasing input through remaining intact afferent fibers. Fuller & Collins (1968) found that re-

peated exposure to bell-ringing at 6-hour or 12-hour (but not 18-hour) intervals delayed the development of convulsability on the stimulated side.

The delay or attenuation of acoustic priming effects during re-peated presentation of the priming stimulus might be due to tempor-ary deafening by loud noise (Henry & Saleh, 1973). However, the an-imals did not appear to be deaf, as judged by their pinnae and star-tle responses to low-intensity clicks (Collins, 1970); furthermore, Bock et al., L974) found that the priming effect was attenuated in BALB/c mice exposed to intermittent white noise which was believed to be too weak to produce temporary threshold shifts on its own (90 db SL 10 minutes/hour for 6 days following priming).

The capacity of noise itself to retard the effects of priming tends to support the disuse hypothesis; however, there are aspects which require clarification. Thus, Fink & Itturian (1970), using a different strain, found that noise following priming may prolong the period of increase seizure susceptibility. Additional experiments are required: It may be that exercise retards the development of seizure susceptibility, but that further sound-induced damage pro-longs the effect, once it develops.

The first direct evidence of sound-induced cochlear damage during priming was obtained by the Australian investigators, Saun-ders et al (1972), who found that cochlear microphonics and audi-tory nerve responses were greatly diminished by priming. It was on the basis of this finding that they suggested the disuse hypothesis (which had also occurred to us on theoretic grounds; Schlesinger & Uphouse, 1972). Since then, the Australian investigators and Henry and associates have amassed a considerable body of data to buttress this concept. As mentioned previously, the auditory pathways from the cochlear nucleus to the medial geniculate shows diminished re-sponses to weak sounds and increased responses to intense sounds after priming, suggesting that the auditory centers experience a paucity of input from normal low-level noise but react explosively to high-level noises (Saunders et al., 1972; Henry & Saleh, 1973; Willott & Henry, 1974). The effect is consistent with damage to the outer hair cells, as Willott & Henry have observed.

If priming were a manifestation of damage-induced disuse super-sensitivity, it might be mimicked by conditions which limit acoustic input without destruction of the neural elements of the cochlea. Gates & associates (1973) tested this by destroying the tympanic membraines of BALB/c mice at 21 days of age. Sixty percent of the an-imals with bilateral destruction of the tympanic membrane exhibited convulsions when exposed to the sound of a loud electric bell one week later; fifty-three percent of the animals with unilateral de-struction showed convulsions; none of the sham-operates convulsed.

Electrophysiological studies in some of the animals indicated substantial hearing loss, although the tympanic membrane had regener-
ated, being thicker than in the normal mouse. The effects of acoustic deprivation were also studied by McGinn et al. (1973), employing ear plugs of cotton and clay to avoid traumatic damage to structures of the ear. The ears of C57Bl/6J mice were plugged at 17 days
of age, and when tested 5 days later, about half of the animals
seized and all showed wild running. Control animals in which the
plug was removed immediately after insertion showed neither. The
effect was age-dependent, since animals whose ears were plugged at
28 days of age (beyond the "critical period") developed little seizure susceptibility.

The Australian group (Chen et al., 1973) reasoned that if sensory deprivation were responsible for seizure susceptibility, it
ought to be possible to induce it by rupturing the tympanic membranes
at an early age, so that the animal enters the critical period with
hearing loss. Normally, it is difficult to prime BALB/c mice at
14 days of age, but the investigators found that destruction of the
tympanic membrane at this age resulted in seizures when the animals
were tested 7 days later. The seizure susceptibility seemed to develop more rapidly in the younger animals. Chen and associates
point out that two factors may contribute to the age-related susceptibility to priming: The structures of the inner ear may be especially fragile and susceptible to mechanical damage at a certain
age, and the auditory pathways themselves may be labile and plastic
only during certain maturational phases. The latter suggestion
would be in line with Scott's view of the critical period, in which
the system is most modifi ble when active processes or organization
are going on (1962). There is little evidence on the course of development of the auditory system in mice, but such as there is indicates that the system is essentially mature by 14 days of age
(See discussion in Chen et al., 1973).

On the whole, the evidence now strongly suggests that priming
is another instance of disuxe supersensitivity in the central nervous system. The catalogue of such phenomena is now quite large,
but the mechanisms underlying such changes are still obscure. Postjunctional spread of receptors in disused neurons similar to that
which occurs in disused skeletal muscle has not been demonstrated
convincingly in the central nervous system; on the other hand, even
in peripheral junctions, disuse seems to alter very basic processes
in excitable cells, which may be maifested in all spheres of cellular function (Sharpless, 1974). At present, we can do little better than appeal to what might be called the "teleological residuum"
of Cannon's law of denervation, namely, the principle of "compulsory
nervous control," according to which various feedback processes
have evolved to insure that the nervous system achieves and maintains
control of excitable elements. Loss of input to such an element in-

itiates changes which tend to restore access, including possibly
collateral growth, competition of endings for available membrane
sites (possible leading to hyperneurotization of the isolated elements), increased transmitter release from disused endings, changes
in postjunctional sensitivity, and changes in energetics and the
capacity to sustain repetitive firing. There is evidence for each
of these changes following periods of disuse or denervation.

REFERENCES

ABOOD, L. G., & GERARD, R. W., A phosphorylation defect in the
    brains of mice susceptible to audiogenic seizure. In: H.
    Waelsch, Biochemistry of the Developing Nervous System.
    Academic Press, New York, 1955, pp. 467-472.

ANTONITIS, J. J., CRARY, D. D., SAWIN, P. B., & COHEN, C. Sound
    induced seizures in rabbits. J. Heredity, 1954, 45:278.

BALLANTINE, E. The effects of gamma-aminobutyric acid on the audio-
    genic seizure. In: Psychophysiologie, Neuropharmacologie et
    Biochemie de la Crise Audiogene. Paris: Centre National de
    la Recherche Scientifique. 1963.

BEACH, F. A., & WEAVER, T. H. Noise induced seizures in the rat
    and their modification by cerebral injury. J. Comp. Neur.,
    1943, 79:379.

BERCEL, N. A. The periodic nature of some seizure states. Annals
    of the New York Academy of Science, 164, 117:555.

BEVAN, W. Sound-precipitated convulsions: 1947-1954. Psych. Bull.,
    1955, 53:473.

BEVAN, W. & CHINN, R. Mc. C. Sound induced convulsions in rats treat-
    ed with reserpine. J. Comp. Physiol. Psychol., 1957, 50:311.

BOCK, G. R., GATES, G. R. & CHEN, C. -S. Priming for audiogenic
    seizures in mice: Influence of post-priming auditory environ-
    ment. Exp. Neur., 1974, 42:700.

BOGGAN, W. O., FREEDMAN, D. X., LOVELL, R. A., & SCHLESINGER, K.
    Studies in audiogenic seizure susceptibility. Psychopharma-
    cologia, 1971, 20:48.

BOGGAN, W. O., & SEIDEN, L. W. DOPA reversal of reserpine enhance-
    ment of audiogenic seizure susceptibility in mice. Physiology
    and Behavior, 1971, 6:215.

BUDAY, P. V., CARR, C. J., & MIYA T. S. A pharmacologic study of
    some nucleosides and nucleotides. J. Pharm. Pharmacol. 1961,
    13:290.

BUSNEL, R. G. Psychophysiologie Neuropharmacologie et Biochemie de
    la Crise Audiogene, Paris, Centre National de la Recherche
    Scientifique, 1963.

BUSNEL, R. G., & LEHMANN, A. Action de convulsivants chimiques sur
    les souris de lignées sensible et résistante a la crise audioge
    gene. Part III. Caffeine. J. Physiol., 1961, 53:285.

CARRIER, O., & JUREVICS, H. A. The role of calcium in "non-specific"
    supersensitivity of vascular muscle. J. Pharmacol. Exp. Ther.,
    1973, 184:81.

CHEN, C. -S., GATE, G. R., & BOCK, G. R. Effect of priming and tym-
    panic membrane destruction on development of audiogenic sei-
    zure susceptibility in BALB/c mice. Exp. Neur., 1973, 39:277.

COHEN, S. A., & FISCHBACH, G. D. Regulation of muscle acetylcholine
    sensitivity by muscle activity in cell culture. Science, 1973
    181:76.

COLEMAN, D. L. Phenylalanine hydroxylase activity in dilute and non-
    dilute strains of mice. Archives of Biochemistry & Biophysics,
    1960, 91:300.

COLEMAN, D. L. & SCHLESINGER, K. Effects of pyridoxine deficiency
    on audiogenic seizure susceptibility in inbred mice. Proc.
    Soc. Exp. Biol. & Med., 1965, 119:264.

COLLINS, R. L. Unilateral inhibition of sound-induced convulsions
    in mice. Science, 1970, 167:1010.

COLLINS, R. L. A new genetic locus mapped from behavioral variation
    in mice: Audiogenic seizure prone (asp). Beh. Genetics, 1971,
    1:99.

COLLINS, R. L., & FULLER, J. L. Audiogenic seizure prone (asp): a
    gene affecting behavior in linkage group VIII of the mouse.
    Science, 1968, 162:1137.

COLLINS, R. L., & WARD, R. Evidence for an asymmetry of cerebral
    function in mice tested for audiogenic seizures. Nature, 1970,
    226:1062.

DARROUZET, J., NIAUSSAT, M. M., & LEGOUIX, J. P. Etude histologique
    de l'organe de corti de souris d'une lignee presentant des

crises convulsives au son. *Comptes Renous Acad. Sci. Paris*, 1968, 266:1163.

DAVIS, W., & WEBB, O. L. A circadian rhythm of chemoconvulsive response thresholds in mice. *Medicina Experimentalis*, (*Basel*), 1963, 9:263.

DAVIS, W. M., & WEBB, O. L. Chemoconvulsive thresholds in mice of differing audioconvulsive susceptibilities. *Experientia*, 1964, 20:291.

DELGADO, J. M. R., & SEVILLANO, M. Evolution of repeated hippocampal seizures in the cat. *Electroenceph. Alog. Clin. Neurophysiol.*, 1961, 13:722.

DENENBERG, V. H., & KLINE, N. J. Stimulus intensity versus critical periods: a test of two hypotheses concerning infantile stimulation. *Canad. J. Psychol.*, 1964, 18:1.

DESMEDT, J., & FRANKEN, L. Long-term physiological changes in auditory cortex following deafferentation. In: *The Effect of Use and Disuse on Neuromuscular Functions*, Edited by E. Gutmann & P. Hnik, pp. 264-276. Czechoslovakian Academy of Sciences, Prague, 1963.

DICE, L. R. Inheritance of waltzing and of epilepsy in mice of the genus Peromyscus. *J. Mammal.*, 1935, 16:25.

DIXIT, B., & BUCKLEY, J. P. Circadian changes in brain 5-hydroxytryptamine and plasma corticosterone in the rat. *Life Sci.*, 1967, 6:755.

DRACHMAN, D. B., & WITZKE, F. Trophic regulation of acetylcholine sensitivity of muscle: Effect of electrical stimulation, *Science*, 1972, 176:514.

ECHLIN, F. A., & MCDONALD, J. The supersensitivity of chronically isolated and partially isolated cerebral cortex as a mechanism in focal cortical epilepsy. *Trans. Amer. Neurol. Assoc.*, 1954, 79:75.

FENTRESS, J., & DOTY, R. Effect of tetanization and enucleation upon excitability of visual pathways in squirrel monkeys and cats *Exptl. Neurol.*, 1971, 30:535.

FINGER, F. W. Convulsive behavior in the rat. *Psychol. Bull.*, 1947, 44:201.

FINK, G. B., & ITURRIAN, W. B. Influence of age auditory condition-

ing and environmental noise on sound-induced seizures and seizure threshold in mice. In: Welch, B. L. & Welch, A. S. (Eds.),
Physiological Effects of Noise. New York: Plenum Press, 1970,
pp. 211-226.

FOGLIA, V. G., MONTANELLI, R. P., LANGER, S. Z., EPSTEIN, R. Action
des drogues psychotrops sur les convulsions audiogenes chei la
souris. Compte Renou Société Biologie (Paris), 1963, 157:1813.

FRIEDMAN, A. H., & WALKER, C. A. Circadian rhythms in rat mid-brain
and caudate nucleus biogenic amine levels. J. Physiol., 1968,
197:77.

FRINGS, H., & FRINGS, M. Development of strains of albino mice with
predictable susceptibilities to audiogenic seizures. Science,
1953, 117:283.

FRINGS, H., & KIVERT, A. Nicotine facilitation of audiogenic seizures in laboratory mice. J. Mammal., 1953, 34:391.

FULLER, J. L., & COLLINS, R. L. Mice unilaterally sensitized for
audiogenic seizures. Science, 1968, 162:1295.

FULLER, J. L., & COLLINS, R. L. Temporal parameters of sensitization
for audiogenic seizures in SJL/J mice. Develop. Psychobiol.,
1968, 1:185.

FULLER, J. L., EASLER, C., & SMITH, M. E. Inheritance of audiogenic
seizure susceptibility in the mouse. Genetics, 1950, 35:622.

FULLER, J. L., & SJURSEN, F. H., JR. Audiogenic seizures in eleven
mouse strains. J. Heredity, 1967, 58:135.

FULLER, J. L., & SMITH, M. E. Kenetics of sound-induced convulsions
in some inbred strains of mice. Amer. J. Physiol., 1953, 172:
661.

FULLER, J. L., & THOMPSON, W. R. Behavior Genetics. John Wiley and
Sons, New York, 1960.

FULLER, J. L., & WILLIAMS, E. Gene controlled time constants in convulsive behavior. Proc. Nat. Acad. Sci., U.S., 1951, 37:349.

FULLER, J. L., & WIMER, R. E. Neural, sensory and motor functions.
In: E. L. Green (Ed.), Biology of the Laboratory Mouse. New
York: McGraw-Hill, 1966, pp. 609-629.

FURUCHI, Y. Clinical and electroencephalographical study of nocturnal
epilepsy. Psychiatria. Neurol. Jap., 1969, 71:101.

GATES, G. R., CHEN, C. -S., & BOCK, G. R. Effects of monaural and binaural auditory deprivation on audiogenic seizure susceptibility in BALB/c mice. Exp. Neurol., 1973, 38:488.

GATES, G. R., & CHEN, C. -S. Priming for audiogenic seizures in adult BALB/c mice. Exp. Neurol. 1973, 41:457.

GELLER, L. M., COWEN, D. & WOLF, A. Effect of the antimetabolite, 6-aminonicotinamide, on sound-induced seizures in mice. Exp. Neurol., 1966, 14:86.

GINSBURG, B. E. Genetics and the physiology of the nervous system. Genetics and the inheritance of integrated neurological and psychiatric patterns. Proc. Ass. Res. in Nervous and Mental Disease, 1954, 33:39.

GINSBURG, B. E. Causal mechanisms in audiogenic seizures. Colloq. Intern. Centre Nat. Rech. Sci. Paris, 1963, 112:227.

GINSBURG, B. E., COWEN, J. J., MAXSON, S. C., & SZE, P. Y. -L. Neurochemical effects of gene mutations associated with audiogenic seizure. Proc. 2nd. Int. Cong. Neuro-Gen. and Neuro-Ophthamol., 1967, 1:695.

GINSBURG, B. E., & MILLER, D. S. Genetic factors in audiogenic seizures. Colloq. Intern. Centre Nat. Rech. Sci. Paris, 1963, 112:217.

GINSBURG, B. E., & ROBERTS, E. Glutamic acid and central nervous system activity. Anat. Rec., 1951, 111:492.

GODDARD, G. V. Analysis of avoidance conditioning following cholinergic stimulation of amygdala in rats. J. Comp. Physiol. Psychol. Monograph, 1969, 68:1.

GODDARD, G. V., MCINTYRE, D. C., & LEECH, C. K. A permanent change in brain function resulting from daily electrical stimulation. Exp. Neurol., 1969, 25:295.

GOODSELL, J. S. Properties of audiogenic seizures in mice and effect of anticonvulsant drugs. Fed. Proc., 1955, 14:345.

GRIFFITHS, W. J., JR. The production of convulsions in the white rat. Comp. Psychol. Monog., 1942, 17:1.

HALBERG, F., BITTNER, J. J., & GULLY, R. J. Twenty-four hour susceptibility to audiogenic convulsions in several stocks of mice. Fed. Proc., 1955, 14:67.

HALBERG, F., BITTNER, J. J., GULLY, R. J., ALBRECHT, P. G., & BRACKNEY, E. L. 24-hour periodicity and audiogenic convulsions in I mice of various ages. Proc. Soc. Exp. Biol. Med., 1955, 88: 169.

HALBERG, F., JACOBSEN, E., WADSWORTH, G., & BITTNER, J. J. Audiogenic abnormality spectra: Twenty-four hour periodicity and lighting. Science, 1958, 128:657.

HAMBURGH, M., MENDOZA, L. A., KRUPA, P., GELFAND, D., & LEHRER, R. The effect of parabiosis on audiogenic convulsions in seizure-susceptible mice. Exp. Neurology, 1970, 26:283.

HAMBURGH, M., & VICARI, E. A study of some physiological mechanisms underlying susceptibility to audiogenic seizures in mice. J. Neuropath. and Exp. Neur., 1970, 19:461.

HANSON, A. Inhibition of brain glutamic decarboxylase by phenylalanine metabolites, Naturwissenschaften, 1958, 45:423.

HARRIS, H. Human Biochemical Genetics. Cambridge: Cambridge University Press, 1962.

HENRY, K. R., Audiogenic Seizures. Unpublished thesis, University of North Carolina, 1966.

HENRY, K. R. Audiogenic seizure susceptbility induced in C57BL/6J mice by prior auditory exposure. Science, 1967, 158:938.

HENRY, K. R., & BOWMAN, R. E. Effects of acoustic priming on audiogenic, electroconvulsive and chemoconvulsive seizures. J. Comp. Physiol. Psychol., 1969, 67:401.

HENRY, K. R., & BOWMAN, R. E. Behavior-genetic analysis of the ontogeny of acoustically primed audiogenic seizures in mice. J. Comp. Physiol. Psychol., 1970, 70:235.

HENRY, K. R., & SALEH, M. Recruitment deafness: Functional effect of priming-induced audiogenic seizures in mice. J. Comp. Physiol. Psychol., 1973, 84:430.

HUDGINS, P. M., & FLEMING, W. W. A relatively nonspecific supersensitivity in aortic strips resulting from pretreatment with reserpine. J. Pharmacol., 1966, 153:70.

HUFF, S. D., & FULLER, J. L. Audiogenic seizures, the dilute locus, and phenylalanine hydroxylase in DBA/1 mice. Science, 1964, 144:304.

HUFF, S. D., & HUFF, R. L. Dilute locus and audiogenic seizures in mice. Science, 1962, 136:318.

ISAACSON, A., & SANDOW, A. Caffeine effects on radiocalcium movement in noraml and denervated rat skeletal muscles. J. Pharmacol., 1967, 155:376.

ITTURIAN, W. B., & FINK, G. B. Conditioned convulsive reaction. Fed. Proc., 1967, 26:736.

ITTURRIAN, W. B., & FINK, G. B. Influence of age and brief auditory conditioning upon experimental seizures in mice. Develop. Psychobiol., 1969, 2:10.

IVERSEN, L. L. The Uptake and Storage of Noradrenaline in Sympathetic Nerves. Cambridge: Cambridge University Press, 1967.

JAMESON, H. D., FALACE, P., PREROST, A. & CLEMONS, G. Acetoxycycloheximide enhances audiogenic seizures in DBA/2J mice. Science, 1971, 173:249.

KARCZMAR, A. G., SOBOTKA, T., & SCUDDER, C. L. Cholinesterases of mice strains and genera. Fed. Proc., 1968, 27:471.

KARRER, R., & CAHILLY, G. Experimental attempts to produce phenylketonuria in animals: A critical review. Psych. Bull., 1963, 64:52.

KELLOGG, C. Serotonin metabolism in the brains of mice sensitive or resistant to audiogenic seizures. J. Neurobiol., 1971, 2:209.

KESNER, R. P. Subcortical mechanisms of audiogenic seizures. Exp. Neurol., 1966, 15:192.

KESNER, R. P., O'KELLY, L. I., & THOMAS. G. J. Effects of cortical spreading depression and drugs upon audiogenic seizures in rats. J. Comp. Physiol. Psychol., 1965, 59:280.

KOENIG, E. The effects of auditory pathway interruption on the incidence of sound-induced seizures in rats. J. Comp. Neurol., 1957, 108:383.

KORNFELD, M., GELLER, L. M., COWEN, D., WOLF, A., & ALTMANN, F. Pathologic changes in the inner ear of audiogenic seizure-susceptible mice treated with 6-aminoninotinamide. Exp. Neurol., 1970, 26:17.

KUFFLER, S., DENNIS, M. J., & HARRIS, A. J. The development of chemosensitivity in extrasynaptic areas of the neuronal surface after denervation of parasympathetic ganglion cells in the heart of the frog. Proc. R. Soc. B., 1971, 177:555.

KURIYAMA, K., ROBERTS, E., & RUBINSTEIN, M. K. Elevation of gamma-aminobutyric acid in brain with amino-oxyacetic acid and susceptibility to convulsive seizures in mice: A quantitative reevaluation. Biochem. Pharmacol., 1966, 15:221.

LAUFER, M. W., DENHOFF, E., & RUBIN, E. Z. Photo-metrazol activation in children. EEG and Clin. Neurophysiol., 1954, 6:1.

LEHMANN, A. Action des hydrazides convulsivants sur l'epilepsie acoustique dite crise audiogene de la souris. J. Physiologie (Paris), 1963, 55:282.

LEHMANN, A. L'acide gamma-amino-butyrique est'il un inhibiteur du systeme nerveux central convulsions et acidé gamma-butryique. Therapie, 1965, 18:1509.

LEHMANN, A. Modification de l'intensite de la crise audiogene par des substances actives sur le metabolisme des amines biogenes due cerveau de souris. C. R. Societe Biologie (Paris), 1968, 162:24.

LEHMANN, A. Psychopharmacology of noise response. In: Physiological Effects of Noise, B. L. Welch & A. S. Welch (Eds.). New York: Plenum Press, 1970. pp. 227-257.

LEHMANN, A., & BUSNEL, R. G. A new test for detecting MAO-inhibitor effects. Int. J. Neurophar., 1962, 1:61.

LEHMANN, A., & BUSNEL, R. G. A study of the audiogenic seizure. In: R. G. Busnel (Ed.), Acoustic Behavior of Animals. New York: Elsevier Publ. Co., 1963, pp. 244-274.

LOMO, T., & ROSENTHAL, J. Control of ACh sensitivity by muscle activity of the rat. J. Physiol., 1972, 221:493.

LYON, J. B., WILLIAMS, H. L., & ARNOLD, E. A. The pyridoxine-deficient state in two strains of inbred mice. J. Nutr., 1958, 66:261.

MACINNES, J. W., BOGGAN, W. O., & SCHLESINGER, K. Seizure susceptibility in mice: Differences in brain ATP production in vitro. Behav. Gen., 1970, 1:35.

MAIER, N. R. F. Some factors which inhibit the abnormal reactions to auditory stimulation. Psychol. Bull., 1942, 39:591.

MAIER, N. R. F., & GLASER, N. M. Studies of abnormal behavior in the rat. II. A comparison of some convulsion-producing situations. Comp. Psychol. Monog., 1940, 16:1.

MAUER, I., & SIDEMAN, M. B. Phenylalanine metabolism in a dilute-lethal strain of mice. J. Heredity, 1967, 58:14.

MCGEER, E. G., IKEDA, H. A., SAKURA, T., & WADA, J. A. Lack of abnormality in brain aromatic amines in rats and mice susceptible to audiogenic seizure. J. Neurochem., 1969, 16:945.

MCGINN, M. D., WILLOTT, J. F., & HENRY, K. R. Effects of conductive hearing loss on auditory evoked potentials and audiogenic seizures in mice. Nature, 1973, 244:255.

NAKAI, K., IDA, H., KAKIMOTO, Y., HISHIKAWA, Y., SANO, I., & KANEKO, Z. A low metrazol threshold in the heterozygote of phenylketonuria. J. Nervous & Mental Disease, 1966, 144:436.

NELLHAUS, G. Experimental epilepsy in rabbits: Observations on a strain susceptible to audiogenic seizures. In: R. G. Busnel (Ed.), Psychophysiologie Neuropharmacologie et Biochimie de la Crise Audiogene. Centre National de la Recherche Scientifique, Paris, 1963.

NELLHAUS, G. Paper read to Am. Acad. Neurology. 1968.

NIAUSSAT, M. -M. Caractére génétique de la dissociation entre le potentiel microphonique cochleaire et le potentiel d'action du nerf auditif de la souris audiogene. Comptes Rendus des Seances de la Societe de Biologie, 1968, 162:21.

NIAUSSAT, M. -M., & LEGOUIX, J. -P. Anomalies des responses microphoniques cochleaires dan une lignee de souris presentant des crises convulsives au son. C. R. Acad. Sc. Paris, 1967, 264:103.

PARTINGTON, M. W. The early symptoms of phenylketonuria. Pediatrics, 1961, 27:465.

PASQUINI, J. M., SALOMONE, J. R., & GOMEZ, C. J. Amino acid changes in the mouse brain during audiogenic seizures and recovery. Exp. Neurology, 1968, 21:245.

PFEIFFER, C. C., JENNEY, E. H., & MARSHALL, W. H. Experimental seizures in man and animals with acute pyridoxine deficiency produced by isoniazid. EEG and Clin. Neurophysiol., 1957, 8:307.

QUAY, W. B. Regional and circadian differences in cerebral cortical serotonin concentration. Life Sci., 1965, 4:379.

RALLS, K. Auditory sensitivity in mice: Peromyscus and Mus musculus. Animal Behavior, 1967, 15:123.

RAUCH, H., & YOST, M. T.   Phenylalanine metabolism in dilute-lethal
    mice. Genetics, 1963, 48:1487.

RUTLEDGE, L., RANCK, J., & DUNCAN, J.   Prevention of supersensitiv-
    ity in partially isolated cerebral cortex.   EEG and Clin. Neuro-
    physiol., 1967, 23:256.

SANDLER, M., & CLOSE, H.   Biochemical effects of phenylacetic acid
    in a patient with a 5-hydroxytryptophan secreting carcinoid
    tumor. Lancet, 1959, 277:316.

SAUNDERS, J. C., BOCK, G. R., CHEN, C. -S., & GATES, R.   The effects
    of priming for audiogenic seizure on cochlear and behavioral
    responses in BALB/c mice. Exp. Neurol., 1972, 36:426.

SCHLESINGER, K.   Experimentally induced seizures in mice.   In:
    Charles Rupp (Ed.) Mind as a Tissue. New York: Harper & Row,
    1968.

SCHLESINGER, K., BOGGAN, W. O., & FREEDMAN, D. X.   Genetics of audio-
    genic seizures: I.   Relation to brain serotonin and norepine-
    phrine in mice. Life Sci., 1965, 4:2345.

SCHLESINGER, K., BOGGAN, W. O., & FREEDMAN, D. X.   Genetics of audio-
    genic seizures: II. Effects of pharmacological manipulation of
    brain serotonin, norepinephrine and gamma-aminobutyric acid.
    Life Sci., 1968, 7:437.

SCHLESINGER, K., BOGGAN, W. O., & FREEDMAN, D. X.   Genetics of audio-
    genic seizures: III. Time response relationships between drug
    administration and seizure susceptibility. Life Sci., 1970, 9:
    721.

SCHLESINGER, K., BOGGAN, W. O., & GRIEK, B. J.   Pharmacogenetic cor-
    relates of pentylenetetrazol and electroconvulsive seizure
    thresholds in mice. Psychopharm., 1968, 13:181.

SCHLESINGER, K., ELSTON, R. C., & BOGGAN, W.   The genetics of sound
    induced seizures in inbred mice. Genetics, 1966, 54:95.

SCHLESINGER, K., & GRIEK, B. J.   The genetics and biochemistry of
    audiogenic seizures.   In: G. Lindzey and D. D. Thiessen (Eds.),
    Contributions to Behavior-Genetic Analysis-The Mouse as a Pro-
    totype. Appleton-Century-Crofts, 1970, pp. 219-257.

SCHLESINGER, K., & SCHREIBER, R. A.   Interaction of drugs and pyri-
    doxine deficiency on central nervous system excitability. Ann.
    N. Y. Acad. Sci., 1969, 166:281.

SCHLESINGER, K., SCHREIBER, R. A., GRIEK, B. J., & HENRY, K. R.
Effects of experimentally induced phenylketonuria on seizure susceptibility in mice. J. Comp. Physiol. Psychol., 1969, 67:149.

SCHLESINGER, K., STAVNES, K. L., & BOGGAN, W. O. Modification of
audiogenic and pentylenetetrazol seizures with gamma-aminobutyric acid, norepinephrine and serotonin. Psychopharm., 1969,
15:226.

SCHLESINGER, K., & UPHOUSE, L. L. Pyridoxine dependency in central
nervous system excitability. In: E. Costa & M. S. Ebadi (Eds.),
Vitamin B_6 in the Central Nervous System, Advances in Biochemical Psychopharmacology, Vol. 4, 1972, 105-140, Raven Press, New
York.

SCHREIBER, R. A., & SCHLESINGER, K. Circadian rhythms and seizure
susceptibility: Relation to 5-hydroxytryptamine and norepinephrine in brain. Physiol. & Behav., 1971, 6:635.

SCUDDER, C. L., KARCZMAR, A. G., EVERETT, G. M., GIBSON, J. E.,
& RIFKIN, M. Brain catecholamines and serotonin levels in
various strains and genera of mice and a possible interpretation for the correlations of amine levels with electroshock
latency and behavior. Int. J. Neuropharmacol., 1966, 5:343.

SHARPLESS, S. Isolated and deafferented neurons: Disuse super-
sensitivity. In: H. Jasper, A. Ward, and A. Pope (Eds.),
Basic Mechanisms of the Epilepsies. Boston: Little, Brown &
Co., 1969. pp. 329-348.

SHARPLESS, S. K. Supersensitivity-like phenomena in the central
nervous system. Fed. Proc. (1974) In Press.

SHARPLESS, S. K., & HALPERN, L. The electrical activity of chronically isolated cortex studied by means of permanently implanted
electrodes. EEG and Clin. Neurophysiol., 1962, 14:244.

SPECTOR, S., SJOEROSMA, A., & UDENFRIEND, S. Blockage of endogenous
norepinephrine synthesis by alpha-methyl-tyrosine, an inhibitor
of tyrosine hydroxylase. J. Pharmacol. Exp. Ther., 1965, 147:86.

SPEHLMANN, R., CHENG, M., & DANIELS, J. Excitability of partially
isolated cortex. I. Macroelectrode studies. Arch. Neurol.,
1970, 22:504.

SPIEGEL, E., & SZEKELY, E. Supersensitivity of the sensory cortex
following partial deafferentation. EEG and Clin. Neurophysiol.,
1955, 7:375.

STAVRAKY, G. W. Supersensitivity Following Lesions of the Nervous
System. Toronto: University of Toronto Press, 1961.

SWINYARD, E. A., CASTELLION, A. W., FINK, G. A., & GOODMAN, L. S.
Some neurophysiological and neuropharmacological characteristics of audiogenic-seizure susceptible mice. J. Pharmacol.,
1963, 140:375.

SZE, P. Y. Neurochemical factors in auditory stimulation and de-
velopment of susceptibility to audiogenic seizures. In: B. L.
Welch and A. J. Welch (Eds.), Physiological Effects of Noise.
New York: Plenum Press, 1970.

TEWS, J. K., & LOVELL, R. A. The effect of a nutritional pyridoxine
deficiency on free amino acids and related substances in mouse
brain. J. Neurochem., 1967, 14:1.

TOWER, D. B. Neurochemical mechanisms. In: H. H. Jasper, A. A.
Ward, and A. Pope (Eds.), Basic Mechanisms of the Epilepsies.
Boston: Little, Brown & Co., 1969.

VICARI, E. M. Fatal convulsive seizures in DBA mouse strain. J.
Psych., 1951, 32:79.

WADA, J. A., TEREO, A., WHITE, B., & JUNG, E. Inferior colliculus
lesion and audiogenic seizure susceptibility. Exp. Neurol.,
1970, 28:326.

WARD, R., & SINNETT, E. E. Spreading cortical depression and audiogenic seizures in mice. Exp. Neurol., 1971, 31:437.

SATSON, M. L. The inheritance of epilepsy and waltzing in Peromyscus.
Contr. Lab. of Vertebrate Genetic, University of Michigan, 1939,
No. 11, 1-24.

WEBB, D. L., & RUSSELL, R. L. Dinural chemoconvulsive responses and
central inhibition. Arch. Int. Pharmacodyn. Ther., 1966, 159:
471.

WEINER, H. M., & MORGAN, C. T. Effects of cortical lesions upon audiogenic seizures. J. Comp. Psychol., 1945, 38:199.

WELCH, B. L., & WELCH, A. S., (Eds.), Physiological Effects of Noise,
New York, Plenum Press, 1970.

WILLOTT, J. F., & HENRY, K. R. Auditory evoked potentials: Developmental changes of threshold and amplitude following early acoustic trauma. J. Comp. Physiol. Psychol., 1974, 86:1.

WITT, G., & HALL, C. S. The genetics of audiogenic seizures in the
    house mouse. J. Comp. Physiol. Psychol., 1949, 42:58.

YEN, H. L., & RITMAN, P. New metabolites of phenylalanine. Nature,
    1964, 203:1237.

ZANNONI, V. G., WEBER, W. W., VAN VALEN, P., RUBIN, A., BERNSTEIN, R.,
    & LA DU, B. N. Phenylalanine metabolism and "phenylketonuria"
    in dilute-lethal mice. Genetics, 1966, 54:1391.

POTENTIAL APPLICATIONS OF MULTIVARIATE ANALYSIS OF VARIANCE

TO PSYCHOPHARMACOGENETIC RESEARCH

Merrill F. Elias, Ph.D.

Department of Psychology and All-University
    Gerontology Center
Syracuse University
Syracuse, New York   13210

CONTENTS

435

INTRODUCTION

Recent advances in computer technology, the development of a variety of computer programs for multivariate data analyses, and new applications for multivariate analyses of variance place useful tools for the organization and analysis of research data at the disposal of the investigator who is concerned with psychopharmacogenetics and the nature of the relationship(s) between drugs, behavior and genotype. Unfortunately, many investigators have not taken advantage of multivariate approaches to data analysis. Reluctance of researchers in experimental psychology and psychopharmacogenetics to utilize these relatively new statistical tools is related to the fact that early descriptions were highly technical and thus difficult for the nonstatistician to readily comprehend. Moreover, the extensive statistical computations necessary to analyze data with multivariate techniques either precluded their application or made it exceedingly time consuming and tedious.

In recent years, there have been excellent nontechnical explanations of multivariate methods, and an increase in the number of large and small computer programs that perform the extensive calculations involved in multivariate analyses. In 1975, most investigators have access to either a large or small computer. Consequently, it seems reasonable to speculate that a major factor contributing to the slow incorporation of these techniques into the research projects of a variety of disciplines, including psychopharmacology, is the failure to make a wide range of researchs aware of: 1) their existence, 2) their usefulness as a tool for organizing and making sense out of

complex multivariate data, and 3) their importance in terms of
precision in hypothesis testing.

The "new" statistical approaches can be broken into two
major categories: (1) multivariate analysis of variance for
nonrepeated measurements (between-subjects) designs, and (2)
application of multivariate analysis of variance to repeated
measurements designs. The reader who is familiar with these
approaches will realize that they are not really new in terms
of their development. Rather they are new in the sense that
the majority of investigators in psychopharmacology, experimental
psychology, and behavior genetics do not make use of them.

The purpose of the present chapter is to call attention to
these statistical techniques. No mathematical or statistical
development is provided. The scope of the chapter is limited
to a brief description of the rationale for their application.
Bibliographical references to computer programs, technical and
nontechnical discussions, and examples from the literature are
provided.

Multivariate analysis of variance is essentially an extension of univariate analysis of variance model to a set of dependent variables (McCall & Appelbaum, 1973; Cole & Grizzle,
1966). Thus, it is necessary to review procedures normally
utilized in application of analyses of variance to factorial
designs.

ANALYSIS OF VARIANCE

Definition of Terms

The terms used in this chapter are similar to those used
by Winer (1971) and McCall & Appelbaum (1973). A factor is a
series of related treatments or experimental conditions. For
example, a drug factor might include the following drug treatments: methyldopa MSD, hydralazine HCI NF, and reserpine. A
dosage factor might include 10, 20, and 40 mg of these drugs.
A single factor analysis of variance involves two or more treatments subsumed under the same factor. A multifactor analysis
of variance involves two or more factors, e.g., drugs and
dosage levels, with various treatments subsumed under each
factor. In contrast, a multivariate analysis of variance refers to either a single factor, or a multifactorial analysis of
variance with more than one dependent variable. The distinction
between a multifactorial and a multivariate analysis is quite
important because the two terms are often confused by those who
are unfamiliar with the latter term.

A <u>nonrepeated measurements</u> analysis of variance refers to
analyses of data for a between-subjects design in which different subjects are assigned to different treatments. In contrast, a <u>repeated measurements</u> analysis of variance, single
factor or multifactorial, involves the analysis of data for a
single dependent variable which has been measured or observed
repeatedly for the same subjects over a period of time. The
experimenter may be interested in the influence of the same
drug administered at several different time periods, or the
influence of different drugs on the same subjects. This is
often referred to as a within-subjects design. A <u>partially</u>
<u>repeated measurements</u> design involves both between- and within-
subjects components.

A <u>multivariate analysis of variance</u> is distinctly different
from a repeated measurements analysis of variance. It involves multiple response variables which are qualitatively and
logically different from each other, e.g., errors, latency of
response, blood pressure, heart rate, respiration. Table 1
illustrates the difference between a multivariate factorial
and a univariate factorial design.

<u>Analysis of covariance</u> may or may not be done in the
context of multivariate analysis of variance. This procedure
involves the measurement of one or more concomitant variables
in addition to the dependent variables of primary interest.
The concomitant variables are often referred to as <u>covariates</u>
while the dependent variables of interest are called <u>criteria</u>.
Covariance analysis is one method of adjusting the criterion
for the influence of the covariate. "In terms of a linear regression, an adjusted criterion mean has the following form,

$$\bar{Y}_j = Y_j - b\,(\bar{X}_j - \bar{X}),$$

where b is an estimate of β, the population linear-regression
coefficient" (Winer, 1962, p. 597). Thus, differences between
criterion means which are adjusted are free of the linear influence of the covariate. The covariance procedure is typically
used when experimental control cannot be built into the design,
e.g., changes in heart rate accompanying changes in blood pressure cannot be controlled.

Good Testmanship

A brief review of the generally accepted rules for testing hypotheses in a single variable (<u>univariate</u>) design is in
order as the logic behind the use of multivariate analyses in
a "protective" sense is similar to that used in the performance

of an overall univariate analysis of variance prior to specific
contrasts (comparisons between means) or probing tests. The
overall univariate analysis of variance protects against the
erroneous rejection of H-1 for a single contrast made in the
context of many other contrasts. Clearly, a significant difference in a contrast between means representing two groups of
subjects exposed to different treatments does not have the
same meaning in the context of twenty contrasts as it does
in the context of one. In the former case, 1 out of 20 contrasts may be expected to be significant by chance ($p < 0.05$).

In multifactor, univariate designs, overall tests of interactions are often followed by tests of simple effects
(Winer, 1962, p. 174; 1971, pp. 347-350) which are, in turn,
followed by multiple contrasts. A variety of contrast schemes
may be utilized depending on the experimental rationale, and
the extent to which the investigator wishes to be conservative
regarding the rejection of H-1. They include individual t tests,
the Duncan test, the Newman-Keul's test, the Tukey (a) and (b)
tests, and the Schaffé test. Individual contrasts, in the absence of overall analyses, are generally only appropriate when
they have been "built into" the design on the basis of a theoretical formulation or a prediction based on previously reported
empirical findings. Regardless of the outcome of overall analyses
of variance, it is appropriate to make these planned (a priori)
contrasts (Winer, 1971, p. 196).

Care should be taken in the selection of tests for a posteriori or "after the fact" contrasts. Winer (1962, 1971), among
others, discusses the advantages and disadvantages of the various
contrasts. Specific contrasts between means for the RI strains
(Eleftheriou & Elias, Chapter 1) provide an example of a case
when the most conservative contrast may not be the contrast of
choice. This is true because testing of any single gene hypothesis
with the RI strains, or selection of congenic lines for linkage
testing, depends on sensitivity to differences which do exist.
In other words, the pattern of differences is of concern. A test
which is overly conservative, or insufficiently conservative, may
not be maximally sensitive to an emerging strain distribution
pattern. For this reason, many of the contrasts done with the
RI strains have utilized the Newman-Keul's test (Winer, 1971,
pp. 191-195). On the other hand, comparison of a progenitor
strain with several congenic lines in the context of linkage
(genetic linkage) testing may more appropriately involve procedures (Winer, 1962, p. 89; 1971, pp. 201-204) for comparing all
means (congenic lines) with a control (progenitor strain). Testing of other hypotheses such as heterosis or maternal effects may
be more meaningfully accomplished in the context of specific individual contrasts. Contrasts in the form of trend analyses a-

Table 1

Examples of a simple partially repeated

measurements design and a simple multivariate design

In the first example all subjects assigned to aldomet treatment or the control condition receive multiple dosage of a drug and heart rate is measured for each dose. In the second example, multiple dependent variables are measured for subjects assigned to aldomet or control conditions. Designs 1 and 2 could be combined so that multiple response measures are obtained for each dosage and drug treatment condition[1].

Repeated Measurements Design[2]

Treatments (Dosage)

	$\underline{S}$s	5 mg	10 mg	20 mg	30 mg	40 mg
ALDOMET	S_1	X_1	X_1	X_1	X_1	X_1
	S_2	X_2	X_2	X_2	X_2	X_2
	.					
	.					
	S_{29}	X_{29}	X_{29}	X_{29}	X_{29}	X_{29}
PLACEBO	S_{30}	X_{30}	X_{30}	X_{30}	X_{30}	X_{30}
	S_{31}	X_{31}	X_{31}	X_{31}	X_{31}	X_{31}
	.					
	.					
	S_{60}	X_{60}	X_{60}	X_{60}	X_{60}	X_{60}

Table 1 - Cont'd

Multivariate Design[3]

Variables

$\underline{Ss}$	Heart Rate	Blood Pressure	Respiration	Errors	Time to Respond
ALDOMET S_1	X_1	X_1	X_1	X_1	X_1
S_2	X_2	X_2	X_2	X_2	X_2
.					
.					
S_{29}	X_{29}	X_{29}	X_{29}	X_{29}	X_{29}
PLACEBO S_{30}	X_{30}	X_{30}	X_{30}	X_{30}	X_{30}
S_{31}	X_{31}	X_{31}	X_{31}	X_{31}	X_{31}
.					
.					
S_{60}	X_{60}	X_{60}	X_{60}	X_{60}	X_{60}

[1] X_1 = a score for subject$_1$

[2] Treatments could be counterbalanced or randomized in design 1 and order of presentation might be treated as a factor if a number of subjects received the same order.

[3] In this design, different dosages might be assigned to different subjects or design 1 and 2 might be combined.

cross blocks of trials, or individual trials are particularly
useful when the RI strains are to be characterized in terms of
learning rather than levels of performance. Trend analyses may
be accompanied by calculations of slope and regression equations
(Guilford, 1965, pp. 366-371). This procedure is quite useful
under circumstances in which dose-response curves for the RI
strains are of concern. In some cases, a strain distribution
pattern based on regression equations or calculations of slope
for each strain is more meaningful than specific contrasts. For
example, the degree of improvement from the beginning to the end
of a learning experiment, or with increasing dosages of a drug,
may be more important than the absolute level of performance on
any given trial or for any specific dosage level.

How Significant is a Significant Difference?

Generally, the practical significance of a statistically
significant difference is based on the judgement of the investigator which is related to his experience with the area and knowledge
of the literature. There is a statistic which aids the experimenter in reaching this decision: ω^2 (Hays, 1973, p. 417). This
statistic is reported infrequently, despite its usefulness in the
context of "meaningfulness" or "practicality" decisions with regard
to drug effects. Greek omega squared (ω^2) represents the strength
of the association between the treatment administered (X) and the
independent variable Y, or the proportion of variance in Y accounted for by X. A difference between two drugs may be statistically
significant, but relatively unimportant relative to the strength
of the association between the treatment variables and the performance variables. It is for this reason that it is advisable
to calculate ω^2.

Assumptions Prerequisite to Analyses

Most researchers appear quite sensitive to the assumptions
which underlie nonrepeated measurements analyses of variance, e.g.,
normality of within cell distributions, homogenity of within cell
variances. Similarly, they seem to be aware of the possibility
of satisfying assumptions underlying nonrepeated measurements
analyses of variance by applying various transformations which
effect changes in the shape of the original distribution (log or
reciprocal), or increase the homogeneity of within cell variances
(square root transformations). Discussions of strategies and
appropriateness in the application of various transformations
may be found in Winer (1962, pp. 218-222; 1974, pp. 400-401). A
variety of transformations are available. No transformation
should be automatically applied prior to inspection of the data.

Latencies are often, but not always, skewed and transformations do
not always accomplish the objectives for which they were intended.
Most important, they are not always meaningful in terms of the
experimental question regardless of their effort on the distribution of scores.

Nonparametric statistics (Siegel, 1956) are available for
treatment of data which do not meet assumptions underlying analysis of variance, although they are often applied improperly. Some
nonparametric tests have quite precise assumptions which must be
met. McCall and Appelbaum (1973) have discussed the issue of nonparametric tests. They point out that:

"The fact that nonparametric tests do not address precisely
the same statistical question as 'comparable' parametric tests
is always true, and it is not unique to the repeated-measures
issue. The same may be said of the relative power of these two
approaches."

"A second liability is that nonparametric alternatives exist
principally for this simple one-factor design, though new advances in the nonparametric analysis of two- and three-factors
designs with one or two repeated dimensions may eventually dis-
count this liability (Puri & Sen, 1967)." (McCall & Appelbaum,
1973, p. 404.)

Appropriate application of nonparametric analyses is relevant
particularly to the discussion to follow because nonparametric analyses have been suggested as an alternative to analyses of variance
when the rather stringent assumptions underlying repeated measurements
analysis are not met (Lana & Lubin, 1963). However, McCall and
Appelbaum (1973) offer an alternative statistical strategy, applications of multivariate analysis of variance technique to repeated
measurements data when failure to meet assumptions underlying conventional parametric methods (Wimer, 1971, p. 305) dictates an alternative strategy.

MULTIVARIATE ANALYSIS OF VARIANCE

Because individual differences play an important role in response to different kinds of drugs and to different dosages of the
same drug, techniques for the most appropriate treatment of repeated measurements data are of major importance to psychopharma-
cologists. Thus, it is important to be aware of the advantages
of the multivariate analysis of variance approach to the treatment of repeated measurements data. Before introducing this important application of multivariate analysis, it is necessary to
describe two useful applications of multivariate techniques in
the context of nonrepeated measurements designs; 1) as a protection scheme, and 2) as a means of analyzing a meaningful composite

Table 2

A sequence of testing for assuring protection against chance
differences due to contrasts involving multiple dependent
variables and multiple treatments

Example Design

Drug	Strain	Heart Rate	Blood Pressure	Respiration	Activity Level	Errors
Scopolamine	C57BL/6J	$\overline{X}$	$\overline{X}$	$\overline{X}$	$\overline{X}$	$\overline{X}$
	DBA/2J	$\overline{X}$	$\overline{X}$	$\overline{X}$	$\overline{X}$	$\overline{X}$
Amphetamine	C57BL/6J	$\overline{X}$	$\overline{X}$	$\overline{X}$	$\overline{X}$	$\overline{X}$
	DBA/2J	$\overline{X}$	$\overline{X}$	$\overline{X}$	$\overline{X}$	$\overline{X}$
Control	C57BL/6J	$\overline{X}$	$\overline{X}$	$\overline{X}$	$\overline{X}$	$\overline{X}$
	DBA/2J	$\overline{X}$	$\overline{X}$	$\overline{X}$	$\overline{X}$	$\overline{X}$

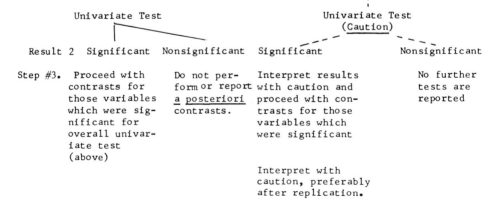

Steps in Analysis

Step #1.   Overall Multivariate Analysis of Variance

Result 1   Significant   Nonsignificant

Step #2. Proceed with Univariate Analy-   Do not perform Univariate Analyses or
         sis of variance if the program   proceed with Univariate Analysis with
         does not automatically perform   caution (or interpret univariate anal-
         univariate analyses.   ysis of variance with caution if the
                                                  program automatically performs this
                                                  analysis). Reader of the research re-
                                                  port should be made aware that multi-
                                                  variate analysis was not significant.

           Univariate Test   Univariate Test
                                                           (Caution)

Result 2 Significant Nonsignificant   Significant   Nonsignificant

Step #3. Proceed with   Do not per-   Interpret results   No further
          contrasts for   form or report with caution and   tests are
          those variables a posteriori   proceed with con-   reported
          which were sig- contrasts.   trasts for those
          nificant for   variables which
          overall univar-   were significant
          iate test
          (above)
                                          Interpret with
                                          caution, preferably
                                          after replication.

of scores.

A "Protection" Scheme

Many research problems in psychopharmacology, when dealing with genetics, require the simultaneous employment of a battery of dependent variables. It is rare that a drug effects only one aspect of behavior and thus, a battery of behavioral tests is used. The investigator may be interested in the effects of these drugs on each test of behavior. Thus, a <u>univariate</u> analysis of variance, followed by <u>a posteriori</u> contrasts, may be done for each response measure.

If, for example, significant differences among treatments were observed for 9 out of 10 variables, a conclusion might be reached that drug effects for each behavior were not due to chance alone. On the other hand, the finding of a single significant difference at the $p < 0.05$ level might lead to a question as to whether this difference might not have occurred by chance. Certainly, testing at the 0.05 level does not afford the same protection against falsely rejecting H-1 when there are ten variables as it does when only one variable is under consideration. If twenty variables have been tested, one univariate test in 20 is expected to be significant by chance alone. Thus, a protection procedure is needed for multivariate analysis, just as a protection procedure is needed for multiple t tests.

For a single dependent variable design, the protection against chance differences resulting from multiple contrasts (contrasts involving multiple treatments) is provided by univariate analysis of variance. For multiple response measures, it is necessary to protect against chance differences for a single dependent variable which may result from the simultaneous testing of multiple dependent variables measured within the context of a single experiment. In this case, the multivariate test may be used in a protection scheme which considers the results of univariate tests context of the results of the multivariate test. Specifically, univariate tests are either not made in the absence of a significant finding for the multivariate test, or univariate findings are reported with a precautionary note to the reader regarding the nonsignificant multivariate finding. Table 2 summarizes a recommended sequence of steps to be followed for hypothesis testing with a battery of measures.

A variety of tests are available for multivariate analysis of variance including Wilks' lambda criterion using Rao's approximate F test (Rao, 1952, pp. 236-272). Hotelling's T^2 test is often used in two treatment (group) designs with multiple measures of performance (Winer, 1962, pp. 632-635; 1971, p. 54, 238, 305,

Table 3a

A table adapted from Elias and Eleftheriou (1973). A multivariate protection scheme was used because four dependent variables were measured for each experimental condition. In this case, the multivariate test[1] was nonsignificant and all the univariate tests were non-significant. In the event that one of the univariate tests was significant, it would not have been reported, or it would have been reported with a note of caution to the reader that the multivariate F ratio was nonsignificant.

Means, Standard Deviations (SD), and Summary of Multivariate Analyses of Variance for the Four Behavior Measures*

	Original Learning**							
	Days-to-Criterion		Error Frequency		Error Trials		Time per Trial (sec)	
	Mean	SD	Mean	SD	Mean	SD	Mean	SD
Quaking (N = 10)	3.90	(0.99)	7.30	(4.42)	4.60	(2.27)	19.96	(7.38)
Littermates (N = 10)	4.40	(1.26)	7.10	(5.06)	4.60	(2.55)	21.04	(15.97)
Univariate Differences (df=1/18)	$F=0.97$ $p>0.05$		$F=0.01$ $p>0.05$		$F=0.01$ $p>0.05$		$F=0.79$ $p>0.05$	

* Univariate Fs are not interpreted unless the multivariate F is significant.

** Multivariate $F = 0.74$, df = 4/14, $p>0.05$.

1 Wilks' Lambda Criterion (likelihood ratio), Rao's approximate F test.

2 Table abstracted by permission of the editor of Physiology & Behavior.

Table 3b

A table adapted from Elias and Eleftheriou (1973). In this example, a significant multivariate F[1] was obtained and two out of four univariate tests were significant. Univariate tests were reported.

Means, Standard Deviations (SD), and Summary of Multivariate Analyses of Variance for the Four Behavior Measures*

| | Reversal Learning** | | | | | | | |
| | Days-to-Criterion | | Error Frequency | | Error Trials | | Time per Trial (sec) | |
	Mean	SD	Mean	SD	Mean	SD	Mean	SD
Quaking (N = 10)	5.70	(1.16)	15.50	(4.47)	12.60	(2.27)	11.25	(2.13)
Littermates (N = 10)	4.00	(1.15)	10.80	(6.10)	6.20	(2.28)	11.14	(4.54)
Univariate Differences (df=1/18)	$F=10.79$	$p<0.004$	$F=3.69$	$p>0.05$	$F=20.03$	$p<0.0004$	$F=0.01$	$p>0.05$

* Univariate Fs are not interpreted unless the multivariate F is significant.

** Multivariate $F = 6.69$, df = 4/14, $p<0.003$.

1 Wilks' Lambda Criterion (likelihood ratio), Rao's approximate F test.

2 Table abstracted by permission of the editor of Physiology & Behavior.

568). If H-1 for the multivariate test is rejected, the investigator proceeds with individual contrasts among treatments for the
various dependent variables. Examples of this particular application of multivariate analyses of variance may be seen in Tables
3a and 3b. (Here H-1 is the null hypothesis.)

Honest and Dishonest "Fishing": Some Ethical Decisions and Possible Consequences

A question frequently raised by investigators when the
multivariate "protection procedure" is utilized is "why can't significant univariate differences be reported despite the outcome
of the multivariate test if my main concern was for a single
specified variable?" Clearly, a significant univariate finding
can be reported in the absence of overall multivariate significance. The important questions is with regard to the meaning
which can be attached to a single significant univariate test
when the multivariate test is not significant. Alpha (α) for
the univariate test is misleading in terms of its indication of
the potential replicability of the finding. In general, then, a
post hoc decision that one variable was of major concern represents little more than justification for a fishing expedition.
However, replication of findings with the single variable which
was significant in a preliminary test of a battery of variables
is quite legitimate and strengthens the probability that the
finding represents a "true" effect.

A Priori Selection of Variables and Covariance Analysis

The stricture against post hoc decisions that one variable
in a battery of tests was of prime concern while others were included for exploratory purposes does not preclude the legitimate
a priori decision to include specific variables as criteria
(dependent variables of interest) and others as covariates. In
this instance, the experimenter may be concerned with the correlation of the covariates with the criteria. In the event of a
significant regression of criteria and covariates, he may wish
to adjust criterion scores with covariance analysis. Covariance
analysis is particularly useful in instances in which variables
contributing to error variance cannot be controlled via experimental manipulation, and yet it is often ignored in studies where it
is applicable. In some instances, adjustments are based on techniques such as simple subtraction of scores, or the generation
of a ratio such as adrenal weight/body weight ratios or heart
weight/body weight ratios in studies of stress. If a priori
knowledge based on theory or prior data suggests that such an
adjustment is meaningful, it can be appropriate. In the absence

of a priori knowledge, the advantage of the covariance approach
to adjustment is that the adjustment is based on the empirically
derived within- and between-class correlations. Reduction in the
magnitude of the error term (increase in $\underline{F}$) for the criterion is
positively related to increase in the magnitude of the square of
the pooled within class correlation (r_w^2) (Winer, 1962, pp. 593-
594). However, data must conform to important assumptions underlying covariance analysis (Tatsuoka, 1971, pp. 39-61).

Composite Scores

Procedures other than multivariate analysis of variance are
available as a protection against erroneously rejecting H-1 for a
specific univariate test made in the context of multiple univariate tests. Formulas are available for calculating the probability
of obtaining a chance difference for more than one dependent vari-
albe (Hays, 1973, p. 611). However, multivariate analysis of
variance provides additional information regarding the effect of
combining several variables and thus answers an important question
which may arise when test batteries are used. Do a number of
differences, small but consistent, indicate a significant treatment effect when they are combined into a meaningful composite?
Winer (1971, pp. 322-340), Tatsuoka (1971), McCall (1970), and McCall
& Appelbaum (1973), among others, describe application of multivariate analysis of variance in this context. Development of the
rationale underlying this procedure is not within the scope of
this chapter. However, a quotation from McCall & Appelbaum (1973)
may provide some insight with respect to the concepts underlying
the application of multivariate analysis of variance when a meaningful composite score is required.

"Multivariate analysis of variance is simply the extension
of the usual univariate analysis of variance model to a set of
response variables (i.e., a vector) rather than just a single dependent measure. In the case of an orthogonal factorial design,
the method essentially combines in a linear fashion, the information in the several response variables in such a way as to detect any existing treatment effects. In effect, this approach
produces, separately for each effect in the design, a set of
weights for the dependent variables such that when the p weighted
response variables are linearly combined the differential treatment effects are maximally represented in this new composite variable. Symbolically, the method determines a composite score Y
(a 'canonical variate') associated with each effect such that

$$Y = c_1 X_1 + c_2 X_2 + \ldots + c_p X_p,$$

in which the X_i are the p dependent variables (the vector of
responses) and the c_i are coefficients determined by the analysis

which are constant across subjects. The composite variable Y max-
imizes what might be conceived as the between-groups variance relative to the within-groups variance. The resulting test statistic
is compared with a sampling distribution that takes into account
the number of levels of the treatment factor, the number of variables, the number of subjects, and the fact that the maximizing
procedure has been used." (pp. 406-407).

A detailed development of the statistical models and rationale underlying the multivariate analysis of variance is not within
the scope of this chapter. McCall (1970) and McCall & Appelbaum
(1973) have provided excellent nontechnical discussions of this
approach and they cite a number of technical papers dealing with
the topic. The reader may also wish to consult publications by
Bock & Darrell, 1966; Cole & Grizzle, 1966; Jones, 1966; Norton,
1963; Smith, 1962; Winer, 1971, pp. 232-240, and Tatsuoka, 1971,
p. 194-237.

McCall & Appelbaum (1973) call attention to the fact that
multivariate analysis of variance is "conceptually related and com-
putationally equivalent to a number of other multivariate procedures." (p. 407). For example, discriminant analysis (Tatsuoka,
1971) produces a weighted linear combination of dependent variables that results in large differences in group means. Thus, a
multivariate analysis of variance for a one factor design is similar to a multiple discriminant problem with multiple experimental
treatments. A two treatment, one factor, multivariate analysis
of variance yields essentially the same information as the Hotelling T^2 procedure for testing the difference between two groups
(treatments). McCall & Appelbaum (1973) caution the user of
these procedures that there are logical differences between them
despite the fact that they are similar conceptually.

Other Multivariate Techniques Applicable to Batteries
of Tests

A multivariate technique which has been used quite extensively in many areas of psychology and the social sciences, factor
analysis, is particularly useful when the object of data analysis
is to reduce a large number of variables in a performance battery
to a smaller number of factors or components based on patterns
of relationships among the original variables. It permits the
construction of new scores (factor scores) for each subject which
are based on the new composite variables (factors), and these
scores may be subjected to further statistical analyses, e.g.,
multivariate analysis of variance or multiple regression analysis.
The factor analytic method of obtaining composite scores for a
large number of dependent variables is statistically superior to

the construction of composite scores based on the simple addition
of the original variables. Detailed descriptions of factor analysis and multiple discriminant analysis may be found in texts by
Harmon (1967), Van de Greer (1971) and Tatsuoka (1971). These
techniques may be particularly useful in the derivation of strain
distribution patterns for Bailey's RI strains (Chapter by Eleftheriou & Elias) when a battery of behavioral or physiological tests
is used.

REPEATED MEASUREMENTS DESIGNS

One of the most useful applications of multivariate analysis
of variance is with respect to repeated measurements data which
fail to meet homogeneity of population covariance assumptions.

Assumptions

Many investigators are aware of the fact that F is relatively
robust to the assumptions underlying nonrepeated measurements
designs. Research by Box (1953) indicates that departures from
normality of distribution and homogeneity of variance are not
damaging to the accuracy of the F ratio when these departures
are not severe. However, it is less well known that an additional
assumption which must be met in order to perform analyses of variance for repeated measurements data, homogeneity of covariances
on the variance-covariance matrix, is quite important. The F
ratio is much less robust with regard to this assumption than it
is with regard to homogeneity of variance assumptions. Moreover,
it is difficult to satisfy this assumption, particulary in learning experiments which often involve a restriction in range of
scores.

Winer (1971, p. 277, 282; 1962, pp. 632-633) and McCall &
Appelbaum (1973) provide a detailed explanation of the nature of
variance-covariance matrices, and they discuss criteria which
permit the investigator to determine whether or not homogeneity
of covariance assumptions are met. Briefly, the rationale is as
follows. In a repeated measurements design, covariances between
repeated measures vary considerably. Correlations between repeated
treatments are thus dissimilar. This variation constitutes a
departure from homogeneity of covariance assumptions underlying
the conventional repeated measurements analysis of variance.

Table 4a provides an example of a variance-covariance matrix
calculated for five subjects that receive four trials in a learning experiment. In this contrived example, correlations between
tratements vary from 0.69 to 0.99. While this is a contrived

Table 4a

Artificial learning scores (errors) for four repeated trials
following administration of a drug. The variance-covariance matrix
for these scores indicates a departure from homogeneity.[1,2]

Raw Data (Errors)			
Ss	Trial 1 (T_1)	Trial 2 (T_2)	Trial 3 (T_3)	Trial 4 (T_4)
---	---	---	---	---
S_1	6	4	3	2
S_2	5	3	2	1
S_3	4	2	1	2
S_4	7	5	3	1
S_5	10	7	4	0

Variance-Covariance Matrix with Variances on the Diagonal

	T_1	T_2	T_3	T_4
T_1	5.30			
T_2	4.40	3.70		
T_3	2.45	2.10	1.30	
T_4	-1.60	-1.30	-0.65	0.70

Correlations

	T_1	T_2	T_3	T_4
T_1	1.00			
T_2	0.99	1.00		
T_3	0.93	0.92	1.00	
T_4	0.83	0.81	0.68	1.00

[1]Covariances are calculated for each trial and each other trial (T).

[2]Normally, this design would include a control group and a second
variance-covariance matrix.

STATISTICS 453

Table 4b

An example of heterongeneity of covariance as inferred from the within cell correlations between repeated measurements treatments in a learning experiment by Elias and Schlager (1975)[1]

	Stages of Testing[2]							
Experimental Groups	H-1	H-2	B_1	B_2	B_3	B_4	B_5	B_6
High BP	2.26	2.10	2.69	2.31	2.18	1.95	1.97	1.92
Low BP	2.18	1.62	2.44	1.91	1.86	1.62	1.48	1.43

	Within Cell Correlations							
	H-1	H-2	B_1	B_2	B_3	B_4	B_5	B_6
H-1	1.00							
H-2	0.44	1.00						
B_1	0.56	0.35	1.00					
B_2	0.35	0.18	0.58	1.00				
B_3	0.37	0.25	0.51	0.62	1.00			
B_4	0.23	0.39	0.38	0.50	0.78	1.00		
B_5	0.21	0.24	0.42	0.45	0.66	0.71	1.00	
B_6	0.09	0.08	0.27	0.42	0.58	0.66	0.78	1.00

[1] H-1 and H-2 refer to two blocks of habituation trials; B-1, B-2, B-3, B-4, B-5, and B-6 refer to blocks of discrimination learning trials. All animals received two blocks of habituation trials and 5 blocks of learning trials.

[2] Scores are $\log_e$ latency of response.

group of scores for a small number of subjects, considerable variation in correlations (heterogeneity of covariance) occurs frequently for real data. Table 4b shows a within-cell correlation
matrix for an experiment in which two Blocks of habituation trials
(H_1 and H_2) were followed by six Blocks of discrimination learning
trials (Elias & Schlager, 1975). The dependent variable was $\log_e$
latency of response. It may be seen that the within cell correlations varied from 0.08 to 0.78.

Departure from homogeneity of covariance assumptions is obvious for the example provided in Table 4b. It is not obvious in
all cases, but there are tests (Winer, 1971, pp. 594-599; Kirk,
1969, pp. 139-141) which enable an investigator to determine
whether his data depart significantly from a condition of covariance homogeneity. These tests should not be confused with the
tests for homogeneity of within-cell variances in nonrepeated
measurements designs. The tests of homogeneity of variance have
come to be considered relatively unimportant because the $\underline{F}$ ratio
is relatively robust with regard to the assumption of homogeneity
of variance for nonrepeated measurements designs.

McCall & Appelbaum (1973) and Appelbaum[1] present a convincing
argument that 1) homogeneity of covariance assumptions are far
less robust than homogeneity of variance assumptions, 2) that
tests are often made with conventional analyses in violation of
the homogeneity of covariance assumptions, and 3) violation of
this assumption can result in a markedly inflated $\underline{F}$ ratio. They
do point out, however, that use of the conventional analysis in
an experiment does not indicate that the conventional analysis
was used in violation of homogeneity assumptions.

Assumptions are even more difficult to meet in multifactor
repeated measurements designs. McCall & Appelbaum (1973) outline
these additional assumptions in more detail than is possible here.

Alternatives to Conventional Analyses

The important question is with regard to alternatives to
the conventional approach to repeated measurements designs (Winer,
1971, Ch. 7) when the variance-covariance matrix departs from a

-----

[1]Personal communication.

condition of homogeneity in a repeated measurements design. Nonparametric statistical approaches provide one alternative solution
to the problem (Lana & Lubin, 1963), but they have limitations
which have been noted in this chapter and in previous papers e.g.,
McCall & Appelbaum (1973).

Greenhouse & Geisser (1959) have provided a correction procedure which may be applied to parametric analyses when they fail
to meet underlying variance-covariance assumptions. Advantages
and disadvantages of the Greenhouse-Geisser correction have been
discussed by McCall & Appelbaum (1973). One disadvantage is that
the procedure has not been explored for complex factorial designs.
However, an easily applied correction (Greenhouse-Geisser lower
bound estimate) is available for repeated measurements designs.
A major drawback of this procedure is that it is highly conservative and leads to considerable error on the side of failure to
reject H-1 when in fact H-1 is false.

A Multivariate Solution

One solution to the problem of heterogeneity in the variance-
covariance matrix which has been suggested by Bock (1963) and by
McCall & Appelbaum (1973) is to apply a multivariate analysis
procedure to the analysis of repeated measurements data. Utilization of this multivariate repeated measurements approach may be
illustrated with the Hotelling $\underline{T}^2$ test. The Hotelling $\underline{T}^2$ test is
usually applied in those situations where multiple dependent
measures are gathered for two treatments (groups) in a single
factor design. The only assumption underlying the use of $\underline{T}^2$ is
that the distribution must be multivariate normal (Tatsuoka,
1971). Moreover, the number of subjects must exceed the number of
repeated measurements treatments. Three times as many subjects
as treatments is often recommended as an arbitrary "rule of
thumb" where concern for power is paramount.

The computation of the Hotelling $\underline{T}^2$ statistic is tedious and
complex and thus it did not represent a particularly practical
repeated measurements solution until computer services became
available to most investigators. Presently, a number of com-
puter programs are available for Hotelling's $\underline{T}^2$ analysis or approximations. Hotelling's $\underline{T}^2$ solution to a repeated measurements
analysis, or any of the multivariate solutions, requires that the
data be transformed into deviation scores or into orthogonal poly-
nominals. Tables 5a and 5b illustrate the nature of the transformation. Any combination of linear independent contrasts can be
made (McCall & Appelbaum, 1973).

Once the raw scores have been transformed, they are treated

Table 5a

Transformation of raw scores into deviation[1] scores as a
first step in the multivariate analysis of variance solution to
a single factor repeated measurements design.

Subjects	Raw Data (Errors on Four Trials)				Transformed Data[a]		
	T_1	T_2	T_3	T_4	T_1-T_2	T_2-T_3	T_3-T_4
1	6	4	3	2	2	1	1
2	5	3	2	1	2	1	1
3	4	2	1	2	2	1	-1
4	7	5	3	1	2	2	2
5	10	7	4	0	3	3	4

[1] The rule for constructing deviation scores was as follows:
(T_1-T_2) (T_2-T_3) (T_3-T_4). These are linearly independent contrasts. The value of one contrast is not fixed by another.
Any set of linearly dependent contrasts can be made, and the
value of F for the Trials main effect will be the same when
the multivariate test is done. Polynominal contrasts would
result in the same F approximation of the multivariate test
(e.g. Hotelling's $\underline{T}^2$).

[a] The number of transformed scores are fixed by the number of
treatments. One less contrast than the number of within treatments (Trials) is made because $DF_{Treatments}$ = Treatments -1.

Table 5b

Transformation of raw scores of table 5a into Polynomial Contrasts[1] in order to create new variables (V_j) as a first step in the multivariate analysis of variance solution to a single factor repeated measurements design.

Polynominals to be Used (see Winer, 1971, p. 878)				
	Number Repeated Treatments			
	1	2	3	4
Linear	-3	-1	1	3
Quadratic	1	-1	-1	1
Cubic	-1	3	-3	1

Raw Data					Transforming the Scores for Subjects
Ss	T_1	T_2	T_3	T_4	
S_1	6	4	3	2	$(-3)6 + (-1)4 + (1)3 + (3)2 = -13$
S_2	5	3	2	1	$(\ 1)6 + (-1)4 + (-1)3 + (1)2 = \ \ 1$
S_3	4	2	1	2	$(-1)6 + (\ 3)4 + (-3)3 + (1)2 = -1$
S_4	7	5	3	1	
S_5	10	7	4	0	

Transformed Data for All Subjects

S_s	V_1	V_2	V_3
S_1	-13	1	-1
S_2	-13	1	-1
S_3	-7	3	1
S_4	-20	0	0
S_5	-33	-1	-1

Information Obtained with MANOVA

Trials Main Effect (Multivariate Solution)

Linear Trend (Univariate)

Quadratic Trend (Univariate)

Cubic Trend (Univariate)

[1]The trials $\underline{F}$ ratio will be the same as that obtained for the deviation contrasts shown in Table 5a.

as if they were discrete independent variables in a true multivariate design and Hotelling's $\underline{T}^2$ is conducted. If this test leads
to rejection of H-1 at a specific alpha level, the investigator
proceeds with a posteriori probing tests using individual univariate contrasts between treatments for the various dependent variables. The advantage of the procedure is that no assumptions need
to be made regarding covariances among the repeated treatments
(McCall & Appelbaum, 1973). The procedure for transforming scores,
and the results of its application in contrast to conventional
analyses, are illustrated in McCall & Appelbaum's review (1973).

Approximations of Hotelling's $\underline{T}^2$ test and other multivariate
tests may also be used for two groups designs. Table 6 shows
transformed scores for a 10 (Strains) x 6 (Treatments) partially
repeated measurements, analysis of variance performed with a computer program which uses the Wilks' lambda criterion (Rao's $\underline{F}$
approximation) for the multivariate test. In this instance, there
are 5 degrees of freedom (DF) for the Trials factor, and thus
the investigators constructed five deviation scores. The deviation scores were then treated as if they were multiple variables
in a conventional multivariate analysis of variance. The Trials
main effect and the Trials x Strain interaction were obtained by
multivariate analysis, and the results were treated in the same
manner as they would be in a univariate analysis. In the absence
of a significant Trials x Strains interaction, the investigators
did not proceed to make univariate contrasts designed to determine
the nature of the interaction.

The Strain main effect involves only a between-subjects
analysis, and thus it was done in the conventional manner. It
utilizes a score for each individual subject which is the mean
of all their scores for six trials. Control cards for the computer program, in this case MANOVA for the IBM 1130 (Hughes, LaRue
& Yost, 1969), allow the experimenter to specify the use of transformed scores for the within-subjects analyses and the between-
subject scores for the Strains main effect analysis. It is also
possible to read in the raw or original nontransformed scores for
each trial (T). In this case a separate analysis for these original scores would provide univariate analyses of variance for
each trial (analysis of simple effects). It is important to note
that polynominal transformations (see Table 5b) would have resulted
in the same $\underline{F}$ values for Trials and the Trials x Strains interaction as did the deviation score transformation (see McCall & Appelbaum, 1973).

Application of multivariate analysis to repeated measurements
data is not limited to the two group-single factor design. It
can be extended to the multifactor repeated measurements design
and the multifactor partially repeated measurements design by

means of the appropriate transformations and subsequent analysis
with multifactorial, multivariate analyses of variance. However,
the calculations necessary to transform scores become even more
complex than they are in the single factor case and the complex
and lengthly calculations necessary to perform the analyses make
the use of computer programs imperative. Examples of the application of this approach may be found in several research reports
(e.g., Delse et al., 1972; Elias & Eleftheriou, 1972; Elias et
al., 1973; Marsh & Thompson, 1973).

                        Computer Programs

     A number of computer programs are available for performing
Hotelling's T^2, approximation of Hotelling's T^2 test and multifactor, multivariate analyses of variance. Some programs perform
the transformations, while others require that a program be written to perform the transformations which are then placed on tape
or cards. We have found that MANOVA, a program originally developed by Bock et al. (McCall & Appelbaum, 1973) is particularly useful for the multivariate approach to repeated measurments designs
and for a variety of multivariate analyses of variance problems.
MANOVA packages are available for IBM 360 series computers with a
minimum core requirement of 256 K memory (Clyde, 1969), the UNIVAC
1108, or for the IBM 1130 computer. For the 1130, a core of 8 K
memory is required (Hughes et al., 1969). The multivariate test
is Wilks' lambda criterion (likelihood ratio test) using Rao's
approximate F test (Rao, 1952). We have made extensive use of
this program in our laboratory and in collaboration with B. E.
Eleftheriou at the Jackson Laboratory. In general, we have found
it an exceedingly easy program to use. Its outstanding virtue is
versatility. It performs multivariate and univariate analyses of
variance, analyses of covariance and regression, and it provides
standardized discriminant coefficients which can be interpreted
as weights in a discriminant function analysis. Options include:
1) contrasts between treatments for main effects and interactions;
2) transformation of variables ($\log_e$, square root, arcsin transformations); 3) orthogonal polynominal contrasts; 4) analysis of
covariance with one or more criteria and one or more covariates;
5) reanalysis with different sets of contrasts, criteria, covariates, and models. The manual provides input and output examples
for a variety of problems. A particularly good example of input
and output for a psychopharmacology study is provided on page
41 of the MANOVA manual (Clyde Computing Service, 1969).

     Other multivariate analysis of variance programs are avail-
able including Multivariance (Finn, 1971) which was written for
the CDS-6400 computer and requires 32 K memory (McCall & Appel-

Table 6

Results of a multivariate approach to repeated measurments
analysis of variance performed on data that have been transformed
with deviation contrasts. Mean deviation scores, shown for each
group of animals, are based on deviation scores obtained for each
subject. The treatments main effect and the trials (T) X strain
interaction represent multivariate F_s based on the transformed
scores. The strain main effect is calculated in the same way as
it is in the conventional analysis. It uses the average score
for all six trials for each subject $(\Sigma T/6)$. Control cards are
used to instruct the program to deal with transformed scores,
or the mean scores for all six trials depending on whether the
between-subjects analysis or the within-subjects analysis is to
be performed. The investigator may also read in the raw scores
for each trial (T) and obtain 6 univariate analyses of variance,
one for each trial.

Battery of RI Strains	Means of Transformed Scores[a]					$\bar{X}$ for all trials[b] $\dfrac{(\Sigma T/6)}{N}$
	$\bar{T}_1-\bar{T}_2$	$\bar{T}_2-\bar{T}_3$	$\bar{T}_3-\bar{T}_4$	$\bar{T}_4-\bar{T}_5$	$\bar{T}_5-\bar{T}_6$	
BALB/cBy	1.090	1.181	0.272	1.272	0.272	1.965
C57BL/6By	2.142	1.000	0.928	0.428	0.214	1.617
CB6F$_1$[c]	2.769	0.307	0.307	0.000	0.384	1.343
D	0.600	1.700	0.400	0.400	-0.100	1.146
E	2.600	0.600	0.900	-0.100	0.200	1.480
G	2.400	1.100	0.500	-0.500	0.600	1.279
H	2.454	0.454	1.000	0.545	0.363	1.722
I	2.090	0.727	0.090	0.000	0.090	0.709
J	0.900	0.400	1.800	0.100	-0.100	1.264
K	1.497	0.727	0.727	0.272	0.272	1.497

Analysis of Variance Table

Source	F	DF	p less than	Solution
Between Subjects				
Strain	1.435	9/101	0.182	Univariate[d]
Within Subjects				
Trials	111.474	5/97	0.001	Multivariate[e]
Strain X Trials	1.061	45/437	0.370	Multivariate

Table 6 - Cont'd

[a]Transformed scores are used for the multivariate calculation of within-subjects effects (Trials and the Trials X Strain interaction). Any set of linearly independent contrasts could have been used.

[b]These scores are used in a conventional analysis of between-subjects effects (Strains main effect).

[c]The battery of RI strains contains 11 groups. The B6CF$_1$ hybrids are not shown because the small computer program used to construct this example (IBM 1130) will only handle 10 groups for a between-subjects factor.

[d]Between subjects contrasts are made with conventional univariate analysis. Scores in the last column are used ($\Sigma T/6$) because they represent a single score for each subject derived by averaging scores for that subject on all six trials and dividing by 6.

[e]Polynominal contrasts could have been used. In this case, additional contrasts would have been available for the Trials main effect and for the Trials X Strain interaction (see the preceeding Tables): Linear, Quadratic, Cubic, and Quartic.

baum, 1973, p. 407), Starmer's MANOVA (Starmer, 1967), and Nybmul
(University of Rochester Computing Center, Rochester, New York).
The BMD statistical package (Dixon, 1973) also contains a multivariance analysis program. We have had no experience with Multivariance. BMD is rather limited in scope, and it will not perform
analyses for nonorthogonal problems. MANOVA-Starmer is not com-
mercially available. Its main attribute is that it is very easy
to set up deviation transformations, contrasts, and to perform
trend analysis. However, it is difficult to test higher order
interactions. Moreover, output is in a form which is relatively
unfamiliar to behavior scientists. Examples of application of
multivariate analysis to repeated measurements designs with
MANOVA and with MANOVA-Starmer (Duke Medical Center) may be found
in the literature (Delse et al., 1972; Elias & Eleftheriou, 1972;
Elias & Kinsbourne, 1972; Elias et al., 1973; Marsh & Thompson,
1973).

Assumptions and Power

McCall and Appelbaum (1973) make it quite clear, in their
nontechnical paper describing the multivariate approach to repeated measurements, that suggestions that the researcher might
profit from the use of the multivariate analysis of variance
approach does not imply that all previous research using the conventional model represents poor methodology or that assumptions
underlying the conventional procedures have been widely abused.
No such statement is possible because no systematic survey was
done to establish this fact. The same comments are apropos to
this chapter.

It is also important to note that under circumstances in which
assumptions underlying conventional repeated measurements are met
the conventional analysis is more powerful than the multivariate
approach (McCall & Appelbaum, 1973). Thus, the conventional approach
results in the same power as the multivariate approach, but with
fewer subjects. Nevertheless, multivariate analysis represents a
useful alternative to nonparametric procedures, transformation procedures, and correction procedures when assumptions of homogeneity of variances on the variance-covariance matrix are not met. It insures that
F ratios will not be inflated and yet it is not over conservative.
Thus, it seemed important to present it to the readers of this text as

---

[2] Dr. C. F. Starmer, Duke University Medical Center, Durham, North
Carolina.

a possibly useful statistical tool with an important application
to psychopharmacology experiments.   We can take absolutely no
credit for the conceptualization of this approach or any aspect
of its development. However, it has been a useful methodological
tool in our laboratory and in our collaborative research at the
Jackson Laboratory. Thus, it seemed appropriate, if not imperative, to briefly describe its application and to urge the reader
to review excellent articles on the topic by McCall & Appelbaum
(1973), Bock (in press), and Finn (1969).

ACKNOWLEDGEMENTS

The preparation of this chapter was supported in part by a
grant from the Public Health Service (National Institute of Child
Health and Human Development) to MFE (HD-08220).

REFERENCES

BOCK, R. D., 1963, Multivariate analysis of variance of repeated
    measurements, in "Problems of measuring change," (C. W.
    Harris, ed.), pp. 85-103, University of Wisconsin Press,
    Madison.

BOCK, R. D., 1966, Contributions of multivariate experimental
    design to educational research, in, "Handbook of multivariate
    experimental psychology," (R. B. Cattell, ed.), Rand McNalley
    & Co., Chicago, pp. 820-840.

BOCK, R. D., in press, "Multivariate statistical method in behav-
    ioral research," McGraw-Hill, New York.

BOX, G. E. P., 1953, Non-normality in tests on variance, Biometrika
    40:318.

CLYDE, D. J., 1969, Multivariate analysis of variance on large
    computers, Clyde Computing Service: Miami.

COLE, J. W. L., & GRIZZLE, J., 1966, Applications of multivariate
    analysis of variance to repeated measurements experiments,
    Biometrics 22:810.

DELSE, F. C., MARSH, G. R., & THOMPSON, L. W., 1972, CNV correlates
    of task difficulty and accuracy of pitch discrimination,
    Psychophysiology 9:53.

DIXON, W. J., (ed.), 1973, Biochmical computer programs, University of California Press: California.

ELIAS, M. F., & ELEFTHERIOU, B. E., 1972, Reversal learning and
RNA labeling in neurological mutant mice and normal littermates, Physiol. Behav. 9:27.

ELIAS, M. F., & KINSBOURNE, M., 1972, Time course of identity
and category matching by spatial orientation, J. Exper.
Psychol. 95:177.

ELIAS, M. F., DUPREE, M., & ELEFTHERIOU, B. E., 1973, Differences
in spatial discrimination reversal learning between two inbred mouse strains following specific amygdaloid lesions,
J. Comp. Physiol. Psychol. 8:149.

FINN, J. D., 1969, Multivariate analysis of repeated measures
data, Multivar. Behav. Res. 4:391.

FINN, J. D., 1971, Multivariate...univariate and multivariate
analysis of variance, covariance, and regression, a
Fortran IV program, State University of New York, Buffalo.

GUILFORD, J. P., 1965, "Fundamental statistics in psychology and
education," McGraw-Hill, New York.

GREENHOUSE, S. W., & GEISSER, S., 1959, On methods in the analysis
of profile data, Psychometrika. 24:95.

HARMON, H. H., 1967, "Modern factor analysis," University of
Chicago Press, Chicago.

HAYS, W. L., 1973, "Statistics for the social sciences," Holt,
Rinehart & Winston, New York, 2nd ed.

HUGHES, E. F., LARUE, R., & YOST, M., JR., 1969, "Multivariate
analysis of variance on small computers," Clyde Computing
Service, Miami.

JONES, L. V., 1966, Analysis of variance and its multivariate
developments, in "Handbook of multivariate experimental
psychology," (R. B. Cattell, ed.), Rand McNally, Chicago.

KIRK, R. E., 1969, "Experimental design; procedures for the behavioral sciences," Brooks/Cole, Belmont, California.

LANA, R. E. & LUBIN, A., 1963, The effect of correlation on the
repeated measures design, Ed. Psychol. Meas. 23:729.

MARSH, G. R. & THOMPSON, L. W., 1973, Effects of age on the contingent negative variation in a pitch discrimination task, J. Gerontol. 28:56.

McCALL, R. B. & APPELBAUM, M. I., 1973, Bias in the analysis of repeated-measures designs: Some alternative approaches, Child Develop. 44:401.

McCALL, R. B., 1970, The use of multivariate procedures in developmental psychology, in "Carmichael's manual of child psychology," (P. H. Mussen, ed.), pp. 1366-1377, vol. 1, Wiley, New York.

NORTON, D. W., 1963, Developments in analysis of variance and design of experiments, Rev. Ed. Res. 33:490.

PURI, H. L. & SEN, K. L., 1967, On some optimum nonparametric procedures in two-way layouts, J. Amer. Statis. Assoc. 62: 1214.

RAO, C. R., 1952, "Advanced Statistical Methods in Biometric Research," Wiley, New York.

SIEGEL, S., 1956, "Nonparametric Statistics for the Behavioral Sciences," McGraw-Hill, New York.

SMITH, H., GNANADESIKAN, R. & HUGHES, J. B., 1962, Multivariate analysis of variance (MANOVA), Biometrics. 18:22.

STARMER, C. F., 1967, A multivariate analysis program for biomedical research, Proceedings of the Sixth Annual Southeastern Meeting of the Association for Computing Machinery and National Meeting of Biomedical Computing, Durham, N. C.

TATSUOKA, M. M., 1971, "Multivariate Analysis: Techniques for Educational and Psychological Research," Wiley, New York.

VAN DE GREER, J. P., 1971, "Introduction to Multivariate Analysis for the Social Sciences," W. H. Freeman, San Francisco.

WINER, B. J., 1962, "Statistical Principles in Experimental Design," McGraw-Hill, New York.

WINER, B. J., 1971, "Statistical Principles in Experimental Design," (2nd ed.) McGraw-Hill, New York.

CONTRIBUTORS

C. Castellano, M.D., Laboratorio di Psicobiologia e Psicofarmacologia, C.N.R., Via Reno 1, Rome, ITALY.

B. E. Eleftheriou, Ph.D., The Jackson Laboratory, Bar Harbor, Maine 04609 U.S.A.

M. F. Elias, Ph.D., Department of Psychology & All-University Gerontology Center, Syracuse University, Syracuse, New York 13210 U.S.A.

P. K. Elias, Ph.D., Department of Psychology, Syracuse University, Syracuse, New York 13210 U.S.A.

E. H. Ellinwood, M.D., Behavior Neuropharmacology Section, Department of Psychiatry, Duke University, Durham, North Carolina 27710 U.S.A.

K. Eriksson, Ph.D., Research Laboratories, State Alcohol Monopoly, Alko, Box 350, SF 00101 Helsinki 10, FINLAND.

W. E. Fann, M.D., Department of Psychiatry, Baylor College of Medicine, Texas Medical Center, Houston, Texas 77025 U.S.A.

J. L. Fuller, Ph.D., Department of Psychology, SUNY-Binghamton, New York 13901 U.S.A.

C. D. Hansult, Ph.D., Department of Psychology, SUNY-Binghamton, New York 13901 U.S.A.

W. Kalow, M.D., Department of Pharmacology, University of Toronto, Addiction Research Foundation, Toronto, Ontario, CANADA

M. M. Kilbey, M.D., Behavior Neuropharmacology Section, Department of Psychiatry, Duke University, Durham, North Carolina 27710 U.S.A.

467

C. R. Lake, M.D., National Institutes of Mental Health, Bethesda, Maryland 20014 U.S.A.

I. P. Lapin, M.D., Ph.D., Bekhterev Psychoneurological Research Institute, Laboratory of Psychopharmacology, UL. Bekhtereva 3, Leningrad, C-19, USSR 65-84-16.

A. E. LeBlanc, M.D., Department of Pharmacology, University of Toronto, Addiction Research Foundation, Toronto, Ontario, CANADA.

R. D. Miller, Ph.D., M.D., Duke University Medical Center, Durham, North Carolina 27710 U.S.A.

A. Motulky, M.D., Division of Medical Genetics, University of Washington Medical School, Seattle, Washington 98105 U.S.A.

A. Oliverio, M.D., Ph.D., Laboratorie di Psicobilogia e Psicofarma-cologia, C.N.R., Via Reno 1, Rome, ITALY.

G. S. Omenn, M.D., Ph.D., Department of Medicine, Division of Medical Genetics, University of Washington Medical School, Seattle, Washington 98105 U.S.A.

B. Richman, M.A., Department of Psychiatry, Baylor College of Medicine, Texas Medical Center, Houston, Texas 77025 U.S.A.

K. Schlesinger, Ph.D., Department of Psychology & Institute for Behavioral Genetics, University of Colorado, Boulder, Colorado 80302 U.S.A.

S. K. Sharpless, Ph.D., Department of Psychology & Institute for Behavioral Genetics, University of Colorado, Boulder, Colorado 80302 U.S.A.

L. Shuster, Ph.D., Department of Biochemistry & Pharmacology, Tufts University School of Medicine, Boston, Massachusetts 02111 U.S.A.

J. L. Sullivan, III, M.D., Duke University Medical Center, Durham, North Carolina 27710 U.S.A.